THE ORGANIZATION OF LANGUAGE

The organization of language

Janice Moulton & George M. Robinson
The University of Kentucky

CAMBRIDGE UNIVERSITY PRESS
CAMBRIDGE
LONDON   NEW YORK   NEW ROCHELLE
MELBOURNE   SYDNEY

Published by the Press Syndicate of the University of Cambridge
The Pitt Building, Trumpington Street, Cambridge CB2 1RP
32 East 57th Street, New York, NY 10022, USA
296 Beaconsfield Parade, Middle Park, Melbourne 3206, Australia

© Cambridge University Press 1981

First published 1981

Printed in the United States of America
Typeset printed and bound by Vail-Ballou Press, Inc., Binghamton, New York

Library of Congress Cataloging in Publication Data
Moulton, Janice, 1941–
  The organization of language.

  Bibliography: p.

  Includes index.

  1. Grammar, Comparative and general – Syntax.
2. Generative grammar.
3. Language acquisition.
I. Robinson, George M., 1942– II. Title.
P291.M6 415 80–19052
ISBN 0 521 23129 9 hard covers
ISBN 0 521 29851 2 paperback

To the memory of Henry David Block, our friend and colleague and teacher. He taught us many things that helped us write this book, but more important, he taught us a way of thinking about scientific problems.

Contents

vii

Contents

Foreword

It is a privilege for me to introduce readers to what I look upon as a gem of scientific theory construction in the field of language, a new and refreshing theory of syntax and syntax acquisition that should command the attention of all those concerned with language and its learning. Moulton and Robinson provide a new and satisfying orientation to many of the issues that have occupied linguists and psycholinguists since the advent of the Chomskyan revolution more than two decades ago. It draws upon the best features of modern behavioral and cognitive approaches.

There are at least three respects in which the Moulton-Robinson theory is distinctive.

First, it emphasizes the language learner's or user's powers of conceptualization as a basis for the organization of language structure, and stresses the role of the nonlinguistic environment in helping language learners to acquire that structure as it is realized in a particular language. These matters have been too long neglected in standard linguistic and psycholinguistic theories.

Second, it is explicit about what kinds of grammatical objects or entities are involved in language use and acquisition. These grammatical objects are structures embodied in the authors' highly original "orrery" and "syntax crystal" models, based on their notions of "scope" and "dependency." The authors specify how these structures are manifested in particular constructions and arrangements in the English language – their "syntax modules." Their proposal that the orrery and syntax crystal models have great generality, applicable to all human languages, is compellingly believable, although of course it remains to be subjected to further investigation and testing with a variety of languages.

Third, the theory provides a credible and viable alternative to the nativist hypotheses about language acquisition that have dominated much discussion in the last few years. Moulton and Robinson show that it is unnecessary to postulate a "wired-in," innate language acquisition device in the child, and that it is more than conceivable that children can learn the syntactical rules and conventions of their native language by noticing how the relations they perceive and recognize among things in their environment, on a "prelinguistic" basis so to speak, can be handled in the construction of the language utterances that they hear and that they try out in their own efforts to communicate.

The style is lively, creative, and readily understood. There are places where the reader will be forced to pay close attention and to study details, but the effort will be rewarding. To aid in the appreciation and full comprehension of their ideas, the authors have provided some "language games" in Appendixes B and C. I highly recommend that the reader or student take the trouble to construct the needed materials for these games: he or she will find them not only instructive but also more entertaining than any Double-Crostic.

A computational parser of English, SCRYP, by Paul J. Gruenewald, is presented in Appendix A. This should be of great interest to computational linguists, because it appears to provide a highly efficient procedure for translating language into conceptualizations – one that follows closely the authors' postulated mechanisms for human language comprehension.

While the authors were at Duke University over several years, I was able – at some remove – to watch them develop their ideas. It is a pleasure to see these ideas become available to a wider audience. Any controversy they may spark will surely enliven the psycholinguistic scene for some time.

JOHN B. CARROLL

Chapel Hill, North Carolina

Preface

This book is an attempt to explain language structure and its relation to language cognition and acquisition. By starting at the beginning and reformulating the questions asked by current linguistic theories, we analyze the essential features of language and language users. From this base we construct a theory that avoids the complexity of many contemporary language theories and requires few presuppositions about innate language abilities. At the same time the theory is able to explain a great variety of language structures and much of the data of human language performance.

Because we start with fundamental questions about the nature of language, the book makes language science accessible to the nonspecialist. In order to provide a background for understanding our theory and its implications, we consider major contemporary theories of language in detail and evaluate related claims about language. These decisions provide a framework for evaluating our own claims. We hope that publication of this book will get other people interested in our approach and solicit help in finding theoretical and empirical consequences of the theory.

Frederik Pohl and Cyril Kornbluth, when asked of a jointly-authored work "who did what?", are reported to have replied that one of them wrote the nouns and the other the verbs. When we are asked the same question, we answer that one of us wrote the vowels and the other the consonants. This reply represents the spirit of our collaboration on this book; even the smallest meaningful unit was a joint effort. We did everything together and together we take responsibility for it; the order in which our names appear on the book cover was determined by a lengthy Alphonse and Gaston routine.

Many friends, colleagues, and students helped us by their suggestions, criticism, and encouragement, especially, Michael Arbib, John Carroll, Herb Crovitz, Ed Matthei, Julie Meister, David McNeill, John Staddon, Lise Wallach, and Robert Weisberg. We are also grateful to Ann Jacobs and to Susan Milmoe and Sophia Prybylski of Cambridge University Press. And we thank Larry Erlbaum, Marc Boggs, and Joan Goldstein for their kindness and confidence. Our parents have graciously agreed to take responsibility for any mistakes remaining in the book.

George M. Robinson and Janice Moulton

1
Introductory perspectives

This book is an attempt to answer the following questions: What are the essential features of language that permit a sentence or string of words to convey a complex idea? and What are the essential features of language users that enable them to produce and understand meaningful strings of words and to learn how to do so? The heart of these problems is syntax, and our answers constitute a new theory of syntax and syntax acquisition.

The goal of a theory of syntax

A theory of syntax must explain how someone can express a complex idea by organizing units of language into an appropriate pattern that conveys the idea, and how another person is able to identify from the language pattern, not only the concepts expressed by the individual units of language, but the relationships among the concepts that make up the idea. A theory of syntax should also explain what essential properties of language and of language users allow this method of encoding to be learned.

In trying to identify the essential features of a phenomenon, a good theory tries to represent the phenomenon as simply as possible without doing injustice to the complexity it is trying to explain. Actual syntax use (and its learning) may involve many redundant operations in order to increase speed and reliability. A theory of syntax will not be directly interested in all the properties and processes that may be involved in syntax use and acquisition, but in those that *must* be involved – the minimally essential features for syntax to work and to be learned.

1

A theory of syntax should apply to any language user, human or otherwise. The actual processes used by different individuals or species may not be the same. But a theory of syntax need not claim that actual language cognition must correspond exactly to the descriptions given by the theory. It need only claim that the properties and processes described by the theory are functionally equivalent to whatever ways humans or others do language, no matter how complex and difficult their way of doing it. The object is first to construct the minimal model and see how it works. If the model fails to account for an important theoretical or empirical aspect of syntax, appropriate alterations or adjustments must be made. Beginning simply, one can keep track of which features of the model are needed for particular aspects of syntax. When such a model succeeds in accounting for syntax encoding and its acquisition, it will represent the basic principles, or essence, of syntax.

What we mean by minimally essential features, or basic principles, can be explained with an analogy. Suppose we were trying to explain the principle of the internal combustion engine. It is not a fault to omit a discussion of camshafts and water pumps even though some engines use them and would fail to operate without them. It would be a fault to suppose that these components were *essentially* involved in the principle of the engine. On the other hand, it would be a fault to *not* mention that fuel and oxidant are mixed and introduced into the engine. Our explanation, if adequate, would apply to any engine regardless of whether it was two or four cycle, rotary or reciprocating piston, air or liquid cooled, fueled on alcohol or propane gas, etc. What we would have explained would be the essential features of a particular method of converting chemical potential energy to mechanical energy.

Similarly, for syntax, we do not want a theory to suppose that some nonessential properties that happen to be part of existing syntaxes are essential. It is not a fault to omit a discussion of nonessential properties. It would be a fault to include them as if they *were* essential. It would also be a fault for a theory to omit essential properties. The theory, if adequate, should apply just as well to any language and to any language user. It would be a fault to limit a theory so that it applies just to English or just to humans, because they happen to be conveniently available for illustration.

Much of what we shall say in the next few sections may seem obvious and even elementary to some readers. But much of it has been ignored by leading researchers on language. And so to put these sections in perspective, let us mention some recent claims about language:

1. It has been assumed by some (e.g., Katz, 1966; Chomsky, 1972) that the nonlinguistic environment is irrelevant, or plays no significant role in syntax learning. Then it is concluded that the *linguistic* data available to a child are insufficient for syntax learning so there must be considerable innate prewiring.
2. In some theories, the proposition is taken as the basic unit of meaning (Davidson, 1967, 1975, where he identifies a theory of meaning with a theory of truth of propositions; H. Clark and E. Clark, 1977). Other theories have claimed that subject-verb-object (Chomsky, 1965), or topic-comment, or agent-action-object (Fillmore, 1969) relations are basic to syntax. Examples of language that do not exhibit these relations are then supposed to be elliptical, or the products of deletion rules.
3. Another assumption has been that a theory of meaning needs to consider only the logical relations among propositions, and not the relations among the concepts that have been expressed (Fodor, Bever, and Garrett, 1974). Only recently has it been argued that a theory of meaning needs to consider more (Partee, 1978).
4. The notional versus formal debate (Skinner, 1957; Chomsky, 1959) over definitions of syntactic categories has made it appear that the *only* alternatives are either (1) that syntactic categories correspond to ontologic categories from the world, such as agent and action, or (2) that information from the world plays *no* role in the development of such categories.

Information processed during language use and acquisition

Linguists have traditionally partitioned their subject matter into three areas: morphophonemics, syntax, and semantics. As a result of changes in theory, the domains of syntax and semantics have shifted and overlapped. We are going to partition the information that must be processed during language use and acquisition in a different way. First, we describe *lexical* information, which involves the representation of concepts by words. Second, we describe *pragmatic* information, which comes from our knowledge of how things are in the world, that is, which concepts may be related and under what conditions. Third, we describe *syntactic* information, which involves the way relations among concepts are represented by relations among the lexemes that name those concepts. We are not going to discuss how particular signal systems are used to transmit lexical and syntactic information – the domain of morphophonemics.

Lexical information

Lexical information involves learning to associate a symbol with a concept and then using this association to interpret the occurrence of a symbol as representing its concept and also to produce the symbol in order to represent its concept. We use the term *lexeme* for a symbol that stands for a concept. Following Lyons (1971), a lexeme is that aspect of a word which stands for a concept, the part without any syntactic information. Thus the words INK, INKY, INKER, INKS . . . are all inflected variants of the same lexeme. The inflections, produced by adding to or changing the form of the word, carry syntactic information that tells in each case how the concept expressed by the lexeme INK can be related to other concepts. (Inflections may also carry semantic information; for example, the suffix -ER, as in INKER, tells us not only that the word is a noun but something about what it might mean in relation to the root.)

We are using the term *concept* to refer to a category that an organism establishes through experience. A thing that belongs to a cognitive category is an *instantiation* of the concept. Some concepts, like "envelope," have many instantiations; others, like "Billie Jean King," have only one.[1]

We intend our use of the term "concept" to be broad enough to include anything that can be considered part of the meaning of a lexeme.[2] Thus an instantiation of a concept may include the referent of a lexeme, an appropriate situation where the lexeme may be used, as well as affective and connotative associations. For example, all these aspects of meaning are probably included in an instantiation of a child's concept expressed through the lexeme BYE-BYE. Such a broad sense of "meaning" also includes the *linguistic* context of a lexeme, how it appears in relation to other lexemes. At least for an adult, most concepts include some linguistic information as well.

We are going to emphasize the role of the environment in syntax acquisition. Here we want to point out that the environment is important in lexeme acquisition as well. The language learner must pay attention to the way things are in the world. Many concepts derive more or less directly from their instantiations in the environment that are perceived and categorized. Some concepts become associated with lexemes by repeated conjunction of an instantiation of the concept with a token of the lexeme. In natural language there is no convenient one-to-one relationship between lexemes and concepts. One concept may be represented by a string of words containing two or more lexemes, for example, THE MAN IN THE MOON. Several lexemes may represent roughly the same concept, for example, BIG, LARGE, HUGE. This synonymy may vary across language users; for example, DRESSER and BUREAU are synonyms for some users of English, but not for all. In addition, the same symbol may be used for more than one lexeme (homonymy): BILL standing for a bird's jaw extension is clearly a different lexeme than BILL standing for a financial instrument. In other cases it is not clear whether to attribute differences in the meaning of homonyms to their symbolizing different lexemes, or different aspects of a concept referred to by the same lexeme, or different syntactic roles. For example, SWELL may mean "to expand," or "wonderful," or "nob." It is not easy to decide whether these are three different concepts or whether the second and third are metaphoric extensions of the first concept. Sometimes it is even hard to decide whether inflected variants of the same root represent a single concept. For example, while INK, INKS, and INKY seem to be derived referentially from the same concept, INKER as one who inks might be conceptually closer to, say, WRITER than INK.

Since we are not trying to explain the nature of concepts and meaning and how lexemes are learned, we ask the reader to be tolerant of the use of "lexeme" in this book, but also to be vigilant that any slack in the correspondence among lexeme, word, meaning, and concept is not used inadvertently to cover a flaw in syntactic theory.

A set of lexemes, each associated with a concept, constitutes a lexicon. When two language users share a lexicon, a simple form of linguistic communication is possible. By uttering a lexeme, a concept is expressed. By making suitable use of nonlinguistic context, one language user can inform another of the presence of an unnoticed thing, request a thing, evoke a shared train of association, etc.

Pragmatic information

In its simplest form, pragmatic information involves the organism's knowledge of its world that is not *essentially* linguistic. It involves learning and making use of information about what concepts or instantiations of concepts can occur in particular contexts, and what concepts and/or their instantiations can be related to each other in particular contexts. Pragmatic information is used by any creature that adaptively interacts with its environment. Although characteristically, pragmatic information can be acquired nonlinguistically, this does not mean that it must be or always is acquired nonlinguistically. Much of our knowledge about the world is mediated by language. Even a bee's knowledge of nectar locations is often acquired, not by direct experience, but through a primitive kind of "language" (von Frisch, 1967).

We are also not suggesting that human children first acquire a concept and then learn how to represent it linguistically. Linguistic information plays an important role in the generalization and discrimination tasks of concept formation. It is important for our purposes only that conceptual categorization can be done independently of language – as it is by dogs and squirrels, for example. This independence permits us to base our explanation of language acquisition on other cognitive capacities.

Pragmatic information is also important for a competent language user in order to understand ambiguous language. Consider the sentence MARY HAD A LITTLE LAMB. The verb HAD expresses so many lexemes and/or differences in sense, that unambiguous interpretation of the sentence depends essentially on pragmatic information. We have to know whether Mary was a pet owner, a gourmet, an obstetric anomaly, a rural sodomite, or a con artist, to name just five possibilities. The disambiguation of this sentence relies on context-dependent pragmatic information that may be supplied either linguistically or nonlinguistically. There is also the general pragmatic information that helps us recognize, for example, that if Mary had a little lamb *to eat*, it was probably a small part of what might have been a large animal, while if she had a little lamb to own, it was small for a baby sheep. In other words, general pragmatic information reflects our understanding of concepts and the ways in which they can be related.

Syntactic information

In addition to lexical information and pragmatic information, syntactic information is important to language. In English the lexeme RED stands for one concept and the lexeme BALL stands for another. But put the lexemes together in a phrase, RED BALL, and suddenly more than the individual concepts is expressed. The phrase not only conveys the concepts expressed by RED and BALL but also conveys that the concepts go together, that they are related in some way. In this case, pragmatic information tells us that RED and BALL apply to the same thing. The lexemes are related in the phrase RED BALL, but not related when they are uttered or written separately, as in a list of independent lexemes. It is the relationship of the lexemes which conveys that the concepts expressed by those lexemes are related.

In our discussion of the essential properties of syntax, we are going to discuss the different ways in which relations of concepts may be conveyed.

Representing relations of concepts by single lexemes

Communication based on the exchange of lexical information alone depends heavily on context and even then is limited in its range and reliability. What is missing is the ability to express relations among concepts. Natural languages do express some relationships among concepts by single lexemes. For example, PENSION stands for "the regular payments to a former employee, or pension plan member, given by the employer, or pension agency, to the employee for his or her lifetime after terminating a period of employment greater than some given number of years or after reaching a given age."[3]

Where the particular combinations of concepts are not numerous and recur frequently, the single-lexeme method of representation does not lead to enormous lexicons and may be worthwhile to save communication time. Western Union discovered that its customers often send essentially the same telegraph messages over and over again, for example: WARMEST WISHES TO YOU AND YOUR FAMILY FOR A HAPPY HOLIDAY SEASON. A telegraph customer willing to forego a choice of the exact wording selects a message from a list. Each message has a numerical "lexeme" written next to it. The clerk transmits only this number to the destination office. There, a second clerk reconstitutes the original message by looking up the number on a duplicate list. Many recipients of such messages never know their well-wishers paid only for a one- or two-digit telegram.

Unlike the limited stock of the canned greeting, the complexity of our environment with the myriad concepts that may be interrelated make it combinatorially impossible to express all important relations of concepts by using only single lexemes. Imagine the lexeme RELK standing for the relation of concepts we would describe in English as: MONDAY AFTERNOON FELICIA REPLACED THE THIRD PISTON ON THE BENTLEY WITHOUT REMOVING THE ENGINE FROM THE CHASSIS. Even confining our communication to the repair shop, consider how many single lexemes one would need to express the several relations of concepts involved with ten half-workdays, ten mechanics, ten auto parts, ten auto makes, and ten repair procedures. The resulting 100,000 lexemes are already more than the average human can handle. Clearly, the single-lexeme method of representing several concepts related together is unworkable for most natural language communication.

The way out of the difficulty is to avoid having to use a completely different linguistic representation for every one of the 100,000 possible combinations of individual concepts. We can keep the lexicon from growing absurdly large by using a lexeme for each one of the individual concepts and finding another method of expressing the relations among the concepts. For the repair-shop example, this reduces the size of the lexicon to 50. We can express the concepts involved in any one of the 100,000 possible events by five lexemes, one representing the appropriate half-workday, one the appropriate mechanic, etc. If we then wish to express "Monday afternoon, *Arthur* replaced the third piston on the Bentley without removing the engine from the chassis," we have only to replace the lexeme standing for "Felicia" with that standing for "Arthur," leaving the other lexemes unchanged. This scheme has another desirable quality – similar messages have similar representations. Now our task is to find a method of expressing the relations among the concepts. This brings us to syntactic information processing, which involves encoding relations among concepts as relations among lexemes. We now describe three different ways of using relations among lexemes to convey information about relations of concepts.

Primitive syntax

Let us first consider the simplest possible method of representing something about the relations among a set of concepts. One method, a kind of *primitive syntax,* would provide a means of encoding *which* concepts are related, even if nothing else about their relationship can be conveyed. One way of doing this is to present the lexemes standing for the concepts in such a way that they will be perceived as belonging together. For example, a language user might utter some lexemes one right after the other, allowing a relatively long silent period before and after the set of lexemes. For example: . . . DRINK(s), MARC, SPILL(s) . . . , where the order may be random or perhaps based on the relative importance or salience of the individual concepts. Taking a clump of lexemes as "belonging together" could be a convention agreed upon by a community of language users, although the Gestalt perceptual law of proximity might be adequate to explain the association. Either way, the clumping together is a relation of lexemes – the relation of being gathered around the same point in time (or in space if the medium is writing). The relation of lexemes signals a relation of concepts, informing the hearer that the set so clumped is to be taken as a unit, to be understood as representing a single multiconcept idea.

Primitive syntax works fairly well as an adequate linguistic representation of many multiconcept ideas. For the SPILL(S), MARC, DRINK(S) example, we have a high probability of correctly interpreting the message using our general pragmatic knowledge of the concepts "spills," "Marc," "drinks" and the ways they are likely to go together. Assuming a coherent, everyday world, we understand the message to describe an event that proper English renders as MARC SPILLS DRINKS. Knowing Marc to be a domestic pet nourished by frequent kitchen accidents might lead us to interpret the message as expressing the conceptual relations proper English would express as MARC DRINKS SPILLS. Our general pragmatic knowledge of how concepts can be related and how likely certain relations are, allows us to rule out in most cases the relation of concepts expressed by DRINKS SPILL MARC.

We can show how well primitive syntax plus general pragmatic information can represent multiconcept ideas without ambiguity by destroying all ordinary syntactic information. This can be done by writing each of the lexemes of a sentence (without their inflections) on a separate piece of paper and presenting them in scrambled order as a puzzle to someone else. The reader might like to try this. In Chapter 3 we describe an experiment that uses this technique to find sentences whose interpretations depend crucially on their syntactic information.

For sentences that are not long and not semantically bizarre, it is often easy to figure out the original sentence using only primi-

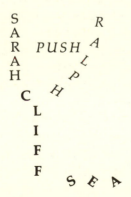

Figure 1.1. Rebus representation of iconic syntax: "Sarah pushes Ralph over a cliff into the sea."

tive syntax and general pragmatic information. But one can never be sure; maybe DRINKS SPILL MARC really does express the intended relation of concepts. Primitive syntax becomes inadequate as the number of lexemes to be related increases, or if several relations among concepts are plausible. Change SPILL(S) to SPOIL(ED) and primitive syntax plus general pragmatic information does not distinguish among SPOILED MARC DRINKS, MARC SPOILED DRINKS, and DRINKS SPOILED MARC. Therefore, we need more information than is available from primitive syntax. We need to know more about the relations of the concepts expressed by the individual lexemes.

Iconic syntax

A simple way of representing more information about the relation of concepts is to make the relation of lexemes *portray* the relation of concepts. The arrangement of lexemes should "look like" the way the concepts are related, an *iconic syntax* (Robinson, 1977). One simple example is a radio announcer naming the cars going by the press box during an auto race. The temporal order and spacing of the names of the racers reflect their order and spacing on the track. The temporal pattern of the names allows the listener to make some of the inferences that would be possible by actually witnessing the race: for example, who might win, and which positions are being challenged. This type of iconic syntax plays some role in natural language communication. When someone tells us: "I went to the fishmarket, Woolworth's, and the welding shop," we cautiously infer that the visits were made in that order.

Other features of the relations among concepts can be represented by iconic syntax. Told that "a carburetor, fuel pump, set of points, distributor cap, and some gaskets" are on a certain shelf, we head toward the middle of the shelf when we need a set of points. An old form of word-picture puzzle, the rebus, illustrates how other types of relations can be represented in a medium that presents simultaneously all the lexemes involved (Figure 1.1). Notice that we cannot derive the correct relation of concepts represented in Figure 1.1 using only primitive syntax and general pragmatic information. Even if we discount the ambiguity of CLIFF, primitive syntax still could not tell us who are the victim(s) and/or perpetrator(s). Many alternative relations of the concepts are possible: "Ralph and Sarah (a bulldozer team) push the cliff into the sea"; "Ralph pushes Sarah into the cliff by the sea"; "The sea pushes Sarah and Ralph against a cliff." Iconic syntax conveys the intended relation of concepts by presenting the lexemes in a similar relation. In this case the similarity shared by both lexemic and concept relations is spatial.

Notice that iconic syntax allows us to derive the correct interpretation of the rebus picture with the help of general pragmatic information. For example, we can assume that Ralph is falling over the cliff because it is in the nature of pushes to propel objects away. If we substitute PULL for PUSH, we are more likely to assume that Ralph is climbing up the cliff away from the sea. Thus a different relation of concepts will be inferred from the same syntactic information if some of the individual concepts are altered. Changing individual concepts changes the general pragmatic information used to infer the relation of concepts. This is an important point: It first arose in our discussion of primitive syntax, is seen again here in iconic syntax, and will make an important appearance again when we discuss the syntax actually used in natural language.

Iconic syntax in language acquisition: semiotic extension.   In a paper entitled "Semiotic Extension" (1975), David McNeill suggested an intriguing version of iconic syntax. He proposed that the motor and perceptual schemata which organize and guide a child's activity come to organize and guide the linguistic representation of that activity. McNeill suggests that the entrainment of word sequence by sensorimotor organization makes language acquisition more understandable as part of general cognitive development. One important feature of sensorimotor organization is the sequence of its components. When some of these components are expressible as lexemes, the child will tend to express them in the corresponding sequence. For example, I PUSH BOX WALL reflects the sequence in which the child processes the components of the activity it is describing: first the *self* as the origin of the intention to perform the act; next the initiation of the motor *pushing;* then the sensorimotor experience of engaging the *box;* finally the contact with the *wall* as immovable obstacle.

McNeill's thesis is supported by data showing that children learning different languages (including those not related historically) tend to order their lexemes in the same ways. In some cases, the order may differ from that used by adults. For our discussion here, the important point is that there sometimes occurs a nonarbitrary correspondence between the sequence in which concepts are organized and the sequence in which the lexemes naming those concepts are expressed, an iconic syntax. For simple ideas conveyed by simple expressions, the iconic correspondence can help in conveying and inferring relations of concepts. Beyond the language acquisition stage, iconic correspondence plays only a small supplementary role. In adult natural language the relations of lexemes, for the most part, have only a *conventional* correspondence with the relations of concepts they encode. One indication of this is that natural languages differ considerably from one another in the syntactic conventions they use. For example, English and French express the same concept as follows: BIRD, OISEAU. They express one simple relation between this concept and another as follows: RED BIRD, OISEAU ROUGE. The expression for the concept "red" is placed before the lexeme expressing the concept "bird" for English and after it for French.

Sequence and inflection codes for syntax

Human natural language communication employs several cues for primitive syntax: punctuation and spacing, gestures, pauses, grouping and changes in pitch, tempo, and loudness. Iconic syntax may also play some role in encoding features like temporal or spatial sequence. But most information about how concepts are related is conveyed by three methods: One is to arrange the lexemes naming the concepts in particular *sequences.* Another is to distribute among the lexemes a set of *inflection* "labels." A third method is by the addition of syntactic *functors* such as TO, OF, etc. Although no language uses one method exclusively, some languages (for example, English) rely mostly on the first method, while others (for example, Latin) rely mostly on the second. Sequence allows us to infer the appropriate relation of concepts from each of the following: THE GIRL LOVES THE WOLF and THE WOLF LOVES THE GIRL. Only the order of lexemes distinguishes one from the other; nothing else differs. Expressing the first of these two ideas in Latin may be done by any permutation of the order of the inflected (i.e., grammatically labeled) lexemes: PUELLA AMAT LUPUM and LUPUM AMAT PUELLA have approximately the same meaning. But THE WOLF LOVES THE GIRL is expressed as LUPUS AMAT PUELLAM or PUELLAM AMAT LUPUS, or AMAT LUPUS PUELLAM, or AMAT PUELLAM LUPUS. The order is not crucial; the terminations of AMAT, LUPUS, and PUELLAM carry all the syntactic information that tells us what relation of concepts is being expressed.

English sometimes uses both encoding methods redundantly. Since proper names are not inflected in the following examples, we rely on sequence coding to understand CHANG PUSHES KIM and KIM PUSHES CHANG. But pronouns *are* inflected and so HE PUSHES HER and SHE PUSHES HIM use both sequence and inflection coding to convey relations of concepts. If we pit sequence against inflection – HER PUSHES HE and HIM PUSHES SHE – we find that most listeners will be swayed by the sequence information. Where sequence information is weaker, as in less frequent forms of expression, inflection information may sometimes be more powerful. For example, most listeners understand CHANG KIM PUSHES to mean that Kim pushes Chang. However, when the pronouns are substituted, HE HER PUSHES, most listeners understand this to mean that he pushes her.

That translations can also be made between English and Latin is one indication that sequence relations and inflection relations are equally powerful and equivalent coding schemes for relations of concepts. Since one of our aims is to describe a general model of syntax and its acquisition, this interchangeability claim, if true, suggests that a single model might be adequate to explain both sequence and inflection encoding. We will return to this claim in Chapter 5. In the following section we are going to examine the method of encoding based on ordering the lexemes in sequence. We concentrate on this method because English relies most heavily on it.

Table 1.1. *Badlish and the English equivalents*

SPIDAH EETS FLIE	SPIDER EATS FLY
EETS PHROG FLIE	FROG EATS FLY
DJOMPS SPIDAH	SPIDER JUMPS
GRENE DJOMPS SPIDAH	GREEN SPIDER JUMPS
SPIDAH DJOMPS PHROG	FROG JUMPS SPIDER
FLIE PHROG GRENE EETS	GREEN FROG EATS FLY
FLIE DJOMPS	FLY JUMPS
SPIDAH PHROG EETS	FROG EATS SPIDER
EETS PHROG SPIDAH	SPIDER EATS FROG

Why sequential lexeme relations need to be systematic

Let us look at methods of encoding relations of concepts that use lexeme-sequence information. First, we consider a method with the fewest possible constraints. In Table 1.1 are some lexeme strings from a made-up language called Badlish along with their English translations. The lexicon of Badlish resembles English; but the syntax is not at all similar. Each relation of concepts is expressed by arranging the appropriate lexemes in a particular sequence. This meets the requirements for a true syntax: Relations of lexemes convey relations of concepts. In Badlish, the correspondence between a sequence of lexemes and a relation of concepts is analogous to the correspondence between a lexeme and a concept. Every relation of concepts is adequately encoded. But, analogous to lexical encoding, almost nothing about the representation of one relation of concepts bears any systematic resemblance to any other. For example, if we learn the new lexemes ELLYFINT and PEENOTZ and wish to express "fat elephant eats peanuts," there is no way for us to use our previous experience with Badlish to figure out how to do this. Badlish has no *systematic* use of sequence information. If we hear a new sentence in Badlish, we have to look it up in a "sentence dictionary" to find out what relation of concepts is conveyed. Since even a few concepts can be related to each other in so many different ways, such an unsystematic syntax imposes an information-storage burden on the language user nearly as cumbersome as the method of using single lexemes to encode entire complex ideas. Natural languages make some use of unsystematic syntactic encoding. Idioms and collocations have unique lexeme relations not systematically generalizable to any other expressions. For example, we can say SHE WAS NOT GONE LONG but not *SHE WAS GONE LONG (Bolinger, 1975, Chapter 5).

Generality in lexeme relations

To avoid the disadvantages illustrated by Badlish, relations of concepts need to be encoded by a system with some generality. Systematic generality enables the language user to learn something from the correspondence between one lexeme sequence and a particular relation of concepts, and to apply that knowledge to new correspondences between sequences and relations of concepts. Goodlish in Table 1.2 is a made-up language with such systematic generality. There are apparent regularities in the sequential syntax used by the set of sentences in this table. Given the set, most people agree on how to encode the new idea, "fat elephant eats peanuts." The syntax of Goodlish provides a basis for generalization. Information about relations of concepts is encoded not by sequences of particular lexemes but by sequences of particular *types* of lexemes. Since these types are classifications for the purpose of syntactic encoding, they are syntactic categories. The traditional set of syntactic categories includes noun, verb, adjective, and the like. Now we take a closer look at how these categories can be determined.

Syntactic categories: notional versus formal

There are two main ways to define syntactic categories: notional and formal. Notional categories are based on the meanings of the words that fall under them. For example, a noun is said to be the "name of a person, place, or thing." Formal categories are determined independently of meaning and depend only on the possible relationship a word may have with words of other categories in a well-formed string. Something is classified as a noun if it can be preceded by articles and adjectives, occurs in phrases of a certain type, and so on.

Table 1.2. *Goodlish and the English equivalents*

EETS SPIDAH FLIE	SPIDER EATS FLY
EETS PHROG FLIE	FROG EATS FLY
DJOMPS SPIDAH	SPIDER JUMPS
DJOMPS SPIDAH GRENE	GREEN SPIDER JUMPS
DJOMPS SPIDAH PHROG	SPIDER JUMPS FROG
EETS PHROG GRENE FLIE	GREEN FROG EATS FLY
DJOMPS FLIE	FLY JUMPS
EETS PHROG SPIDAH	FROG EATS SPIDER
EETS SPIDAH PHROG	SPIDER EATS FROG

Notional syntactic categories

Notional categorization is appealing because it is based directly on nonlinguistic ontologic categories – actions, animate and in-animate things, and so on. If one could explain syntactic categories in terms of such nonlinguistic categories, then the learning of syntactic categories and rules would be a simple ex-tension of nonlinguistic learning.

B. F. Skinner (1957) relied on notional categories in his descrip-tion of how syntax works. By definition, if syntactic categories were notional, then the concepts associated with words in each category would have some similarities. These similarities would then serve as the basis for generalization, permitting new words to be included under a category. Thus a language user could as-sociate every word with a category as long as the meaning of the word had been learned. The sequence of syntactic categories in a sentence, the "autoclitic frame," controls the interpretation of (Skinner would say "the response to") a string of words, just as a discriminative stimulus cue controls the response to the presence of a lever in an operant chamber. Through reinforcement, the language user learns to use the autoclitic frame as a discrimi-native cue to the relations of concepts named by the lexemes. For example, using Goodlish, the language user learns to associate strings like EETS SPIDAH FLIE; DJOMPS PHROG PEENOTZ; EETS PHROG SPIDAH with events in the environment. Generalizing across words, the language user recognizes the presence in each string of the autoclitic frame given by the syntactic category sequence:

verb noun noun. Generalizing across the three events that accompany these strings, the language user learns that this autoclitic frame is a cue associated with events in which, speaking loosely, the first noun does the verb to the second noun. This learning can then be applied to new situations and new language strings. For example, BUTZ GOTE PHENTS can be interpreted by recognizing BUTZ as a verb and GOTE and PHENTS as nouns. The string is accompanied by (is in the format of) the autoclitic frame: verb noun noun. This enables the language user to respond to the string as signaling the relation of concepts expressed in English as GOAT BUTTS FENCE. Skinner also considered inflections and functors as autoclitic cues to supplement the sequence cues.

Using a model developed by H. D. Block for language acquisition by a robot, L. Harris (1972) presented a heuristic procedure for abstracting syntax from a training set of well-formed sentences. The procedure requires that each sentence in the training set first be represented as a sequence of syntactic categories. In Block's model this is based on the design principle: "the parts of the robot are the parts of speech." The robot determines the syntactic category of each word while it learns its "meaning." Its ability to do this is "prewired" by classifying as a noun any word that reliably accompanies an input to the robot's visual or touch sensing devices. In a similar way verbs are those words that correlate with the operation of the robot's motors or the detection of motion external to itself; adjectives are those words that correlate with the detection of properties of physical objects such as size and color; adverbs, with properties of the motions such as fast and slow.

Skinner's and Harris's proposals for a notional syntax are plausible when applied to a limited set of simple sentences. Problems with this method are revealed by trying to extend its range of application. One problem is that, even using inflection and functor cues, the language user could not determine the syntactic category of many words by treating them in isolation. For example, SWIM fits several syntactic categories: DID YOU HAVE A GOOD SWIM? (noun), WE SWIM IN THE OCEAN (verb), WHAT COLOR SWIM SUIT DID YOU BUY? (adjective).

One cannot *define* nouns or verbs or other syntactic categories in terms of the things they express because there are too many exceptions. There may be a tendency to try to include exceptions by broadening what is meant by "thing" in "name of a thing" or what is meant by an "action" or a "state of being." So one might try to say that the noun HELP, in HELP IS ON THE WAY, is a thing, while the verb HELP, in YOU CAN HELP ME BY NOT DOING A THING, is a word for an action or state of being. But if so, what is meant by a word that describes an action or a state of being is *any* word that functions in a particular way in a string (i.e., as a verb) and what is meant by the name of a person, place, or thing is any word that functions in another way in a string (i.e., as a noun).

As Lyons says, the definition of a noun:

> cannot be applied without circularity to determine the status of such English words as TRUTH, BEAUTY, ELECTRICITY, etc. The circularity lies in the fact that the only reason we have for saying that "truth," "beauty," and "electricity" are "things" is that the words which refer to them in English are nouns. [Lyons, 1968:318–319]

Lyons goes on to recommend that the definitions be taken as giving characteristics of typical members of syntactic categories rather than as defining their membership.

Probably, notional classification plays some role in language learning. Even if we do not first classify a concept into a broader category such as an action and then use it in language, concepts that are similar in meaning can be related syntactically to many of the same concepts. For example, knowing that DENNIS can be related to HOPS in the string DENNIS HOPS, the child who is aware of the similarity between hopping and jumping may generalize and produce the string DENNIS JUMPS. Thus, semantic similarity allows the second word to acquire the syntactic properties of the first. However, this does not require the formation of some broader concept that includes both hopping and jumping, nor that the syntactic properties shared by the two words be associated with any broader concept.

The difficulties of notional categorization can be overcome by specifying the category of each word in a string in terms of its relation to the categories of the other words in the string. This is formal categorization.

Table 1.3. *Formal syntactic categorization*

(a) The sentences of Goodlish abbreviated							
ESS	EFF	EPP	DSS	DPP	DFF	ESP	EPS
ESF	EPF	EFP	DSG	DPG	DFG	DSP	DPS
DPF	DFP	DSF	DFS	ESG	EPG	EFG	EFS

(b) Production rules for Goodlish

$C_1 \rightarrow \{E, D\} \qquad C_2 \rightarrow \{S, P, F\} \qquad C_3 \rightarrow G$

$S \rightarrow C_1 C_2 \{C_2, C_3\}$

Standard linguistic notation is used. The arrow means "is rewritten as"; braces mean that only one of the elements inside is to be selected; C is the abbreviation for syntactic category; S is the symbol for a string.

Formal syntactic categories

Formal syntactic categories depend, not on the meaning of the words that belong to them, but on how the words belonging to them can be related to those of other categories in the strings of a language. Ignoring for the moment inflections and functors, formal syntactic categories depend on the sequential relations their members can have with those of other categories. We can illustrate these sequential relations using a set of 24 three-word sentences from the artificial language Goodlish. To eliminate the possibility of using notional properties, we abbreviate each word by its initial letter in Table 1.3(a). We gave this sample of letter strings to people and asked them to find the syntactic categories and production rules that characterized three-element strings from abbreviated Goodlish. Since they did not know either the meaning of individual letters or the whole strings, they could not use any notional properties. All subjects came up with the analysis in Table 1.3(b) based only on the sequential properties of the strings.

The three formulas for the syntactic categories plus the formula for the string describe the generalizable, formal properties of three-element strings of Goodlish. For such a simple lexicon, the formal syntactic classification corresponds to a notional classification. The reader who turns back to the preceding sections will see that C_1 is the verb category, C_2 the noun category, and C_3, the adjective category.

The set of formulas is an elegant and economical means for representing the sequential properties of the strings of a language. As we discuss in the next two sections, the rules can be followed to generate all and only the sequences belonging to the language. Since the sequences of symbols in natural language carry information about relations of concepts, we want to look carefully at the psychological properties of symbol sequences to understand how a language user can learn to recognize, discriminate among, and produce them.

Inferring and using sequential properties: underlying structure

Some of the psychology of how people handle generalizable symbol sequences can be illustrated by another little experiment using abbreviated Goodlish. This time we gave people only a list of the elements of the language: D, E, F, G, P, and S. Their job was to try to discover which 24 of the 216 three-element strings were the well-formed sentences in an artificial language. They guessed one string at a time and we told them whether or not the guess was a well-formed string. In effect, this was a standard concept-learning task.

The expected value of the number of trials required to randomly pick 24 items from a pool of 216 is 208. However, none of our subjects required more than 110 trials; one person succeeded in 55 trials. Therefore, our subjects were not just picking strings at random.

It is clear that our subjects were learning more than just a list of the individual well-formed strings. They were learning something about the sequential properties of the strings that they were able to generalize and use to produce new examples. What they learned about the well-formed strings is a generating principle, or algorithm, which might be represented as shown in Figure 1.2. It is very much more economical than the list of 24 strings. This means it is easier to remember and easier to use. Note that the graph contains the same information as the set of production rules derived by our subjects in the first experiment. Our subjects, since they were able to produce nonrandomly the remaining strings of Goodlish from a partial sample, must have

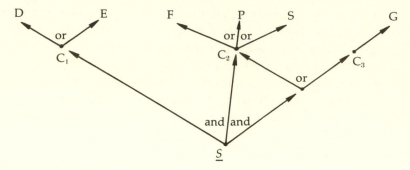

Figure 1.2. Graph generating all the well-formed three-symbol strings of abbreviated Goodlish.

been using a generating algorithm. Some subjects, in fact, are able to describe such an algorithm. A traditional account would claim that subjects generalized from previously learned to novel Goodlish strings. But to avoid circularity, such an account then must specify the dimensions of similarity between old and new strings along which the generalization occurred. A description of the similarity turns out to be a restatement of the algorithm. Because the graph provides information about connections that are not overtly present in the set of well-formed strings themselves, it is an example of an *underlying structure*.

Natural language learners do the same thing as our subjects except on a grander scale. From a limited sample of strings they are able to generalize the sequential properties and produce new, well-formed strings. They are also able to determine whether a novel string is well formed or not. Natural language users, then, must be using an underlying structure.

But how do language users abstract from symbol sequences the regularities that can be portrayed in underlying structure? Our subjects in the two experiments told us what they were doing, and from this we were able to get a fair idea of how they went about their task. But abbreviated Goodlish is an extremely simple language. What happens when more complex sequential properties are used?

Miller and Stein (Miller, 1967) tried to discover what procedures people use to abstract regularities from incomplete samples of artificial language sentences. Although they were able to distinguish "about nine different strategies," their subjects appeared to be using a great deal of unspecifiable intuition: "There is more psychology here than we know what to do with" (p. 165). Recently, more formal descriptions of language rule inference have been attempted. Harris (1972) developed such a description in the form of a computer program that used a heuristic procedure to find the "best" set of production rules describing a partial sample of English sentences.

In his review, Miller says that he and Stein were surprised at how poorly their subjects did in the rule inference task (Miller and Stein, 1963). Because it was so difficult, Miller concludes that people are not very good at inferring rules on the basis of sequential information alone. He suggests that for natural language learning, people must be using another source of information to supplement that available from the symbol sequences themselves. We believe that Miller is correct. Our model for syntax acquisition works by combining sequence information with semantic information (see Chapter 6).

Some psychologists, notably Skinner (1957), are reluctant to involve underlying structure in explanations of language use, preferring instead to deal with input and output "surface" data, which are directly observable. The ability to produce and understand (behave appropriately in response to) novel sentences is attributed to generalization. But as we argued, to go further and identify the dimensions of similarity along which generalization occurs, the behaviorist is forced to confront the equivalent of underlying cognitive structure.[4]

Underlying structures are widely used by linguists and psychologists as formal descriptions of language data without considering how such structures (generating algorithms) might be acquired by the principles of learning. In fact, many linguists, believing that such structures are innate and impossible to learn, assume that the learning theorist should *not* have an interest in underlying language structure. Lakoff critically summarizes the arguments by some of his fellow linguists (Chomsky in particular) that underlying linguistic structure should not be in the domain of the learning theorist:

> There are at present no general learning theories that can account for this [linguistic structure]. It is hard to imagine what any such theories

> could be like. Therefore, it is plausible to assume that there can be no
> such theories. But the argument is fallacious: Nothing follows from a
> lack of imagination. [Lakoff, 1973:34]

However, the argument is not as simple as that. It has been
supposed that formal definitions of syntactic categories require
that only syntactic information can be used to learn the formal
classifications. The possibility that nonlinguistic sources can provide information other than notional categories for the learning
of syntax has not been adequately considered.

Production rules and the generation
of language strings

The underlying structure in Figure 1.2 and the equivalent set of
production rules are an economical means of describing regularities across the sequences of well-formed Goodlish strings. Since
people can infer new strings from old ones, the structure and
rules might also represent the information used in the inference.
That is, the rules and structure might represent the information a
Goodlish speaker uses to generate and parse strings. The set of
production rules may or may not describe the actual cognitive
operations carried out by a language user. We shall return to this
question in Chapter 3.

Each production rule by itself describes an operation that can
be carried out automatically; that is, independently of any other
rule and without information not explicitly part of the rule. Each
production rule is a *local* rule that does not require information
from other rules, structures, or strings and performs an independent and isolable operation in which everything to be done is
specified within the rule itself. A *global* rule, in contrast, does
require information from other rules, structures, or strings and
depends on the operations of other rules or on other parts of the
structure.

Although the individual production rules given earlier are
local, the way they are combined is governed by global instructions, for example, the instruction allowing syntactic category
rules to be used after the string rule. Although global rules may
be more general and less tedious to state, specifying underlying
structure in terms of local rules guarantees that one has not ig-

nored crucial and difficult steps in the process. Therefore, it is an advantage for a cognitive theory to express as much as possible in terms of local rules, because their mechanical clarity helps to make a theory clear, explicit, and testable. This point is discussed further in Chapter 5. This approach is argued for by Miller, Galanter, and Pribram (1960); Chomsky (1965 and elsewhere); and Arbib (1972).

However, it is impossible to present a complete theory of language use entirely in terms of local rules. We also have to specify how and when to use the local rules and, sometimes, the order in which they must be used. For models of language cognition, we often have to first specify some goal state and then specify how to apply the local rules until that goal state is reached. It is an advantage for a cognitive theory of language to describe the global procedures it requires as clearly and completely as possible. One indication of the clarity and completeness of a global procedure is that it has the mechanical preciseness of a local rule. A guarantee of such preciseness is that the global rules be specifiable in terms of a computer program, to be operated automatically. In some cases, however, it may only be possible to describe a global procedure in a less rigorous way.

Presenting a syntactic theory in terms of a formal mechanical analogy whose parts and operations are explicit and simple ensures that the theory does not inadvertently rely on vague or magical properties. In addition it will be easier to find out if any essential features have been omitted or any errors committed. A theory presented in terms of a mechanism to do syntax has this advantage: "Nothing reveals our ignorance about a phenomenon more clearly than an attempt to define it in constructional terms" (Walter, cited by Block [personal communication]).

There are three different things we can do with a set of production rules: (1) we can generate strings at random; (2) we can generate a particular string, i.e., one expressing particular relations among particular concepts; (3) we can parse a particular string. The same set of local production rules may be involved in all three language tasks, but the global procedures required will be different. The set of global rules required to generate random strings is much simpler than the sets required for the other processes. However, natural language users do not generate sentences randomly. But because random generation is simple we will use it to illustrate how global rules guide the application of local production rules.

For convenience, here is a copy of the production rules for abbreviated Goodlish from Table 1.3:

$$C_1 \rightarrow \{E, D\} \qquad C_2 \rightarrow \{S, P, F\} \qquad C_3 \rightarrow G$$
$$\underline{S} \rightarrow C_1\ C_2\ \{C_2, C_3\}$$

First we need a global rule that tells what to do with the other rules. This is the executive procedure. Then we can give the remaining global rules in the form of a program that calls in and uses the local production rules.

> EXECUTIVE:
>
> Perform the following procedures in numerical order unless directed otherwise.

1. Call in string rule $\underline{S}$.
2. See if there are any elements on the right of the $\underline{S}$ rule that correspond to elements on the left of any C rule. If *yes*, select one such C rule; if *no*, go to 5.
3. Perform the operations on the right side of C rule and substitute the resulting elements in $\underline{S}$ rule.
4. Go to 2.
5. Output transformed right side of $\underline{S}$ rule.
6. Terminate program.

Except for the executive rule and the "go to" steps that order the execution of the rules, the steps in the program are local with respect to each other: Their operation does not require information about the operation or internal structure of the other steps. They only use information about the results of the other steps. However, the program steps are global with respect to the operations of the production rules. Their operation depends on the operation or structure of the production rules.

Even though programs of global procedures for parsing and generating are complicated, with many more "go to" and other control operations, they can be described as exact procedures. For very simple strings, every time the program is followed, exactly the same sequence of operations will be performed. However, for more complex strings there will be many alternative sequences of operations that could eventually complete the parse or generate them. The alternative sequences are likely to differ as to how many steps in the program are needed to reach the goal. A model of linguistic performance should also provide some way to select the more efficient sequences of global procedures and local rules. Such ways to improve efficiency are often difficult to specify as rigorously as ordinary global procedures. In computational linguistics and cognitive theory they are generally referred to as heuristic procedures. In Appendix A we will suggest some heuristic procedures for improving parsing and generating efficiency that are also consistent with what is known about how people actually do these tasks.

Hierarchical and recursive properties of underlying structure

In this section we want to look at some important characteristics of the sequences involved in language string generating and parsing, in other words, the characteristics of the underlying structure of sequences. Two important characteristics of symbol sequences in language are that their underlying structures are (1) hierarchical and (2) recursive.

The production rules for Goodlish and the tree graph of underlying structure in Figure 1.2 carry equivalent sorts of information. Both representations can be characterized as hierarchically organized. This means that elements at one level describe (or control) elements at another level. Each individual production rule is itself hierarchically organized. A string is described in terms of syntactic categories and a syntactic category is described in terms of individual symbols. The relationship of the syntactic category rules to the string production rule is also hierarchical: The category rules operate on products of the string rule, resulting in elements at still a different level.

Notice that for all the rules, the element on the left of the arrow is rewritten in terms of elements on a different level. The tree graph portrays the different levels. The rule corresponding to the lower portion is related hierarchically to the rules corresponding to the upper portion. The rules corresponding to the upper portion operate on the elements produced by the rules for the lower portion, producing the terminal elements. On the tree graph, this compounding of hierarchical organization is shown as nodes that lead to other nodes.

One characteristic of language often discussed in connection with hierarchies and production rules is the absence of a definite limit to the number of strings that can be generated. Sometimes this is described as the "infinite use of finite means" (Bolinger, 1975). The "finite means" are the set of production rules. Each production rule frequently has several alternative products, and there are very many rules needed to even approximately describe a natural language. This means that they can be hierarchically combined to generate a very much larger number of sequences of terminal elements, or strings. But a very much larger number is not an unlimited number. What allows the number of possible strings to expand without bound is that one or a set of the production rules is *recursive:*[5] the same rule or set of rules can be used over and over again. For example, the following set of rules is recursive: $C_1 \rightarrow D\ E$; $C_2 \rightarrow (S)\ F$; $S \rightarrow C_1\ C_2$. The C_2 rule, by electing to produce the optional $\underline{S}$, calls for the $\underline{S}$ rule to be applied all over again. The $\underline{S}$ rule then allows the C_1 and C_2 to be applied and so on. Thus an unlimited number of different strings can be generated, such as:

                    DEF
            DE   DEF   F
    DE   DE   DEF   F   F

Recursion is just a special case of hierarchical organization. It occurs whenever an element can appear on both the left and right sides in a production rule set. The element may appear on both sides of the arrow in a single rule or on the left side in one rule and on the right side in another.

In this chapter we have used examples from simple artificial languages to illustrate hierarchical organization and recursion. But the same characteristics can be found in the structure of natural language sentences as well. Consider a set of simple sentences where the subject of one sentence is the object of another: THE ENGINE PUMPED THE WATER. THE WATER QUENCHED THE FIRE. THE FIRE BURNED THE WOODS. English grammar allows us a great economy by combining the simple sentences into a more complex sentence. We can combine two: THE FIRE (THAT) THE WATER

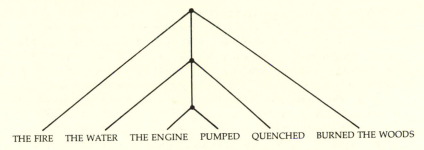

Figure 1.3. A hierarchical sentence with three levels.

QUENCHED BURNED THE WOODS, or we can combine all three: THE FIRE (THAT) THE WATER (THAT) THE ENGINE PUMPED QUENCHED BURNED THE WOODS. Notice how similar this sentence is in form to the string we recursively generated above. Connecting each of the subjects to their respective verbs (Figure 1.3) illustrates the hierarchical nature of the sentence's structure.

There have been several arguments made for the hierarchical organization of language other than the ones presented here (Lashley, 1951; Miller, Galanter, and Pribram, 1960; Lenneberg, 1967; Neisser, 1967). All contemporary views of language cognition include hierarchical organization as a basic principle of syntax. Theories differ as to what is hierarchically organized and how the organization, the underlying cognitive structure, is involved in the generating and parsing of sentences. Much of the remainder of this book is devoted to this dispute and to our model for the acquisition and use of underlying structure for language cognition.

Now we are going to describe some characteristics of the language user that are basic to our model of syntax.

Characteristics of the language user

The acquisition and use of language requires certain cognitive abilities of the language user.

1. We assume that the language user is an organism with enough cognitive apparatus to perceive aspects of its environment and to form cognitive categories and deal with relations of these categories. In other words, language users must be capable of processing pragmatic information.

2. The organism must be capable of perceiving and producing the signals that carry linguistic information. For most humans this means the perception and production of speech and writing, but using language does not involve these media necessarily. Although it may be possible for language to be acquired and understood by an organism that receives but never produces linguistic signals, the organism would have to be capable of producing some nonlinguistic behavior as evidence of its understanding even if only to receive appropriate input from its teachers. For our purposes, the important role of competent other language users is not to communicate information about the world *through* language, but to serve as a source of information *about* language. It is important that language data provided by competent language users correlate with the learner's nonlinguistic experience.

3. As well as acquiring concepts and processing linguistic signals, the language user must be able to combine these two skills by forming associations between the linguistic signals and the concepts (lexical information processing).

4. Finally, the language user must be able to form associations between relations among linguistic signals and relations among concepts associated with these signals (syntactic information processing).

Our focus is on the fourth ability, associating relations of concepts with relations of linguistic symbols, and how this ability can be learned. We are interested only in the cognitive skills that serve language acquisition and use, not in how language is used in the service of other cognitive processes. This means that we are not going to discuss topics like the use of language for explanation, phatic interaction, or to achieve human and esthetic goals in poetry and literature.

Our model of syntax

There is a trend in modern linguistics and psycholinguistics to invest syntax with more and more semantic richness.[6] In contrast, we are going to present a model of syntax that is simpler than other models. The simplicity derives from our presupposition that language and thinking are far from identical; that considerable cognitive processing goes on that is not essentially involved in syntax. We take the position also that syntax use and acquisition do not work in an information vacuum, that nonsyntactic information is crucial for understanding and generating language strings and for learning how to do so.

In our view, language is merely a blueprint for thought, a code that carries the bare essentials of the relations of concepts in ideas. To attempt to explain how language works does not entail trying to explain all cognition. Concepts can be related to each other in extremely varied and complex ways. Relations of lexemes signify that these conceptual relations are present. But we do not believe that understanding these conceptual relations is essentially syntactic. Consider the nature of the ontologic relations expressed by the following strings: BAG OF GOLD, BRICK OF GOLD, LOVE OF GOLD, CHLORIDE OF GOLD, DENSITY OF GOLD, BEAUTY OF GOLD, PURCHASE OF GOLD, VALUE OF GOLD, PURIFICATION OF GOLD, MELTING OF GOLD, TRANSMUTATION OF GOLD. A language user understands that the following types of relationships are involved: filled with, made of, affect for, chemical compound, quantified physical property, positive esthetic property, economic transaction, comparative trade property, process of contaminant removal, change of state, change of atomic identity.

All these relations are encoded syntactically by relating GOLD and one of the other lexemes through the preposition OF. In each case syntactic information tells us that the other concept is related to "gold." We do not believe that additional information about the nature of the ontologic relationship must be provided by syntax. Understanding the relationships expressed by connecting GOLD to BRICK or to VALUE or to BAG, is part of our understanding of the concepts named by these lexemes, part of our pragmatic knowledge.

It is the job of syntax to encode these relationships. If syntax encoded all the unique aspects of every relation that could be expressed, the syntactic encoding system would get out of hand. The syntactic information in each of the strings appears to be basically the same: noun followed by preposition OF, followed by GOLD. The strings each use sequence information and the insertion of the functor OF. We could, as some theories do, distinguish different types of noun. There are count-nouns and abstract nouns, nouns that express animate concepts, and nouns derived from verbs by nominalizing inflections, and so on. But even these distinctions in syntactic categories cannot distinguish, say, BAG OF GOLD and BRICK OF GOLD, which respectively can express the different relationships "filled with" and "made of." It would be impossible for syntax to distinguish each kind of relationship in a unique way. The problem is that the range of relationships that can be expressed is so complex while the linear order of language strings is so relatively simple.

There must be an economical basis (underlying structure) for the syntactic code. Syntax will not be able to encode the information required to uniquely distinguish every possible relation of concepts; it is reasonable to assume that the relations can only be partially distinguished.

To distinguish alternatives in a practical way, the alternatives must be grouped into categories. That is, conceptual relationships must be describable in terms of a small set of general relations or features. These general features could then be encoded by syntax. Since there should be far fewer of these general features than there are unique relationships, there is far less information that needs to be carried by syntax. Every model of syntax makes this assumption. However, there is considerable disagreement about just what features of conceptual relationships need to be encoded, how many there are, and the logical and psychological bases for them.

We posit that there are just two very simple features of conceptual relations that must be encoded by relations among lexemes. When expressing a complex idea, only these two features are needed in order to use syntactic information to arrange the lexemes in a well-formed sequence with function words and inflections inserted where needed. When presented with a language string, the syntax gives information about these two features that, combined with lexical and pragmatic information, allows the complex idea to be decoded. These two features, which are not exclusively linguistic, permit the language learner to differentiate the grammatical categories on a formal rather than notional basis.

The two features are *scope* and *dependency.* They are not new to linguistics; most theories include a form of scope, some theories use dependency. Our model is unique in that it takes scope and dependency to be the only essential features for the development of syntactic structure.

Two concepts that are directly related, directly connected, are said to be in each other's scope. Scope only includes the *fact* that two concepts are related, not anything about the nature of the relationship they share. For example, in the phrase BIG HOUSE, the scope of BIG is HOUSE and the scope of HOUSE is BIG. Scope is also compounded hierarchically. For example, for one meaning of the phrase BIG HOUSE SALE, the scope of BIG is HOUSE SALE as a unit, while HOUSE and SALE are in each other's scope.

Dependency is a feature imposed on each scope relationship. It describes which of two connected concepts, or sets of concepts, is the main one and which is the dependent. Using the lexemes to represent the concepts, BIG is conceptually dependent on HOUSE in the phrase BIG HOUSE, and in the phrase HOUSE SALE, HOUSE is conceptually dependent on SALE. We explain scope and dependency in more detail in Chapter 2.

The processes involved in language use

Figure 1.4 shows a simplified overview of the processes we think are involved in understanding and generating language strings. Understanding is represented by the information flow in the upward direction; generation by the flow in the downward direction. Let us follow the diagram through from the top down. We begin with an idea. We do not pretend to have a complete understanding of what ideas are, but we can say that an expressible idea consists of concepts that are related in some way. The idea, or underlying semantics, in the topmost box is what we intend to express.

The second stage is to construct an internal representation of those features of the idea that are essential for syntax to work on. This representation must contain enough information to construct the idea when the information flow is in the upward direction. This representation portrays the idea in terms of more general features. As mentioned above, different theories of language posit different kinds of features for this step. Our model uses only scope and dependency.

Now, going down to the third box, we need a mechanism that can correlate the scope and dependency information with information about lexeme order, functors, and inflections. It must be able to take any representation in the second box and turn it into a language string in the bottom box, but not just any string; it

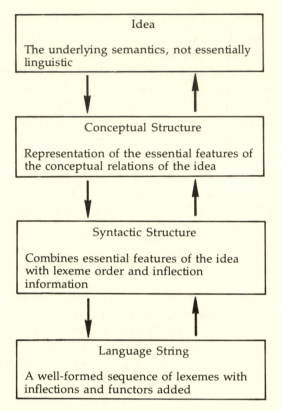

Figure 1.4. Overview of language generating and understanding.

must be a string to which other language users can apply their own syntactic mechanisms and have a good chance of coming out with an idea at the top that is functionally similar to the idea originally expressed.

The reader should not take the diagram in Figure 1.4 to be a claim that actual language processing is so simple. In particular, parallel processing, interactions, and lexical interpretation are not shown in the figure.

What is needed for syntax acquisition

We are going to make as few assumptions as possible about the cognitive processes required for syntax acquisition and the environment in which it occurs. We assume that a language learner has an environment rich enough to provide language with enough semantic complexity to be interesting, at least one competent language user present (a teacher) for the learner to interact with, and the ability to perceive instances of concepts and the utterance of its teacher and be able to produce utterances of its own. In addition, we presume the abilities to associate, discriminate, and generalize – abilities granted to all creatures who are able to interact with their environment in interesting ways.

We require that the language learner be able to determine (and remember) scope and dependency. Determining scope amounts to first connecting two concepts together, then treating them as a unit to be joined to a third concept. The way in which the first pair is connected to the third concept incorporates the dependency relations. In other words, we require for syntax acquisition the ability to form hierarchical associations among concepts and to include dependency in the hierarchy. We are going to demonstrate that this type of hierarchical structure can serve as the basis for an adequate and interesting semantic representation and also for a powerful syntactic mechanism that can convert the semantic information into language strings and vice versa.[7]

Outline of the following chapters

Chapter 2 develops our representation of the essential features of conceptual relations that underlie syntax: the orrery model. We compare our representation to some of the current case grammar models and with the semantic system of transformational grammar.

Chapter 3 describes empirical work on the "psychological reality" of the different versions of underlying conceptual structure. We review earlier studies and present some of our own.

Chapter 4 discusses theories of syntax. We explain the rationale behind some current linguistic methodology and criticize the attempt to represent semantic properties as syntactic rules. The criticisms of phrase structure grammars are discussed. Then the basic operations of transformational grammar are compared and evaluated.

Chapter 5 presents our own model for syntax: the syntax crystal. The rules are represented by modules whose properties are described. Then the application of the modules is illustrated in detail with a variety of constructions, particularly those of concern to other theories.

In the first part of Chapter 6, the arguments supporting an innate, specifically linguistic, acquisition device are discussed and criticized. In the second part, the acquisition of syntax crystal rules is described – first in theoretical terms and then in the form of an algorithm for the production of syntax crystal modules.

The Appendixes include a description of SCRYP, the computer simulation of syntax crystal operations; the language acquisition game, a simulation of language acquisition; the syntax crystal game, a simulation of the generating and parsing of grammatical strings using syntax crystal modules; and further syntactic constructions with syntax crystal modules.

2
Underlying conceptual structure

In the preceding chapter, we looked at some of the properties of language strings. We examined the relations among morphemes that are available to carry information about the relations of concepts. We considered several lines of argument converging on the conclusion that language strings have an organization beyond their sequential structure. The organization is hierarchical, that is, organized at several different levels simultaneously, and the organization can be recursive, which allows parts of the organizing principle to be used over and over again.

The organization does not appear explicitly in language strings, but its existence can be inferred from the strings and how they are handled by language users. No contemporary account of the psychology of language or linguistics denies such organization (although a few may ignore it, e.g., Winokur, 1976).

The organization is the basis for the syntactic code that enables language strings to carry information about the relation of concepts. To understand a string, the language user must convert the sequence of morphemes (inflected lexemes plus function words) into something from which the idea may be extracted. When expressing an idea, the process is reversed. The cognitive operations involved can be described as the syntactic mechanism of the language user. A description of and a model for this mechanism are given in Chapter 5.

In this chapter we are going to study the contents of the second box in the flow chart of Figure 1.4: underlying conceptual structure. Formally, it is the end-product of the syntactic mechanism in the process of expressing an idea. This does not mean that conceptual structure participates in the same cognitive operations for both generating and parsing – the structure may be the same, the way it is used is clearly different. We will discuss the generating and parsing processes in Chapters 4 and 5.

The thought which one attempts to express by a language string could never be *completely* specified.[1] To even approach a strong sense of "complete," such a description would include at least a detailed selection from one's biography. It is clear that a language string could not be expected to carry information about *every* detail of the idea it expresses. And yet language strings do succeed, more or less, in carrying some information about ideas. Lexemes express concepts. Relations of lexemes express relations of concepts. What we want to know is how much and what sort of information about relations of concepts is expressed by the relations of lexemes in language strings. In the spirit of our approach, we first want to find out what there is about relations of concepts that *must* be encoded by syntax in order to sufficiently account for the information passed between language users. In other words: What are the essential features of relations of concepts that syntax must encode?

First, we are going to present the arguments for our own account of the features that best describe the relations of concepts for syntactic encoding. Then we will describe our model, the orrery, in terms of these features. After that we will consider some alternative models that also claim to represent conceptual relations. Then we will critically compare and contrast the different approaches. The next chapter will review empirical research on language use and acquisition to help us assess the psychological plausibility of each model.

Scope and dependency as features of conceptual structure

Our working principle is to try to abstract the minimally essential features of conceptual relations that could provide an adequate basis for syntactic encoding. We need not require the syntactic mechanism to handle information that is independently provided to the language user from other sources. The other sources of information are (1) lexical – what concepts are involved in the idea expressed by the language string; and (2) pragmatic – the

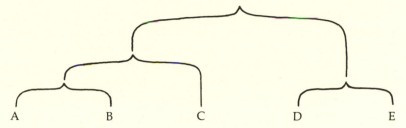

Figure 2.1. One possible scope hierarchy among five concepts.

language user's knowledge of how concepts can be related to one another, and where more than one relationship is possible, the relative likelihood of the alternative relationships.

As we said in Chapter 1, we believe that two features of conceptual relations must be encoded by relations of lexemes: *scope* and *dependency*. Two concepts that are directly related, directly connected, are said to be in each other's scope. The scope of a concept may also be a set of concepts that in turn are in each other's scope. Scope thus describes the hierarchical connections among concepts. Concepts A and B may be joined together in each other's scope to form a unit. That unit in turn may be joined with concept C to form a still larger unit. And that larger unit can then be joined with the unit formed by connecting concepts D and E. What we have just described can be easily shown in a diagram. Figure 2.1 illustrates each of the scope connections by a brace.

Scope information tells only that concepts are connected, not anything about the nature of the connection. In other words, scope describes which concept or set of concepts is connected to (i.e., operates on) each other concept or set of concepts. Determining the scope relations in a complex idea involves determining which concepts are most directly related to other concepts to form a unit, which in turn is directly related to another concept or set of concepts. Treating scope as a binary feature greatly simplifies the representation of the relations of concepts. However, the pairwise connections are not essential to our model. Later we relax the binary assumption and allow three or more units to combine in one scope relationship.

Dependency is the other feature of a representation of conceptual relations that must be extracted from an idea for syntactic encoding. Dependency is a feature that is imposed on each scope relationship. It describes which of two connected concepts, or sets of concepts, is the main member of the pair with respect to the remaining concepts in the idea. It divides each scoped pair into main and dependent components. Since dependency is superimposed on scope, dependency cannot be represented without scope.

For simplicity in presentation, we are going to consider the dependency feature to have only three values. For example, if concepts A and B are scoped together, then either A is the main component, or B is the main component, or they are of approximately equal importance where each depends on the other. This third alternative we will rarely need. Thus, for nearly all cases, dependency is a binary feature. With respect to their connections as a unit to the remaining concepts in the idea, one of each connected pair will be dependent on the other.

Using only scope and dependency provides for a relatively simple representation of the relation of concepts in an idea. Such a simplification provides an important advantage. Look again at Figure 1.4. The representation of conceptual relations (the second box) is connected to the language string (the fourth box) by the syntactic mechanism (the third box). Other things being equal, the simpler the representation of conceptual relations, the simpler it is going to be to construct a syntactic mechanism to map its contents onto language strings. The power and economy of the syntactic model described in Chapter 5 owes much to the simplicity of the representation of conceptual relations described here.

Scope and dependency can be found in other theories of the conceptual structure underlying language strings. Most theories employ a hierarchy of scope, at least implicitly. A few theories (e.g., that of Schank, 1973) employ dependency. But our model uses scope and dependency exclusively to represent underlying conceptual structure. In our model, the syntactic mechanism operates directly on this representation of conceptual relations to generate language and produces the representation of conceptual relations when parsing language strings. Therefore, the syntactic mechanism is also described by the features of scope and dependency. Now we are going to take a closer look at how the conceptual structure of ideas can be represented.

Representing the conceptual structure of a sentence using scope and dependency

Imagine that we are watching some children at play on the frozen surface of a pond. Suppose we are a team of security people assigned to protect the children of visiting United Nations diplomats. A second team is just over a small hill with another group of children. Each team has a walkie-talkie. A plump little fellow is scraping cautiously over the ice on double-runner skates. Nearby, another child is practicing for a speed-skating competition at her school. Her skates flash as she circles the perimeter of the pond. Suddenly she arcs close to the plump beginner, raises her arms, and pushes him over the ice. The little one screams in panic before he realizes his sister is just playing with him. The scream has carried over the hill. The other team asks over the walkie-talkie, "What's going on?"

We know what is happening. We wish to inform the other team about the event over the walkie-talkie and to do so quickly. That is, we want them to know the main features of the event; we want to communicate to them the important part of the knowledge we have about what is going on. We can identify the main concepts involved in the event. One possible set of main concepts is "push," "boy," "fat," "girl," "fast." We can associate a lexeme with each of them: PUSH(ES), BOY, FAT, GIRL, FAST. By speaking these words into the walkie-talkie we can inform the other team of *what is involved in what is going on*. However, with these five concepts, the person with the other walkie-talkie could imagine any of at least twelve events: For example, a boy could be pushing a fat girl fast. We also need to communicate the proper relation of the concepts in order to eliminate the ambiguity. What is the minimum information about the relation of the concepts that needs to be communicated?

Figure 2.2(a) shows each of the concepts, represented by a circle containing the name of the concept. The concepts may be located randomly on the figure.[2] Identifying the individual concepts means that we have perceived and classified the entities, attributes, and actions in the event we wish to describe. However, Figure 2.2(a) gives us no more information about how the concepts are related. It tells us only that they are related. The large oval drawn around the set of concepts shows that they belong to one complex idea. This oval represents the information carried by *primitive syntax* as discussed in Chapter 1.

Figure 2.2(b) shows how we can begin to represent some information about how the concepts are related. The two smaller ovals represent our extracting from the idea of the event the information that "girl" and "fast" are closely and directly related to each other; the same is true of "boy" and "fat." This relation we could further describe as "object-attribute," but we are deliberately not going to do so. The information represented by the two ovals tells us that the two concepts included in each oval are scoped together. BOY-FAT and GIRL-FAST now function as units to be scoped together with other concepts. Figure 2.2(c) adds one more oval to represent this added information. Dependency information is also included. One of the components inside each scope oval is marked with an asterisk. This is the main, or major, component. It is the member of each pair inside an oval that is more important with respect to the concepts outside that oval. Most of the time, we can decide which is the main component by seeing which one, if omitted, would cause the idea to lose more of its content. For example, BOY is the main component of the pair BOY-FAT.[3]

Although clear for simple ideas, representing the scope relations of an idea by a set of nested ovals becomes confusing as the number of concepts in an idea increases. We now present another way of representing scope and dependency relations that is much less confusing and also has heuristic advantages.

The orrery model of conceptual structure

We can think of the concepts in an idea as joined together in a way analogous to the way celestial bodies are joined in a planetary system. In both, a complete description of the interrelationships is enormously complex. However, for both, a description of the essential features is remarkably simple. The representation of a planetary system is called an *orrery* mobile, a

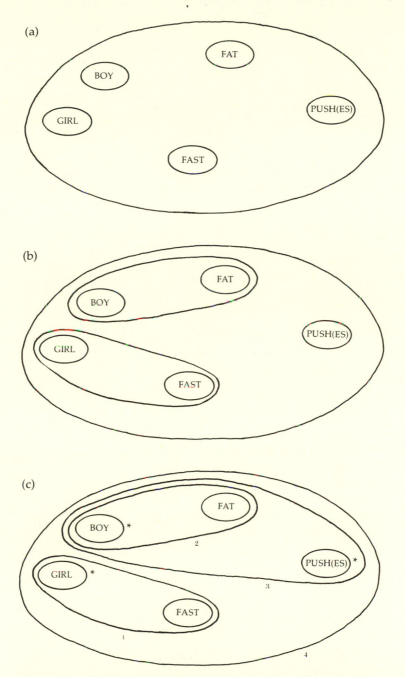

Figure 2.2. (a) The five main concepts of the skating incident. (b) Adding some scope information to the concepts. (c) All the scope information added to the concepts. Dependency information is indicated by
asterisks next to main components.

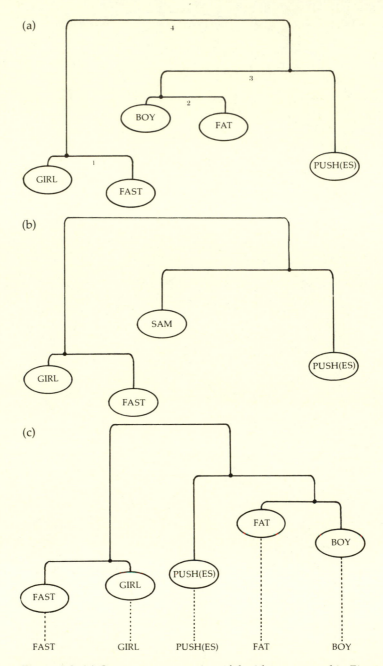

Figure 2.3. (a) Orrery representation of the idea portrayed in Figure 2.2. (b) Substituting SAM for FAT and BOY. (c) The orrery rotated by the syntactic mechanism to place the lexemes in the proper sequence.

mechanical model named after the inventor's sponsor Charles Boyle, fourth Earl of Orrery (d. 1731). Using the analogy between gravitational attraction and concept relatedness, Figure 2.3(a) illustrates the scope and dependency relations of the idea portrayed in Figure 2.2(c) using a "conceptual orrery" representation.

Each one of the numbered brackets joins two concepts together to form a subsystem that functions as a unit with respect to the remaining concepts. The numbers on the brackets correspond to the numbers on the ovals in Figure 2.2(c). For example, bracket 1 joins GIRL and FAST into a conceptual subsystem. The solid dots are the points at which one bracket is attached to another. Since the concepts are not arranged in any left-to-right sequence, we can think of the dots as swivel joints in a hanging mobile that allow one bracket to rotate about its point of attachment. As in any well-designed mobile, each attachment point is at the conceptual "center of gravity." That is, the attachment point is closer to the main "planet," or "heavy" concept and farther from the dependent "satellite," or "light" concept. Thus, for example, suspended from bracket 2 closer to the balance point is BOY. The dependent concept, FAT, is attached farther from the balance point. If there were a single concept equivalent to BOY and FAT joined by bracket 2, that concept could be substituted for bracket 2 and everything suspended from it. For example, if SAM were the fat boy and this fact were known by the speaker, the idea could then be portrayed as in Figure 2.3(b).

The orrery, as a representation of the essential features of the relations of concepts in an idea, describes a cognitive structure that is prelinguistic. It involves concepts and their relations without regard for how the idea might be expressed in natural language. The names of the concepts appear in orrery diagrams just for convenience; we could use pictures or number codes instead (cf. Norman, Rumelhart, and the LNR Research Group, 1975). The order in which the concepts appear in an orrery diagram need have nothing to do with the order in which they would be expressed by lexemes in a well-formed string. The orrery representation could even apply to an organism that did not use language, as long as it was cognitively complex enough to recognize and anticipate a variety of entities and events.

Relation of the orrery model to syntax

For a language user, the orrery represents the information that must be extracted from an idea in order to express it. The information in the orrery is then operated on by the syntactic mechanism to produce a language string. For the idea of the ice-skating incident, the syntactic mechanism must convert the orrery of Figure 2.3(a) into a string that can be spoken into the walkie-talkie: FAST GIRL PUSHES FAT BOY. We can think of the role of the syntactic mechanism as rotating the brackets of the orrery around the attachment swivels so that lexemes placed directly under the concepts they express appear in the proper order. The syntactic mechanism must also insert function words and inflections. Figure 2.3(c) illustrates how the orrery from Figure 2.3(a) is rotated so that lexemes written below their concepts appear in the correct order.

The structural variety allowed by the orrery model

Scope and dependency together permit many alternative conceptual structures for any set of concepts. Three concepts may be connected to form six different structures. With four concepts the number of different possible structures jumps to 84. Figure 2.4 illustrates a small sample of these structures along with a description of their scope and dependency relations.

Thus the orrery has the potential to structurally resolve a great number of distinct relations among concepts.[4] Now we want to apply the orrery principles to some real sets of related concepts in order to show how the system can work.

Different ideas from the same set of concepts: the resolving power of the orrery model

We will begin with a simple set of concepts: "truck," "tomato," and "farm." These three concepts can be combined into several different ideas, some of which are "sensible" given our pragmatic information.[5] Figure 2.5 illustrates how both scope and dependency work together to structurally resolve the more commonsense relations of the three concepts. Each orrery diagram is

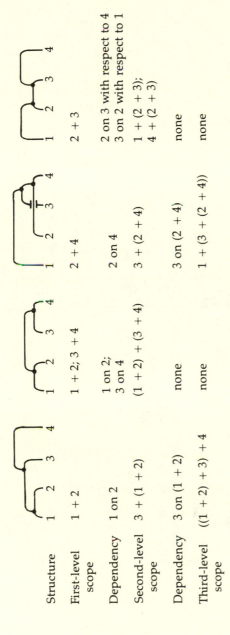

Structure			
First-level scope	1 + 2	1 + 2; 3 + 4	2 + 4
Dependency	1 on 2	1 on 2; 3 on 4	2 on 4
Second-level scope	3 + (1 + 2)	(1 + 2) + (3 + 4)	3 + (2 + 4)
Dependency	3 on (1 + 2)	none	3 on (2 + 4)
Third-level scope	((1 + 2) + 3) + 4	none	1 + (3 + (2 + 4))

Structure	
First-level scope	2 + 3
Dependency	2 on 3 with respect to 4 3 on 2 with respect to 1
Second-level scope	1 + (2 + 3); 4 + (2 + 3)
Dependency	none
Third-level scope	none

Figure 2.4. A sample of the 84 structures made possible by connecting four concepts in a scope hierarchy with dependency.

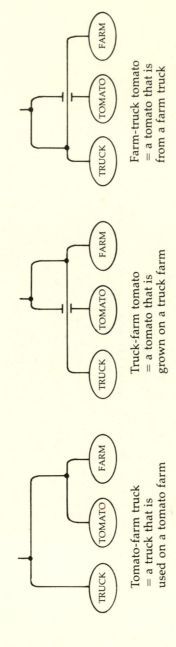

Tomato-farm truck
= a truck that is
used on a tomato farm

Truck-farm tomato
= a tomato that is
grown on a truck farm

Farm-truck tomato
= a tomato that is
from a farm truck

Figure 2.5. Orrery diagrams illustrating different scopes and dependencies among three concepts.

accompanied by a short phrase that expresses the relations of concepts in English. To avoid ambiguity, hyphens are used and a paraphrase is also provided. The left-to-right sequence in the orrery is arbitrary; the only critical information is carried by which concept is connected to which other (scope), and which of two connected concepts is closer to the point where they are connected to a third (dependency). When the idea portrayed by an orrery is expressed in a string, the scope and dependency information is converted to sequence information by the syntactic mechanism.

To avoid any further ambiguity, the dependency relations of the second-level scope bracket are indicated by a truncated attachment closer to the main component. We can think of the truncated attachment as representing a potential connection to one or more other concepts. For example, if we were to connect the concept "red" to the rest of the structure, above TRUCK, the left orrery would then represent the idea of a red (tomato-farm) truck.

Although scope connections alone distinguish the left orrery of Figure 2.5 from the other two, they do not distinguish the center one from that on the right. In this case, the dependency is crucial to distinguish the two different relations of concepts. For the middle orrery, TOMATO is connected more closely to FARM in the unit TRUCK + FARM, indicating that FARM is the main component and TRUCK the dependent component. For the right orrery, FARM is dependent on TRUCK with respect to that pair's connection to TOMATO.

Elaborating on the conceptual structure expressed by simple strings

A very simple idea made up by combining only two concepts can be further elaborated by adding additional concepts. The connection between the two basic concepts that form the core of the idea is not destroyed by the additional structure. It still appears by tracing the orrery through the main component of each scoped pair. The process of gradual elaboration is illustrated in Figure 2.6.

In the second orrery shown in Figure 2.6, CARS is connected to

(a)

(b)

(c)

(d)

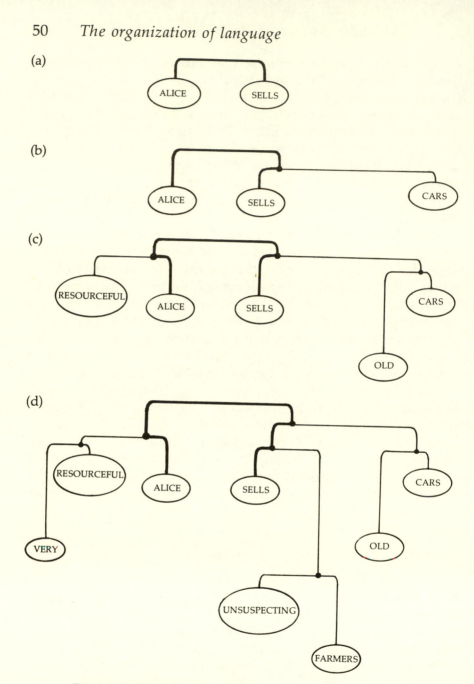

Figure 2.6. Orrery for a simple idea that is elaborated in three stages. Heavy line indicates the original conceptual connection. Concepts are shown in the order they would be expressed.

(a)

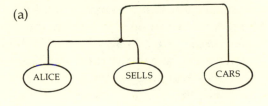

(b)

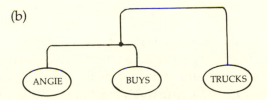

Figure 2.7. (a) Alternative orrery structure for ALICE SELLS CARS. (b) Orrery for ANGIE BUYS TRUCKS that is structurally consistent with (a).

SELLS to form a unit which in turn is connected to ALICE. With respect to ALICE, SELLS is the main component, with CARS dependent upon it. However, there is an alternative method of connecting the concepts: ALICE and SELLS could first be connected as a unit and then CARS connected to them in turn. This is shown in Figure 2.7. How do we choose between them?

Alternative conceptual structures for a given string

Theoretically, it is not necessary that one of the above orreries rather than the other be considered the "true" representation of the conceptual structure underlying the string ALICE SELLS CARS. It is even possible that language users may differ as to which version better describes their conceptual structure. However, it is likely that each language user would maintain some degree of consistency across different orreries. For example, someone whose conceptual structure is better described by Figure 2.7(a) than by Figure 2.6 would most likely conceive the relations underlying the string ANGIE BUYS TRUCKS as shown in Figure 2.7(b).

One reason for favoring the version in Figure 2.6(b) over that in Figure 2.7(a), with SELLS and CARS joined first as a unit, is implied by the series of orreries in Figure 2.6. Each of the lower three orreries is formed by substituting a larger, more complete set of concepts in the place of a single concept in the version above it. Following Miller (1962), we can also look at it the other way around. If we start with the second orrery, we can replace the unit SELLS + CARS by SELLS and still get the main idea across. However, for the orrery in Figure 2.7, it is very difficult to find a single concept that can be substituted for the unit ALICE + SELLS and still represent the basic idea. Thus we might say that the orrery in Figure 2.6(b) is based on more "natural" units. Furthermore, grouping SELLS and CARS together, as in Figure 2.6(b), corresponds to the classic distinction between subject and predicate. Chapter 3 describes some experimental methods that may aid in deciding which of alternative conceptual structures is a better approximation to the cognitive structure of human language users.

The representation of sentence modes

Up to this point we have used very simple examples to show how the orrery represents the relations of concepts that make up an idea. Each of the ideas in our examples would be expressed in English by a simple affirmative declarative sentence. But there are other sentence forms, such as negatives, questions, and sentences in other tenses. Each of these forms can have many variants, each with its own set of grammatical regularities. These different forms of sentences do more than just provide variety in the language. The form of the sentence is an important cue to the relations of concepts expressed by the sentence. There appears to be a relationship between the idea expressed by a simple affirmative declarative sentence and other sentence forms expressing the same set of concepts. For example, a negative sentence may express a denial of the relation of concepts expressed by the corresponding simple affirmative sentence; a question typically expresses a request for information about the truth value, or some other feature, of the relation of concepts expressed by the corresponding simple affirmative sentence. Other sentence forms may express ideas that add to the idea of the basic form, some indication that it occurred in the past or future, that it is a continuing event, involves a conditional, or conveys some other sort of information encoded by *tenses*.

We can follow a tradition in language theory and adopt a simplification, dividing up the complex idea carried by such sentence forms into *conceptual relations* and *mode*. Conceptual relations are what we have been discussing all along – the relations of concepts portrayed by the orrery. Mode is like a very general concept, one that typically would operate on the whole set of related concepts that form an idea. Also a mode is something that would rarely, if ever, stand alone; characteristically it is an operator on a complex idea. Distinguishing between ordinary concepts and modes is a convenient oversimplification we shall use cautiously without any theoretical commitment to the existence of such a distinction.

Where does the information that determines the mode come from? Let's take the case where the mode is *past*. Sometimes the mode can be determined from lexical information, for example: YESTERDAY I PUT OIL IN MY CAR. The lexeme YESTERDAY tells us that the event took place in the past. More often, the mode is not carried by lexical information but is conveyed by one or more syntactic morphemes. For example, in TERRY ARGUED THE CASE, the +ED verb inflection informs us that the event took place in the past. In the previous example, the verb inflection was ambiguous – the past or present form of PUT is PUT. If the mode information is carried by the syntax, it should be represented in the orrery diagram.

Here is a sample of different modes and how they are represented. Let's begin with a simple idea expressed by the string PEOPLE EAT FISH OFTEN. Figure 2.8(a) shows its orrery representation.[6]

Questions represented in the orrery. Suppose now that instead of wishing to express this relation of concepts as a proposition, we want to express a query about it. In English we might say, DO PEOPLE EAT FISH OFTEN? Ignoring the punctuation cue, we can tell that this string expresses a query from its form – the syntactic functor DO is added to the simple affirmative declarative string.[7] In this string, DO is not a lexeme; it does not stand for a concept

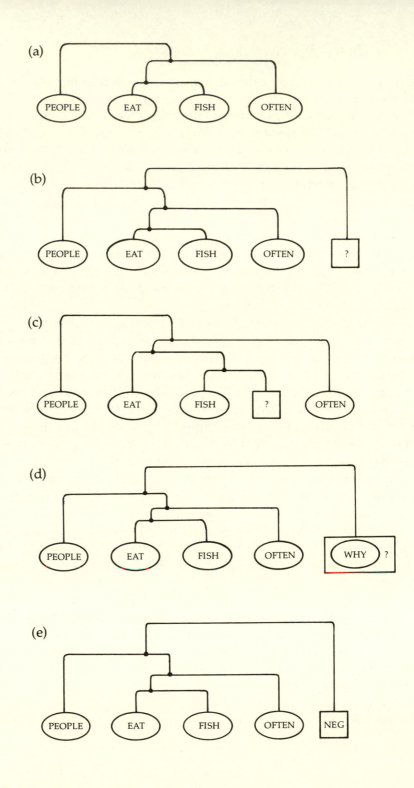

(f)

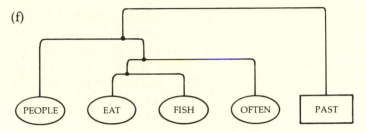

Figure 2.8. (a) Orrery for PEOPLE EAT FISH OFTEN. (b) Orrery for DO PEO-
PLE EAT FISH OFTEN? showing the use of the interrogative mode indica-
tor. (c) Orrery for DO PEOPLE EAT FISH OFTEN? (d) Orrery for WHY DO
PEOPLE EAT FISH OFTEN? (e) Orrery for PEOPLE DO NOT EAT FISH OFTEN. (f)
Orrery for PEOPLE ATE FISH OFTEN.

like FISH stands for a concept. Its job is to indicate the *interrogative* mode of the idea expressed by the sentence. Therefore, no
concepts are added to the basic orrery shown in Figure 2.8(a).
What is added is the mode indicator. Figure 2.8(b) illustrates
how this is portrayed.

The scope of the indicator, indicated by a "?" in a box, is the
entire relation of concepts. This is shown by its point of attachment, above the original structure. Since DO plays a grammatical
role only, it does not appear in the representation of conceptual
structure.

Now, if someone were to say, DO PEOPLE EAT FISH OFTEN?
stressing the word FISH, we take them to be asking a somewhat
different question than if the word FISH were not stressed. We
might paraphrase the new question as IS IT FISH (RATHER THAN
SOMETHING ELSE) THAT PEOPLE EAT OFTEN? Philosophers dispute
the logical status of the difference between the two questions.
But whether we claim they differ in implication or "implicature"
(Grice, 1975), we all can tell there is a difference between the two
questions. This difference can easily be portrayed by the orrery
as a difference in the scope of the interrogative indicator. Figure
2.8(c) illustrates the second version of the question. Compare it
with Figure 2.8(b).

In each of the above questions, what is expressed is a query as
to the truth value of the proposition, or a part of it, respectively.
It is also possible for a sentence to express a much more restricted
form of interrogative: for example; WHY DO PEOPLE EAT FISH

OFTEN? The truth of the proposition expressed by PEOPLE EAT FISH OFTEN is assumed; the questioner wants to know *why* this proposition is true. What is added to the basic proposition is more than an interrogative mode; it has some specific semantic content. In other words, the WHY has both syntactic and lexical information. Figure 2.8(d) shows how this hybrid component is added to the basic conceptual structure. Since the WHY is asking the purpose of the entire proposition, the orrery shows it attached to the top of the basic structure as a unit. Other WH questions (who, what, when, where, how) can have their underlying structure represented in a similar way. Since they replace substantive concepts expressed in affirmative sentences, WHO, WHAT, and the rest appear in orrery diagrams in place of the concepts they question.

Negation represented in the orrery.   Another mode in which sentences appear is the negative. Negative sentences express a denial of the whole proposition or some particular part of it. For example, PEOPLE DO NOT EAT FISH OFTEN denies the entire proposition; NO PEOPLE EAT FISH OFTEN says that there are no people of whom it is true that they eat fish often; and PEOPLE EAT NO FISH OFTEN, can be interpreted to mean that there is no particular (type of) fish that people eat often. Figure 2.8(e) illustrates the orrery for the first of these examples; the reader might try to draw orreries for the other two.

Tense represented in the orrery.   Similarly, a string that expresses an event in some other mode (e.g., the past or future) may have its underlying conceptual structure marked appropriately. For example, one interpretation of PEOPLE ATE FISH OFTEN would be represented as shown in Figure 2.8(f).

By having the indicator for the past mode marker take the whole proposition for its scope, the orrery represents that the entire event took place in the past. If the idea involved people of the present who formerly ate fish often, one might want to represent this idea with the past mode indicator only having (EAT + FISH) + OFTEN in its scope. This distinction, like some of the others discussed earlier, may be too subtle to be of much importance at this stage in the development of underlying conceptual representations. All we want to show is that these distinctions can be easily represented as differences in scope.

Other operators on conceptual structure and an evaluation

Pluralization might be handled by joining a plural indicator to a singular concept to represent a plural idea. However, pluralization is not a simple problem; it is often idiomatic, language specific, and bears a complex relationship to numerosity. For example, we say of a law graduate who sits for a *single* examination that SHE TAKES HER LAW BOARDS. For simplicity, we will not bother to use pluralization indicators in future examples. Thus we would represent BOARDS as one concept, treating numerosity as in the domains of lexical and pragmatic information processing.

A related problem is that of *determiners* and other particles. In the string FRANCESCA BROUGHT THE VIAL AND A BEAKER, there is something different about the two objects she brought, which is indicated by THE and A. Just what the difference is has been the subject of philosophical debate. But, in a simplified sense, we would say that what is referred to by THE VIAL has been directly or indirectly referred to before, while the referent of A BEAKER has probably not been. There are other related uses of THE, for example, to "particularize" and to increase salience. Like the complexities of pluralization, the way in which particles such as THE contribute to conceptual relations often depends on the concept(s) it operates upon. Rather than try to isolate a set of functions which each performs, we shall include THE and other particles in orreries where they affect conceptual relations.

We have considered so far three sources of information indicating the mode of the relation of concepts underlying a natural language string. In the first, the information is carried by a lexeme, within one of the concepts in the underlying conceptual structure. This was shown by the example YESTERDAY I PUT OIL IN MY CAR, where YESTERDAY tells us that the sentence expresses the past mode. At the other extreme, the information about mode is not found in a lexeme or set of lexemes but appears only in the syntactic code. In the string DO PEOPLE EAT FISH OFTEN? the morpheme DO and its position in the string is the (main) cue for the interrogative mode. We then described a hybrid method of carrying mode information where the carrier is part concept and part syntactic morpheme. This was illustrated by the WHY in the string WHY DO PEOPLE EAT FISH OFTEN?

We presented these three methods separately just for didactic clarity. There are probably very few "pure" mode indicators: Mode indicators have overlapping and fuzzy domains. Even the apparently simple ones, such as *interrogative* and *negative*, may have substantial areas of overlap. Consider how sentences in the interrogative mode range from genuine queries, to expressions of uncertainty, to skepticism, to ironic denial, to rhetorical repudiation. For example, in the last category: DOES THE PRINCIPAL EXPECT ME TO BELIEVE THAT MY DAUGHTER IS NOT COLLEGE MATERIAL? The subtlety and richness of the ideas that may be shared through language do not depend upon every nuance being conveyed by a discrete piece of syntactic code; they depend upon the shared ideational structure that is part of general and context-specific pragmatic information processing. Thus, we would claim, it is often unnecessary to codify precisely the mode of the underlying structure that syntax converts into a language string.

Compounds and frozen forms in conceptual structure

How to indicate mode information and how to decide the contribution of individual concepts and abstract mode indicators are not the only problems a model of underlying conceptual structure must face. A related problem is trying to determine whether a given piece of a complex idea is to be represented as a single concept or as a relation of individual component concepts. In other words, is a given piece of an idea conveyed by lexical information alone or by syntactic information as well? For example, does ICE CREAM express a single concept or a compound made up of two individual concepts? Probably, nearly all users of English familiar with the confection conceptualize ICE CREAM primarily as an unanalyzed whole concept. Gleitman and Gleitman (1970) call such compounds *frozen forms* (although they did not use the above example).

A frozen form contrasts with compounds that are composed of two or more individual concepts that operate on each other to produce the whole idea, for example KNEE SURGERY. In this case the principle by which the compound is formed is clear and generalizable. That is, it can be paraphrased as "surgery *performed upon* the knee." Other compounds can be generated and understood on the same basis: BRAIN SURGERY, EYE SURGERY, and even metaphorical extensions such as SYLLABUS SURGERY.

Although many compounds can be analyzed in terms of generative principles, the number of such principles seems not to have a finite limit. The problem of compounds is a special case of the problem of trying to categorize the relations among any set of concepts that form an idea. We have already considered this problem using the set of strings of the form x OF GOLD. We will return to the general problem later in the chapter when we discuss case theory. For the specific problem of analyzing compounds, Marchand says:

> It is no use trying to exhaust the possibilities of relationship; many combinations defy an indisputable analysis. . . . We will always try to classify, but it should be borne in mind that the category of compounding is not one that fills the need for classification. . . . In forming compounds we are not guided by logic but by associations. We see or want to establish a connection between two ideas, choosing the shortest possible way. What the relation exactly is, very often appears from the context only. [Marchand, 1966:22]

Although the ontologic nature of the connections among concepts may not be classifiable in terms of a finite set of categories, *something* about the conceptual structure expressed by language strings can be specified. Which concept is most closely connected to which other can be indicated and often the dependency of one upon the other with respect to the remaining concepts can also. The orrery, as a representation of this much less ambitious analysis, provides a means to explore systematic correspondence between the inferred conceptual structure and our intuitions about the meaning of language strings. Compounds and phrases with more than one modifier, because they are smaller than complete sentences, are a good way to begin the analysis.

Hierarchical conceptual structure in a phrase with several modifiers

Since the examples we have used so far have been hierarchical, let us start with one of this type. A favorite example of Gleitman and Gleitman (1970:67) is VOLUME FEEDING MANAGEMENT SUCCESS FORMULA AWARD. We don't get much help in figuring out the conceptual structure from syntactic cues since each of the words in the compound is a noun. But with a bit of effort and our pragmatic information we arrive at the structure shown in Figure 2.9(a). In other words, "the award given for discovering a formula for succeeding at managing the feeding of people in large volumes" (Gleitman and Gleitman, 1970:67; that it was later discovered to mean something different, is not relevant to our example). The structure is a simple, stepwise hierarchy. Even hierarchical monstrosities can be understood with effort, for example, PLUM TOMATO FARM TRUCK AXLE BEARING GREASE SEAL BUSHING FLANGE ASSEMBLY TOOL CATALOG ORDER NUMBER REVISION DATE POSTPONEMENT CLEARANCE PROCEDURE COMMITTEE. The monotonic left-to-right order is not essential to hierarchical structures. For example, here is a phrase taken from a monograph by a well known linguist: "THE READING EXPRESSING THE TERM WRITTEN SLIGHTLY BELOW THE SEMANTIC MARKER(S) REPRESENTING THE PREDICATE CONCEPT(S) ASSOCIATED WITH THE POSITION," which has both left and right hierarchical steps.

Heterarchical conceptual structure: nonbinary scope

In contrast, an idea may have its component concepts connected in a *heterarchical* as opposed to a hierarchical structure. In a heterarchy, many concepts are connected to a single concept. The relationship of that single concept with each of the heterarchical concepts is independent from the others. Each of the heterarchical concepts is directly connected to the single concept. For example, Figure 2.9(b) shows the heterarchical structure of

(a)

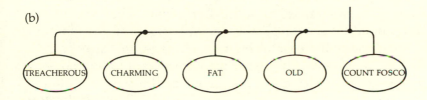

VOLUME · FEEDING · MANAGEMENT · SUCCESS · FORMULA · AWARD

(b)

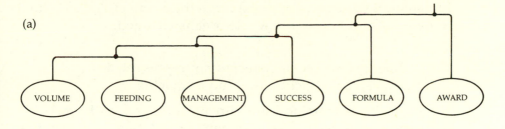

TREACHEROUS · CHARMING · FAT · OLD · COUNT FOSCO

(c)

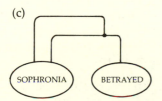

SOPHRONIA · BETRAYED

Figure 2.9 (a) Orrery for the compound VOLUME FEEDING MANAGEMENT SUCCESS FORMULA AWARD. (b) Orrery for the string TREACHEROUS, CHARMING, FAT, OLD COUNT FOSCO. (c) Orrery for the string SOPHRONIA BETRAYED HERSELF, where the same concept is referred to by more than one word.

the orrery for the string TREACHEROUS, CHARMING, FAT, OLD COUNT FOSCO.

We could remove any one or more of the modifying concepts and those that remained would still operate on COUNT FOSCO in roughly the same way. In contrast, this would not work for the hierarchical structure. For example, in the string of Figure 2.9(a), if we remove FEEDING, the whole idea is changed.

Interactions across concepts not represented in conceptual structure (i.e., nonsyntactic)

Although the heterarchical structure portrays each of the modifying concepts as having an independent relationship with the single modified concept, this independence is limited to the syntactic realm. The several modifying concepts still interact at the levels of lexical and pragmatic information. For example, the way we understand someone to be CHARMING given that we are also told that they are TREACHEROUS differs from what our understanding would be *without* the second piece of information. Given the general increase in weight with age, the threshold for labeling someone FAT is higher if we know them to be OLD. And this is just the beginning of an analysis of the possible interactions among the modifying concepts. This is another indication that concept relations do not lend themselves to an analysis in terms of a priori features. Much of the meaning of a language string is configurational (a Gestalt). Only the basic structure of meaning can be delineated as we have tried to do in terms of the scope and dependency relations among concepts.

Repeated reference to a single concept within a string

A special problem for representing conceptual structure occurs when a single concept is referred to more than once in the same string, for example, SOPHRONIA BETRAYED HERSELF. Both SOPHRONIA and HERSELF refer to the same concept. Although it is not necessary, we can represent the concept by a single appearance in the orrery. Figure 2.9(c) shows how this is done.

Conceptual structure across related strings: orreries for discourse

We can extend this method of representation to include examples where the same concept is referred to by more than one string.

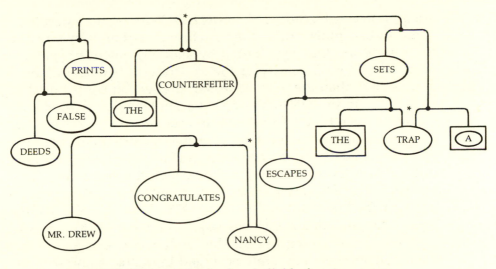

Figure 2.10. How orreries for four individual sentences are combined into one structure.

Up to this point in the chapter we have discussed how concepts combine to form the underlying conceptual structure of individual language strings. Our treatment included units no larger than sentences. Now we want to extend the analysis of conceptual structure to show how it can be used to portray the combining of concepts from more than one string. For simplicity, the following example uses the narrative present tense. Here are some sentences about a related series of events: THE COUNTERFEITER PRINTS FALSE DEEDS. THE COUNTERFEITER SETS A TRAP. NANCY ESCAPES THE TRAP. MR. DREW CONGRATULATES NANCY. We could represent the underlying conceptual structure of each of the sentences individually as separate orrery diagrams. However, by realizing that the COUNTERFEITER in the first sentence is the same as the COUNTER-FEITER in the second sentence, we can combine both mentions of the concept into one, and likewise for NANCY in the third and fourth sentences. Figure 2.10 shows how the four orreries are combined.

The whole diagram represents the conceptual structure of the entire scenario. The orreries for the four individual sentences are joined where they have concepts in common. The joining points are indicated in Figure 2.10 by asterisks. Without the asterisks, it is not so easy to tell where the structure contributed by one sentence ends and that contributed by another sentence begins. In other words, the integrity of the structure as a whole is much more salient than the discreteness of the section contributed by each of the individual sentences. We can take this to model the cognitive operations of underlying structure. Thus, once a language user has converted a set of incoming strings to the corresponding underlying conceptual structure, it will be relatively difficult to assess which pieces of the structure came from a single sentence. This fits very well with the results of a well-known experiment by Bransford and Franks (1971). Their subjects memorized a list of simple sentences like those we used to construct Figure 2.10. The sentences could be combined to form a few short scenarios but were randomly arranged in the list so no scenario was intact. In a recognition test including the original sentences and novel ones as well, subjects claimed to recognize test sentences in proportion to how much of the scenario the test sentence expressed. Thus subjects ranked as most familiar sentences that combined the information from an entire set of related simple sentences. Using our example above, subjects would most often claim the following sentence as one they had memorized: MR. DREW CONGRATULATES NANCY, WHO ESCAPES THE TRAP SET BY THE COUNTERFEITER WHO PRINTS FALSE DEEDS. Test sentences combining the information from three of the original sentences were claimed to be familiar next most often and so on, even though subjects had never seen them before. Language theories that take the sentence to be the basic unit of syntactic organization cannot explain this result.

We suggest therefore that the orrery is a useful representation of the conceptual structure underlying units of language larger than sentences. In addition to its service in a theory of language, the orrery may also be useful as a representation of the basic structure of human information storage. Compared to other models, for example Anderson and Bower's HAM (1973) or Lindsay, Norman and Rumelhart's LNR Structural Network (Norman, Rumelhart, and the LNR Research Group, 1975) the orrery is extremely simple.

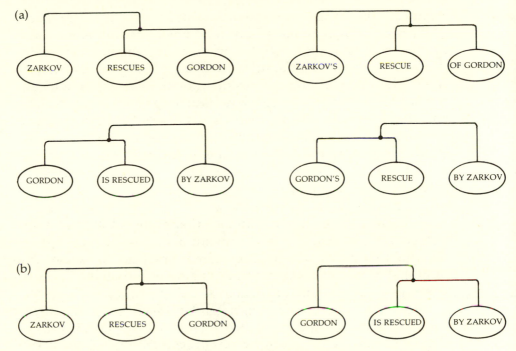

Figure 2.11. (a) Paraphrase similarity illustrated by similar topology in the orrery structure. (b) Alternative orrery diagrams for active and passive forms.

Paraphrase similarity and underlying conceptual structure

It is characteristic of natural language that approximately the same thing can be said in more than one way. Alternative expressions of the same relations of concepts are paraphrases. In addition, there are types of strings that are not paraphrases but noticeably contain the same relations of concepts – such as related declarative and interrogative forms. A model of underlying conceptual structure should provide similar representations for similar relations of concepts. The orrery shows the similarity in meaning of paraphrases of different grammatical forms in terms of the similarity in scope and dependency relations. Figure 2.11(a) gives possible orreries for four paraphrase forms that other theories have considered similar in underlying structure.

Although the orrery can provide similar structures for paraphrases and other similarities in relations of concepts, we claim
neither that all strings with the same orrery relations are paraphrases, nor that all paraphrases will have the *same* orrery relations. The first point recognizes that not all differences in meaning are determined by those relations among concepts that can be
encoded by syntax. Many theories acknowledge that the same
syntactically encodable relations can be expressed by syntactically different forms. However, there may be important semantic differences in the ideas expressed by the different forms. Consider the following pair:

A HIGH WIND (a near-gale)

A WIND THAT IS HIGH (in altitude, such as the jet stream)
A theory could distinguish the meanings of the two strings by
denying that the underlying representations were the same. The
combination HIGH WIND could be considered idiomatic or a frozen form, and consequently treated as a single concept. However,
it would be more accurate to consider HIGH WIND at most a
"slushy" form, not completely frozen into a single concept. Considering strings such as HIGH WIND to be frozen forms too easily
gets out of hand. Treating a combination of concepts as a single
concept ignores the central property of natural language – the use
of known individual concepts in combination to express an unlimited number of different ideas.

Alternatively, a theory might claim that HIGH in the first string
expresses a different concept than HIGH in the second. The two
concepts HIGH₁ and HIGH₂ would then be distinguished in the
underlying representation. Again, there is no limit to making
such distinctions. The danger in this approach is that it commits
the theory to providing a different underlying representation for
every possible cognitive distinction that might obtain when two
or more concepts are related. And this would defeat the purpose
of the underlying representation: to be a more general representation of the idea for syntax to work on.

The second point, that approximately the same idea may be
represented in underlying structure in more than one way, may
be more controversial. Many theorists (Katz and Fodor, 1963;
Katz and Postal, 1964; Chomsky, 1965; Fillmore, 1968; Lakoff,
1968; Matthews, 1968; among others) have assumed that there is

a one-to-one correspondence between meaning and underlying representations. Consider the following pairs of strings:

FLEDGEBY LENDS TO MANTALINI

MANTALINI BORROWS FROM FLEDGEBY

HARMON BEQUEATHS TO BOFFIN

BOFFIN INHERITS FROM HARMON

Since the two sentences of each pair describe the same event, they have essentially the same meaning. According to this view, they should therefore have the same underlying representation. As we will discuss later in the chapter, this is usually done by representing both verbs in terms of supposedly more basic concepts. In one theory (Schank, 1973), for example, the above strings would be analyzed as instances of the concept TRANSFER, with additional differentiating features.

The assumption that there is a one-to-one correspondence between elements on adjacent levels of language organization is not supported by a look at other aspects of language. There may be more than one source for a single representation: Different spellings produce the same sound sequences (ALOUD and ALLOWED); different concepts can be expressed by the same word (SPELL a word and cast a SPELL), and so on. We suggest that the same kind of exceptions to one-to-one encoding may occur between the representation of the conceptual structure of ideas and the meaning of a language string.[8] There is not always a one-to-one correspondence between the relation of concepts in an underlying representation and the meaning of the language string. Even without attempting precise definitions for meaning, concepts, and their relations, we can make the position clear with an analogy. In chemistry, elements can combine, sometimes in different ways to form more than one chemical compound. But it never happens that two different sets of elements combine to form the same chemical compound. If concepts are analogous to chemical elements, then the view we are challenging takes sentence meanings to be analogous to chemical compounds.

But our position is that sentence meanings do not fit the analogy of chemical compounds. Rather, sentence meanings are analogous to classes of chemical substances that are defined by the functions they serve and the ways they interact with other substances: for example, polystyrene solvent, red dye, sugar. Each of these classes of compounds can be produced by more than one structuring of chemical elements. Thus, if we take FLEDGEBY LENDS TO MANTALINI and MANTALINI BORROWS FROM FLEDGEBY to be (functionally) equivalent ideas, we need not represent their conceptual structures in identical ways.

Now if the relations expressed by different concepts (hence by different underlying representations), such as LEND TO and BORROW FROM, can have the same meaning, then perhaps different forms of a single verb can express different relations to other concepts (different underlying representations) yet have the same meaning as well. For example, in the strings of Figure 2.11(a), RESCUES expresses approximately the same meaning with its subject ZARKOV as does IS RESCUED BY with its object ZARKOV; and similarly for RESCUES with its object GORDON, and IS RESCUED BY with its subject GORDON. That is, RESCUES and IS RESCUED BY behave like the different concepts LEND TO and BORROW FROM.[9] Therefore, it is possible that the similarity in meaning between the active and passive forms of a sentence does not require that these two forms have the same underlying representation. If the relations between passive and active forms can be explained this way, then the orreries for these two forms might be those illustrated in Figure 2.11(b) instead of the identical orreries in Figure 2.11(a). However, pending a more thorough investigation of this possibility, we shall conservatively follow other theories in portraying active and passive forms by orreries of the form in Figure 2.11(a).

The orrery model and syntax: more detail

Now that we have sketched the basic design of the orrery model of underlying conceptual structure, we will describe the relationship between the orrery representation and syntactic information processing.

Recall from Figure 1.4 that syntax mediates between underlying conceptual structure and the strings of symbols that make up natural language. When expressing an idea, the formal process goes like this: first, the essential features of the idea are abstracted. This consists of a set of concepts, possibly a mode indicator, and their structure in terms of scope and dependency relations. This is represented by the orrery. Up to this point the process is prelinguistic, or at any rate not essentially linguistic. Next, the information in this representation is mapped onto a language string using the syntactic code appropriate to the particular language being used. For English, the scope and dependency hierarchy of the concepts is converted to a sequence of the lexemes that express those concepts. In addition, inflections and functors may be distributed in the sequence.

The orrery itself contains no sequential information. The location of concepts on the diagram might portray the distribution of the concepts in semantic space, but this would only occasionally mimic the one-dimensional distribution of the lexemes in the corresponding language string.[10] This means that sequence and inflection information must be derived from the scope and dependency hierarchy.[11] The role of syntax, then, is to transform the information in the hierarchy into a linear sequence from which another language user can reconstruct the hierarchy.

We can also express this role in terms of the orrery metaphor: Syntax rotates the randomly ordered arms of the orrery mobile to place them in a certain left-to-right order. The lexemes that name the concepts are produced in a sequence corresponding to this order to express the relation of concepts in a language string. The lexemes may be matched to the concepts after the sequence is established or, more likely, the processes are concurrent. The syntactic mechanism must also insert inflections and functors where they are necessary for a well-formed string. The details of which inflections and functors are used depend upon the particular lexemes selected to express the concepts. The lexemes along with the inflections and functors comprise the morphemes that make up the words of the string.

For parsing a language string, that is, deriving the relation of concepts that it expresses, the process goes in reverse. Lexical information processing identifies the concept or concepts each lexeme expresses. Probably concurrently, the syntactic mechanism begins trying to connect each of the morphemes together into a scope and dependency hierarchy. Since there are ambiguities in words, identifying the morphemes in a given word might also involve other processing. For example, consider the string WET WOOD FIRES SMOKE HEAVILY. It is important that FIRES be identified as the pluralized form of the lexeme expressing "combustion with flames" and not the third person singular of the lexeme expressing "to disemploy." In this case pragmatic information would easily effect the disambiguation. When all of the morphemes are connected together, the resulting structure is an orrery giving the scope and dependency relations among the concepts expressed by the lexemes. The details of the syntactic mechanism during generating and parsing will be given in Chapter 5.

Comparing theories of conceptual structure

In the following section we sketch out a comparison between our model of underlying conceptual structure and those proposed by a sample of currently influential theories. We will concentrate on two "families" of theories: *transformational theory*, based on the ideas of Chomsky, and the more recent *case theories*, based on work by Fillmore. There are now many versions of theories about underlying conceptual structure; see Leonard (1976), for example, who provides a very helpful review of 16 different theories of contemporary interest. We are going to introduce transformational and case theory representations of underlying structure and compare them with the orrery model. This will not be a complete discourse on transformational and case theories, but we will try to be faithful to the spirit of each theory. Within each theory there are many variants. Where they diverge from one another on underlying conceptual structure, we will concentrate on one version. In transformational theory, we will discuss that branch running from Katz and Fodor (1963) through Chomsky (1965) through Fodor, Bever, and Garrett (1974) through Chomsky (1975), Brame (1976), and Bresnan (1978). In case theory, we will deal with the branch running from Fillmore (1968) through Lindsay, Norman, and Rumelhart (Lindsay and Norman, 1972, 1977; Norman, Rumelhart, and the LNR Research Group, 1975).

Consider in Figure 1.4 how the language-using process goes from an ordered string to the idea it expresses. For all theories, a syntactic mechanism operates on the language string to produce a structure, the parse. The parse, in turn, is converted into a representation of the relation of concepts expressed by the string. This contains the essential features of the idea expressed by the string. From the representation of the essential features, the language user constructs the idea; in other words, derives an interpretation of the thought conveyed by the string. Understanding this last step is not a problem for language cognition in particular but for cognition in general. Perception, memory, imagination supply us with essential features of ideas just as language does. How we build upon them, flesh them out, derive implications, and attach associations is a huge and challenging problem, but not one to be solved by the language theorist alone.

Thus the representation of underlying conceptual relations mediates between the language string and the idea it expresses. For all theories of language, the representations are based on general principles that combine a limited number of features. Chomsky (1957) interpreted this to mean that similar strings have similar representations because they share similar principles and features of construction, and made it a criterion by which to judge the adequacy of models of underlying structure. In effect, it requires representations of underlying structure to serve as a basis for generalization and discrimination across ideas and language strings. The criterion says, strings that express similar relations of concepts (paraphrases and different modes, interrogative and declarative, for example) must have similar underlying representations; and strings that express different relations of concepts (including different readings of ambiguous strings) must have distinct underlying representations.

In order for the mechanism of underlying structure to resolve differences in the ideas expressed by different strings, the mechanism must be sufficiently detailed. It should have an adequate number and range of features to provide the discriminability. Every theory posits some set of features for its representations of underlying conceptual structure. There are important differences across theories as to the nature of the features, and the level of detail that each theory holds must be incorporated in the underlying representation. These differences serve as the basis for our comparison of the representative theories.

Transformational model for underlying representation

Not all versions of transformational theory make claims about how the syntax is related to the underlying conceptual structure. We will describe the version of transformational theory (Chomsky, 1965) that pays the most attention to the relationship between conceptual structure and other components of language competence.[12]

A portion of transformational theory's underlying representation for the string DARIA TAUGHT KATE TO PROGRAM THE COMPUTER is diagrammed in Figure 2.12. Aspects of this underlying representation that are important for the theory are: (1) the string is recast in terms of simple active declarative (SAD) sentences, (2) a grammatical tree structure connects the lexemes in the SAD sentences, (3) lexemes and other parts of the underlying representation are further classified by "features," indicated by square brackets. (These features will be discussed further in Chapter 4).

Transformational theory assumes that the basic relation of concepts expressed in a language string is analyzed in terms of SAD sentences and the relations among them. Consequently, the morphemes that are the terminal elements of the tree structure often do not correspond exactly to the morphemes that appear in the original string. The order may also be different. There may be additional morphemes in the underlying representation. The SAD sentences for DARIA TAUGHT KATE TO PROGRAM THE COMPUTER are shown in Figure 2.12 branching from the nodes labeled S1 and S2. The main underlying sentence is constructed from the S1 node: DARIA TAUGHT KATE (S2). The embedded underlying sentence, constructed from the S2 node, is KATE PROGRAMS THE COMPUTER. The morpheme KATE is both the object in the S1 sentence and the subject of the S2 sentence.

In 1963 Katz and Fodor proposed that the underlying representation be converted into the idea by a set of *semantic projection rules.* In terms of Figure 1.4, projection rules would map the con-

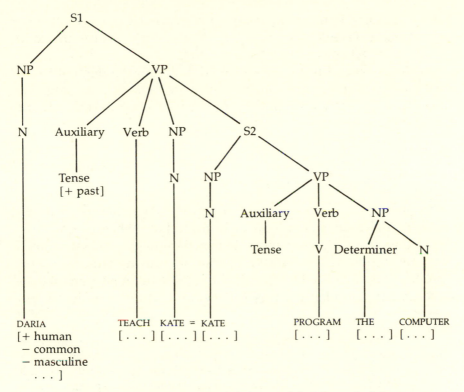

Figure 2.12. Transformational theory model of the underlying representation of the string DARIA TAUGHT KATE TO PROGRAM THE COMPUTER.

tents of the second box into the first box. The projection rules would employ the information contained in the structure and the features of the underlying representation, as well as the simple sentences themselves. It was assumed that the underlying representation would contain sufficient information to allow all the logical entailments of the sentence to be computed. For example, the proposition (idea) expressed by DARIA TAUGHT KATE TO PROGRAM THE COMPUTER implies the following:

ONE HUMAN TAUGHT KATE TO PROGRAM THE COMPUTER

DARIA TAUGHT SOMEONE SOMETHING

AN INANIMATE OBJECT WAS PROGRAMMED BY A HUMAN

The goal was to develop the system so that it could be shown how even more distant entailments could be computed, for example:

AT ONE TIME DARIA KNEW SOMETHING THAT KATE DID NOT
KATE EITHER LISTENED TO OR WATCHED DARIA OR READ
SOMETHING THAT DARIA WROTE

and so on. Thus, on this transformational view, understanding a language string depends on the ability to construct the underlying representation with all the features necessary to compute the logical entailments.

Comparing the transformational model of conceptual structure with the orrery model

The underlying representation of conceptual structure of transformational theory stands in a similar relationship to syntax as does the orrery representation. During language production, it is the starting point for syntactic operations; during language comprehension, it is the final product of syntactic operations. However, the two models are very different in a number of important respects:

1. According to transformational theory, the labels on the nodes of the tree graph and the features attached to the lexemes and grammatical markers and functors contain essential information. Both the semantic projection rules, which map the representation into an idea, and the syntactic rules, which map the representation into a language string, require this information in the underlying representation. In the example of Figure 2.12, that DARIA is the first morpheme dominated by a *noun* node is a datum essential to the understanding of the sentence and also to its expression as a language string. None of this is true of the orrery. The relations of concepts are represented only by the topology of the diagram using the features of scope and dependency.[13]
2. The left-to-right order of the nodes of the transformational model is an essential piece of information. This order is required both for the semantic projection rules and for the syntactic rules. In contrast, there is no left-to-right order constraint upon any nodes, terminal or intermediate, in the orrery model.[14]
3. The simple active declarative (SAD) sentence is the basic structure of the underlying representation of transformational theory. Language strings of other forms are analyzed into SAD sentences with features that would allow the logical entailments to be computed. Figure 2.12 illustrates how a complex sentence was broken down into two atomic SAD sentences. Strings smaller than sentences are often filled out and reanalyzed as SADs. For example, THE PEELING OF POTATOES would be represented in underlying structure as (SOMEONE) PEEL(S) POTATOES.

In contrast, the orrery does not require that the SAD sentence, or any other grammatical unit, be basic to the underlying representation. The only essential thing is that concepts be related. Language strings such as BEAUTIFUL HOUSE! YOUR NAME? AFTER LUNCH, do not have to be analyzed as more complex underlying sentences.[15]

4. The orrery model does not try to reduce meaning to conditions for logical entailment. The orrery presupposes that ideas are better represented as complex associations among a set of concepts where the nature of the relations between concepts depends upon the pragmatic and contextual information available to the language user. In contrast, transformational theory wishes to make its underlying representation independent of any other source of information. Rather than relying on the fact that language processing takes place in an organism that can interact with its environment in complex ways, the transformational approach attempts to produce a self-sufficient program that can determine the acceptability of utterances and generate the basis for a complete account of meaning and understanding.

5. Finally, the nature of the properties of the underlying representations of the orrery and of transformational theory are different. In the orrery, scope and dependency are necessary for syntax but are also present in relations of concepts that are nonlinguistic. Therefore, these relations are not essentially syntactic. In contrast, the properties of the underlying representation of transformational theory were intended by their developers to be syntactic. The claim is only that the representation contains the information that is both necessary and sufficient to produce the semantic interpretation. It does not claim to represent conceptual structure per se. Certainly, the labels used in the transformational underlying structure are syntactic: noun phrases and other grammatical entities, and subclassification features (e.g., can take an object), which are defined functionally rather than notionally (see Chapter 1).

However, the underlying representation of transformational theory is comparable to the orrery model because, although its labels are syntactic, the underlying representations themselves are assigned to language strings on the basis of their semantic similarities. To see that this is true, recall that one of the goals of transformational theory is to give an account of the similarities in the conceptual relations of such strings as:

THE RESCUE OF GORDON BY ZARKOV

ZARKOV RESCUES GORDON

In the first string, ZARKOV and GORDON are both objects of prepositions. However, transformational theory notes that the semantic relations among ZARKOV, GORDON, and RESCUE are the same for both strings. Since a one-to-one correspondence between meaning and underlying structure is assumed, both strings are assigned the *same* underlying structure. Because the SAD sentence form is considered basic, ZARKOV is the subject and GORDON the object in the underlying representation of both strings. Subject and object are defined in purely syntactic terms: the subject is the main or first noun phrase of a SAD sentence; the object is the main or first noun phrase of the verb phrase.

While the syntactic categories that label the underlying representation are defined syntactically, the underlying representation itself is assigned to a string on semantic grounds: For THE RESCUE OF GORDON BY ZARKOV, it is the semantic similarity of its relation of concepts to that of ZARKOV RESCUES GORDON.[16]

Semantic criteria for underlying structure leads to case theory

A problem with transformational theory's use of semantic criteria to select underlying representations is that there is no reason not to extend it beyond where the theory is willing to go. Just as different forms of language strings are analyzed in terms of SAD sentences to bring out the underlying differences in their meanings, so also might other expressed relations be analyzed in different ways to bring out differences in their meanings. For example all the X OF GOLD examples could be assigned different underlying structures corresponding to the paraphrases that bring out differences in the relations of concepts they each express. Thus the underlying structure for BAG OF GOLD would be based on BAG CONTAINS GOLD, and CHLORIDE OF GOLD would be analyzed as GOLD COMBINES CHEMICALLY WITH CHLORINE. To some extent, the radical wing of the transformational school, generative semantics, accepts this extension. But the standard version of transformational theory rejects it.

Chomsky's criterion, that the underlying representation should reflect similarities and differences in the relations of concepts of language strings, was used to argue for the superiority of transformational theory over prior systems. Syntactically ambiguous strings became test cases for the criterion. Since transformational theory analyzed strings in terms of SAD sentences that were their paraphrases, it was frequently able to resolve ambiguities as differences in underlying structure. For example, THE SHOOTING OF THE HUNTERS has two possible meanings. Linguistic accounts prior to transformational theory failed the criterion on such ambiguous strings because they could provide only a single structural representation. Transformational theory analyzed the two interpretations of the noun phrase as different SAD sentences: THE HUNTERS SHOOT (unspecified object) and (SOMEONE) SHOOT(S) THE HUNTERS (unspecified subject) (Chomsky, 1957:89).

Case theory model of conceptual structure

As transformational theory used Chomsky's criterion to demonstrate its superiority over earlier accounts, case theory, based on the work of Charles Fillmore (1968, 1969), appealed to the same criterion to demonstrate its superiority over transformational theory. Fillmore claimed that the simple subject-predicate form of the underlying sentences used by transformational theory was not adequate to represent what appeared to be important differences in underlying conceptual structure. Consider, for example, pairs such as THE CHILD OPENS THE DOOR and THE KEY OPENS THE DOOR. Transformational theory would have the same structural representation for both strings (except for their terminal nodes): the same topology and same intermediate nodes, making no distinction between the relations of concepts in the two strings (Chomsky, 1968). Case theory claimed that the relation of THE CHILD to OPENS is fundamentally different from the relation of THE KEY to OPENS. Transformational theory classifies both relationships as *subject-verb*. Case theory, claiming that it is important to distinguish the two relationships, classifies the first as *agent-action-object* and the second as *instrument-action-object.*

Case theories can account for some additional regularities of language. For example, the relations between noun phrases and certain verbs that can be both transitive and intransitive can be explained easily by analyzing them in terms of the basic case categories. When intransitive, these verbs take noun phrases in the instrument role that would be in the object role in the transitive form. If the object is not specified, the relation of the verb to the subject is understood in a different way. Here are some examples:

THE BIRD CRACKED THE WINDOW
implies: THE WINDOW CRACKED
but not: THE BIRD CRACKED

THE BIRD OPENED THE DOOR
implies: THE DOOR OPENED
but not: THE BIRD OPENED

THE ORPHAN GREW THE TOMATOES
implies: THE TOMATOES GREW
but not: THE ORPHAN GREW

In addition, the subject of the transitive form can be either an instrument or an agent. Thus THE BIRD BROKE THE WINDOW WITH A SHELL and A SHELL BROKE THE WINDOW state roughly the same relationship among shell, window, and breaking. The syntax of a case theory will have different sorts of rules to order the instruments, agents, and objects of each verb.[17] Its task is to discover the general semantic categories and then derive rules to correlate the concept relations in terms of those categories with the sequence, functors, and inflections of the language string.

There are many variants of case theory. What they have in common is an underlying conceptual structure that attempts to describe the nature of the relationship between concepts in terms of a well-defined set of ontological categories. That is, each concept in an idea expressible by a language string is to be classified by the way it is related to the other concepts. These classifications are metaphysical; they represent basic categories of the world. They are prelinguistic. Some theorists have even suggested that they are innate (Fillmore, 1968). We are going to discuss a version of case theory based on the work of Lindsay, Norman, and Rumelhart (Lindsay and Norman, 1972, 1977; Norman, Rumelhart, and the LNR Research Group, 1975). We selected their version because it is clearly described and is at the same time cohesive and broadly eclectic.

The underlying conceptual representation in the LNR model is organized around a set of cases that are attempts to categorize the parts of an event. Table 2.1 lists these cases along with a brief description and an example of each from Lindsay and Norman (1977). In other versions, *beneficiary* and *purpose* are also used. In

Table 2.1. *The basic categories in the LNR version of case theory*

Action	The event itself. In a sentence, the action is usually described by a verb: The diver was *bitten* by the shark.
Agent	The actor who has caused the action to take place: The diver was bitten by the *shark*.
Instrument	The thing or device that caused or implemented the event: The *wind* demolished the house.
Location	The place where the event takes place. Often two different locations are involved, one at the start of the event and one at the conclusion. These are identified as *from* and *to* locations: They hitchhike *from La Jolla to Del Mar*.
Object	The thing that is affected by the action: The wind demolished the *house*.
Recipient	The person who is the receiver of the effect of the action: The crazy professor threw the blackboard at *Ross*.
Time	When an event takes place: The surf was up *yesterday*.

Adapted from Lindsay and Norman (1977, Table 10.1).

addition to the basic cases, there are other components of the underlying representation that are more like operators on entire sections of the representation (even though the LNR Group refers to some of them as cases). These additional ones are: *truth* (value), which is primarily used to indicate false statements; *conditional*, which is a logical relation across events; *mode*, which describes the mode of the string expressing the idea, e.g., interrogative; and *cause*, which indicates causal relations across events.

The concepts that fill the basic case categories can be modified or operated on by still other concepts. The LNR representation provides for several categories of modification, each one indicated by a specific operator. There are many of these operators. A sample of them is: *isa, class, has-as-part, name, applies to, property, example*, and in earlier versions, *quality*. Figure 2.13 shows how the cases and operators work to connect concepts in the underlying representation.

Now we will compare the LNR version of case theory with transformational theory and with the orrery model. In the LNR representation the concepts are arranged heterarchically rather

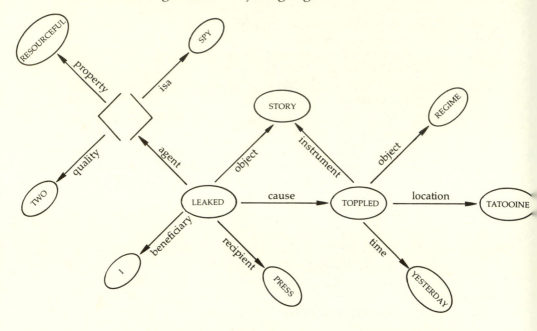

Figure 2.13. The string TWO RESOURCEFUL SPIES LEAKED THE STORY TO THE PRESS FOR ME THAT TOPPLED THE REGIME ON TATOOINE YESTERDAY represented by the LNR model of underlying conceptual structure.

than hierarchically. In addition, the LNR underlying representation has no left-to-right order. In this respect, it is similar to the orrery but unlike transformational theory.

Like transformational theory, the underlying representation of case theory contains essential labels in the structure. In transformational theory, it is the nodes of the tree graph that contain information thought to be crucial for determining the relation of concepts expressed by the string. In the LNR model, the connecting lines of the graph (edges) carry the information that specifies the nature of the relations of concepts. Because they carry so much information, the LNR model and transformational theory provide "rich" underlying representations.[18] In contrast to both of these models, the orrery is strikingly "lean": The orrery carries only one bit of information at each node – that which determines dependency.

Richness is not a virtue in a semantic representation. A lean model is formally more parsimonious, a theoretical advantage. There is no advantage to positing a rich array of properties where fewer can serve as well. Advocates of rich representations are, hopefully, aware of this. They advocate a rich representation because they believe it is necessary to capture the complexity of human thought. The search for general semantic categories to appear in the representations is an attempt to explain something of the cognitive operations of language users by showing how the meaning carried by language strings articulates with the "knowledge structure" of the language user (Norman, Rumelhart, and the LNR Research Group, 1975). Thus a successful theory with a rich semantic representation would accomplish two things: It would explain how relations of concepts can be expressed as relations of lexemes, and it would explain how the concepts and relations of concepts are organized in our thoughts.

Case theory and the problem of universality

Some theorists have assumed that a theory about the structure of thought should apply universally: If the semantic representation of a language theory is part of the structure of the mind, it must be equally applicable for all people and for all languages. Different languages might use different rules to arrange in a string the lexemes that express each semantic category, but the categories and the relations across categories should be universal across all language users.

In the article that launched case theory, Fillmore (1968:24) proposed that "the case notions comprise a set of universal presumably innate concepts which identify certain types of judgments human beings are capable of making about the events that are going on about them." Although the innateness claim is not supported by all theorists who argue for rich representations (e.g., Brown, 1973), most do believe that cases are cognitive universals. But universality may be an unwarranted assumption. Whorf argued strongly against such universals:

> Segmentation of nature is an aspect of grammar – one as yet little studied by grammarians. We cut up and organize the spread and flow of events as we do, largely because, through our mother tongue, we are

> parties to an agreement to do so, not because nature itself is segmented in exactly that way for all to see. Languages differ not only in how they build their sentences but also in how they break down nature to secure the elements to put in those sentences. . . . And it will be found that it is not possible to define "event, thing, object, relationship," and so on, from nature, but that to define them always involves a circuitous return to the grammatical categories of the definer's language. [Whorf, 1956:215, 240]

In case theory there is a fundamental distinction between an *action* "usually described by a verb" (Lindsay and Norman, 1977:397) and those entities that can fill the cases of *object, instrument*, and so on. In the LNR version, this is shown by the heterarchy of the case diagram (see Figure 2.13), where the action is at the center and the concepts filling the other case roles are attached to it.

But Whorf presents evidence that people of other cultures do not segment the world in this way. He points out that in Hopi, "lightning, wave, flame, meteor, puff of smoke, pulsation" and other entities of transient nature are expressed as verbs and treated by the Hopi in the same way as "strike, turn, run" (1956:215). In Nootka, the distinction between actions and objects is even more lacking. Nootka expresses the concept of a residential building as " 'a house occurs' " or " 'it houses' . . . exactly like . . . 'it burns' " (1956:215–216). Although few accept the strong version of the Sapir-Whorf hypothesis – that language *determines* thought – most would agree that language forms tend to reflect cognitive structure. That some languages outside the Indo-European family show forms of organization that do not seem compatible with case notions, at least should make us suspicious of the universality claimed for them.

An additional reason to be skeptical of the universality of case notions is that theorists do not agree upon a basic set of categories (see Leonard, 1976, for a comparison across theory variants), and further, that they have to change their lists of categories (e.g., Fillmore, 1968, 1969; Lindsay and Norman, 1972, 1977). Disagreements about what constitutes the correct set of categories may well be a sign of healthy dialectic but it also indicates that the case categories are not a priori clear and distinct notions.

Criteria to be met by case categories

Although proponents of rich underlying conceptual representations might be willing to give up on cross-language universality, they must maintain that, although languages may differ in the categories they use, within a language, the categories must be universal across all speakers. In order for this to be true, the categories of concepts and concept relations must satisfy certain conditions:

1. There must be a manageable number of general concepts with which to build the semantic representation. It would not do to have an enormous number of general concepts, for then one might as well suppose that syntactic rules operate directly on specific concepts (this argument was given more completely in Chapter 1).
2. Specific concepts or relations of concepts as expressed in a particular language string should not belong to more than one general category (except in the case of ambiguities).
3. It must be clear that a specific concept or relation of concepts belongs to its general category by virtue of its *meaning* and not its syntactic role in a particular string. Otherwise the classification of case categories on a semantic basis is just a disguised syntactic classification.
4. It must be easy to tell what general category each concept or relation of concepts belongs to. If the relation of specific to general is vague, unclear, or difficult to determine, then classification into general categories will not be helpful for an analysis of the conceptual structure underlying language.

Criticism of case theory and semantic categorization
of rich models of conceptual structure

In what follows we shall argue that rich semantic representations fail on all of these conditions. Many of these failures are ignored or consigned to the list of unsolved problems for the theory. These criticisms alone may not condemn case theory. But we are also offering an alternative model that avoids the problems of a rich representation.

Both Bolinger (1965) and Labov (1973) have argued convincingly against the possibility of categorizing lexemes: that if the categories are to make the required distinctions, their number increases unmanageably; and that the boundaries between categories are fuzzy, interpenetrating, and context-dependent to such an extent that the usefulness of categorizing is called into question. Bolinger's method of arguing reexamined the example selected as a paradigm by the advocates of categorization: the concept "bachelor" used by Katz and Fodor (1963). We will reexamine the concept expressed by the verb BREAK, the paradigm that Fillmore (1968) used to show the advantages of case theory.

Using the LNR version (Lindsay and Norman, 1977), this is how case theory would describe the relations expressed in: THE HAMMER BROKE THE WINDOW and THEY BROKE THE SPY ON THE RACK.

> HAMMER-BROKE: instrument-action
> THEY-BROKE: agent-action
> WINDOW-BROKE: object-action
> SPY-BROKE: recipient-action
> RACK-BROKE: location-action,
>   or more probably instrument-action

These categorizations are straightforward except for the RACK-BROKE one. But now consider the string, THE TEMPERATURE BROKE A RECORD. Case theory would analyze the relation between TEMPERATURE and BROKE as instrument-action. Notice, however, that if the definition "a thing or device" is intended to be so broad that it includes temperature, it also will include processes, events, and actions (see Table 2.1). Thus the case definition of *instrument* cannot serve to distinguish instruments from members of other categories. We must conclude that instrument is not purely a semantic notion but is a syntactic category (subject of transitive verb) minus a semantic category (animate, or alive).

Similarly, the definition of *object* ("the thing that is affected by the action") is not adequate to characterize what are counted as objects. Agents, instruments, locations, beneficiaries and recipients are often affected more by the actions than many of the things that are considered objects. Consider such objects as:

> BREAK THE BANK   BREAK THE CODE
> BREAK A TEN-DOLLAR BILL   BREAK RANKS

The variety of relations that can obtain between BREAK and its objects is enormous. To say that a ten-dollar bill or the code are "affected by the action" stretches the sense of what is meant by being affected so that almost anything, no matter what its case category, that is related to breaking will count as being affected by the action. The sense of "affected" is so broad as to fail to distinguish semantically the nature of the relationship. The only way to distinguish what are classified as objects from the other case categories is a syntactic one: An object is the grammatical object of a verb and/or the grammatical subject of an intransitive verb, with the further semantic provision that it not be animate.

But even the syntactic definitions run into trouble. For example, there are some objects that can only be used to express the object-action relations in the active transitive verb form. Using the above example, we cannot say, without changing the sense of BROKE:

        ★A TEN-DOLLAR BILL BROKE   ★THE CODE BROKE

Moreover, there are intransitive forms in which the grammatical subject is more plausibly classified as an agent or instrument:

    WE BROKE FOR LUNCH

    THE WEATHER BROKE IN THE AFTERNOON

    SPOTS BROKE OUT ON THEIR ARMS

    A WAIL BROKE FROM THE CROWD

    WE BROKE INTO LAUGHTER

These problems are recognized by case theorists.[19] Fillmore, when revising his list of basic case categories (1968), made an effort to eliminate syntactic definitions and replace them by semantic ones (1969). The LNR group tries to eliminate some of the problems by giving an analysis of each sentence in terms of concepts and relations not referred to explicitly. For example, WE BROKE FOR LUNCH might be represented as something like THE MEETING, WHICH WE COMPRISED, BROKE FOR LUNCH. Then THE MEETING can be classified as an object. We could represent THEY BROKE JAIL as THEY BROKE THE CONFINEMENT OF THE JAIL, allowing CONFINEMENT to be classified as object since it was affected by the action. In the original version, THEY BROKE JAIL, JAIL is not affected by the action in any specific enough sense to be classified as an object.

Some rich representations try to avoid the problems of classifying the concepts expressed in language by analyzing concepts into atomic semantic primitives. Roger Schank's (1973, 1975) model is one of the most ingenious. Actions in the physical world are not represented directly in the underlying structure but in terms of semantic primitives like the following: *move, ingest, physical transfer, propel, grasp,* and *expel.* There are also sets of semantic primitives for mental actions and other classes of entities. Schank illustrates this analysis using the following sentence: "I THREATENED HIM WITH A BROKEN NOSE." Schank then gives a diagrammatic representation for the conceptual structure, which he renders as: "I COMMUNICATED TO HIM THE INFORMATION THAT I WILL DO SOMETHING TO BREAK HIS NOSE WHICH WAS INTENDED TO MAKE HIM BELIEVE THAT IF HE DOES SOME PARTICULAR THING . . . , IT WILL CAUSE ME TO BREAK HIS NOSE." Schank (1973:213) goes on to say: "If it was ever any wonder as to why people chose to speak in words and not primitive concepts, that last paraphrase ought to give some idea." We would say about rich representations as models for the cognitive structure underlying language use, that if it was ever any wonder as to why people chose to *think* in concepts and not in semantic primitives, that last paraphrase ought to give some idea.

The difficulties involved in trying to decide which case category a specific concept in a string belongs to are very fundamental ones. Consider the following series of examples:

LIGHTNING DAMAGED THE POWER STATION

CARELESS ENGINEERING DAMAGED THE POWER STATION

THE ABSENCE OF FORESIGHT DAMAGED THE POWER STATION

THE MOB GONE BERSERK DAMAGED THE POWER STATION

SABOTEURS DAMAGED THE POWER STATION

At each end of the series the classification is fairly clear: LIGHTœ NING is an *instrument* and SABOTEURS fills the role of *agent.* But the examples in between them suggest that agent and instrument are not exclusive dichotomous categories. Rather, the subjects of the sample strings seem to lie on a continuum. How one classifies things as agents or instruments may well be determined in some cases by one's beliefs involving the issues of free will, whether machines could have minds, etc. The following series of examples suggests a continuum from agent to instrument that lies along a complex philosophical issue:

THE GIRL FED THE CATS

I UNINTENTIONALLY FED THE CATS BY SPILLING MY LUNCH

THE DECEREBRATE CHIMPANZEE FED THE CATS

THE ROBOT FED THE CATS

THE AUTOMATIC TUNA DISPENSER FED THE CATS

Other boundaries such as that between *recipient* and *object* are
also overlapping and unclear. Here are some examples:

SMEDLEY LOVED <u>KENDRA</u>

SMEDLEY PUSHED <u>KENDRA</u>

SMEDLEY TRIPPED OVER <u>KENDRA</u>

SMEDLEY USED <u>KENDRA</u> TO COUNTERWEIGHT THE BEAM

SMEDLEY EMBALMED <u>KENDRA</u>

Both Bolinger and Labov have argued against categorization of
individual concepts: (1) If the categories are to be precise, their
number increases unmanageably; and (2) that the boundaries between categories are characteristically interpenetrating and very
context dependent. We have argued that the same is true for trying to fit relations of concepts into case categories: The boundaries between categories are poorly defined and they depend on
context and complex presuppositions of the individual language
user; in order to improve the category fit, the concepts participating in the relation need to be analyzed into finer and finer
subcategories resulting in implausibly complex analyses of simple language strings. In Labov's words:

> Categorization is such a fundamental and obvious part of linguistic ac-
> tivity that the properties of categories are normally assumed [by
> linguists] rather than studied. . . . Scholars then typically argue how
> many categories exist, and what items are assigned to what categories.
> But in many areas of linguistics, we have extracted as much profit as
> we can from these debates, and we can turn to the resolution of long-
> standing questions by examining the correspondence of the categoriz-
> ing process to linguistic activity. . . . we discover that not all linguistic
> material fits the categorical view: there is greater or lesser success in
> imposing categories upon the continuous substratum of reality.
> [Labov, 1973:342, 343]

And Bolinger claims there is only a restricted range of things
that lend themselves to categorization, namely those things that
owe their meanings to human-imposed convention.

> It is something different to find markers [category defining labels] in
> anything that has a life history independent of our naming-operations.
> A bachelor is a bachelor because he is unmarried, and marriage is an
> arbitrarily defined social ceremony; we impose the conditions. A bird
> or a fish is something that we take as we find it, and the markers are
> adjusted like a suit of clothes, often badly. The fit is crude, metaphori-
> cal, subject to revision, and above all subject to change as the entity it-
> self grows or decays through time. [Bolinger, 1965:567]

The arguments of Labov and Bolinger are supported by recent work in semantics by experimental psychologists. These studies require people to make quantified judgments of the similarity between concepts and to select which of two concepts is more similar to a third. The time it takes subjects to make these decisions is also recorded. From the results of these experiments, a picture of the mental structure of semantics is beginning to emerge. Features (attributes) and categories appear to play no straightforward or essential role in the psychological structure of semantics. In a recent paper, Hutchinson and Lockhead (1977:660) suggest that "people do not organize their [concepts] into well defined formal categories. Instead the general [holistic] similarity between items may be the best structural principle currently available."

The difficulty of categorizing the relationships of concepts is intrinsic to the richness of the world and the enormous range of ways in which things can be related to one another. Categorization works fairly well for the sounds of a language and perhaps its syntactic form classes, but as Whorf, Bolinger, Labov, and Hutchinson and Lockhead remind us, meaning does not lend itself to category analysis. We confront a problem opposite to that which accompanied the birth of modern physics. Physicists presumed a continuum and were forced to acknowledge the categories of discrete quantum levels; scholars of language presumed categories and are forced to confront a continuum.

Conclusion

The problem is that linguists, philosophers, and psychologists of language have, in their enthusiasm for their subject, appropriated too much territory. Language, because it is an accessible part of cognition, is treated as the mechanism of thought rather than a commodity of thought. As Whorf (1956:239) says: "My own studies suggest, to me, that language, for all its kingly role, is in some sense a superficial embroidery upon deeper processes of consciousness, which are necessary before any communication, signaling, or symbolism whatsoever can occur." To develop a representation of the conceptual relations underlying a language string is not to propose representing the complete thoughts of one who utters such a string. Language is a blueprint of thought, a sparse, terse code that evokes rather than portrays ideas. Like blueprints in engineering or genetics, it is the richness of the shared contexts between origin and destination that is responsible for the fidelity of construction at the receiving end. We have argued that a lean representation is closer to that blueprint.

3

Experimental evaluation of models of underlying conceptual structure

In the preceding chapter, we described and criticized the transformational and case models of underlying conceptual structure. Then we introduced the orrery model of underlying structure and compared it to the transformational and case models. Table 3.1 summarizes these comparisons. In this chapter we are going to present some experimental evidence suggesting that the features characterizing the orrery are supported by data on human language performance. That is, we shall support our claim that underlying structure is *hierarchical, unordered,* contains *dependency* information, and is *lean.*

First we discuss the distinction between structure and function as it pertains to experimental verification of models of language. Then we review some evidence to indicate that underlying structure is organized hierarchically rather than heterarchically. These findings favor the orrery and transformational models over the LNR version of case theory. Next we describe the work of Levelt, which supports hierarchical organizations, providing that the feature of dependency is present in the structure. These data favor the orrery model alone. Next we describe an experiment by Weisberg suggesting that left-to-right sequential information is not rigidly fixed in underlying structure. This finding favors the orrery and LNR version of case theory and makes difficulties for both the standard and case versions of transformational theory.

Next we examine the lean-rich dimension, comparing the orrery to the case model. All other things being equal, a simple model is better than a more complex model to explain the same thing. But in order to prefer the simpler model, one has to show that all other things *are* equal: that the simpler model really can

90

Table 3.1. *Characteristics of the orrery, transformational, and case models of underlying conceptual structure*

Feature	Model		
	Orrery	Transformational (standard and case variants)	Case (LNR version)
Topology of structure	Hierarchical	Hierarchical	Heterarchical
Dependency in structure?	Yes	No	No
Left-to-right sequence	Unordered	Ordered	Unordered
Quantity of information in structure	Lean	Rich	Richer

handle everything that the more complex model does. In the preceding chapter we used a range of examples to argue that the orrery could represent underlying conceptual structure as adequately as the much richer case model. In this chapter we supplement these arguments with experimental evidence that scope and dependency alone can do the work of a heterarchy of case categories, at least for human language users.

There have been a few experiments reported that attempt to determine the extent to which case categories might be available for use in language understanding. We review the most important of these and critically evaluate their implications. Then we consider how underlying structure plays a role in syntax acquisition. We describe a study that suggests that scope and dependency information might be more useful for syntax acquisition than case category information. The results are then compared with a recent experiment by Braine and Wells.

At the end of the chapter is a section on the directions future research might take. We describe two pilot projects we have started. One of them attempts to see whether scope and dependency might be features that are general enough to support translation from one language to another; in other words, whether the orrery could serve as a universal model of underlying conceptual structure. The second study is to determine whether some properties of representations of underlying structure might serve as predictors of parsing performance. This project is a cautious attempt to predict basic characteristics of function from structural considerations.

Structure and function claims by models of language

Fodor, Garrett, and Bever (Fodor, 1971; Fodor, Bever, and Garrett, 1974) have distinguished two sorts of claims made by models of language. Although some of the implications of their distinction have been challenged (see J. B. Carroll, 1971), the basic idea is a useful one to consider before going on to the experimental results reviewed in this chapter.

A cognitive model of language makes claims about the psychological reality of the theoretical constructs used by the model. These claims, according to Fodor, Garrett, and Bever, can be divided into strong and weak claims:

> The "weak psychological reality" position . . . specifies the structures that the performance model must recognize and integrate. But . . . [the position] is neutral concerning the character of the psychological operations involved in sentence processing. In effect, the weak view claims that psychological reality exists for the structural descriptions . . . but for nothing else. . . . What might be called the "strong psychological reality" position holds that not only the structural description . . . but also . . . the operations [that the models] employ in the specification of structural descriptions, are directly realized in an adequate performance model. [Fodor, 1971:121]

For our purposes in this chapter, the essential point is that a model may claim either to represent only the structure of underlying conceptual relations, or may go further and claim to represent both the structure and function, i.e., the operations involved in using that structure to parse and generate language strings. The first claim is only to represent the information that must be present; the second claim also predicts the operations required to use the information. An example of a weak psychological reality concern is a model's position on the rich/lean dimension: how much information must be present in an adequate representation of underlying conceptual structure. An example of a strong psychological reality concern – structure and function – is a model's prediction about the relative difficulty of understanding or producing certain language strings because they differ in the number and/or complexity of theoretical operations involved.

The psycholinguistics literature contains many studies of the second kind, most of them based on predictions of strong psychological reality for transformational theory. According to an extensive review by partisans of transformational theory (Fodor, Bever, and Garrett, 1974), the studies do not yield unambiguous support for the strong predictions of the model. Their explanation is that language and language users are very complex. Any reasonable language material is going to provide lexical information as well as syntactic, which, along with pragmatic information, provides powerful clues that are *redundant* to syntactic information. Thus the subject in these experiments can always "guess ahead" and do operations in parallel using a number of heuristics whose nature is still speculated on (see, for example, the list of parsing heuristics suggested by Clark and Clark, 1977:57–84). This makes it extremely difficult to predict real-time language performance on the basis of the number and/or kinds of operations proposed by the model.

Nearly all the studies we review in this chapter are attempts to test the weak psychological reality – i.e., structure alone – of models of underlying structure. In other words, they are based on the model's predictions of what information must be present and how that information is organized. We are not trying to provide an extensive or representative review of experimental psycholinguistics. Rather, we have selected a few studies from the literature and added a few of our own, both completed and in progress, that have not been reported elsewhere.

Hierarchical organization in underlying structure

The orrery, transformational theory, and its case variants (e.g., Stockwell, Schachter, and Partee, 1969) have underlying structures that are organized hierarchically. In contrast, the Lindsay, Norman, and Rumelhart version of case theory has a heterarchical underlying structure. There is an experimental literature which suggests that the organization of language strings during perception, production, and memory is hierarchical. Since we are primarily concerned with underlying conceptual structure, experiments involving memory for language strings are most directly relevant. This is because perception and production also involve the processing of surface forms so the contribution of underlying structure may be confounded.

N. F. Johnson's famous (1965) experiment was extremely simple; the method of analyzing subjects' responses is the ingenious part. Subjects memorized sentences and were later given a recall test. The hypothesis was that memory for sentences would show a hierarchical organization rather than the serial organization such as would be demonstrated for recall of words in a list. Johnson analyzed the recall data for Transitional Error Probabilities (TEPs). This is a measure of how likely subjects are to make an error in recalling word N in a sentence, given that they correctly recalled word $N-1$, where N is any word in the sentence except the first. Johnson used strings of two different structural types. Figure 3.1(a) shows an orrery diagram for a sample sentence from one of the two types. Each transition is indicated by a brace. Below the orrery is the mean TEP score for all the sentences of that structural type.

The important finding in the study is that the highest TEP comes at the major constituent break, the place where the two adjacent words are connected by the most distant path through the nodes of the hierarchy (shown by level 4 bracket in Figure 3.1(a). And there is a tendency for words connected more directly in the hierarchical structure to have lower TEP scores.[1] Thus Johnson's experiment demonstrates that memory for words in sentences is organized in clumps that correspond roughly to scope components, the constituents controlled by nodes in a tree graph. Results of experiments like Johnson's are more difficult for a heterarchical model to accommodate. Figure 3.1(b) shows a Lindsay, Norman, and Rumelhart case diagram for the same sentence. From the structure alone, the difference in TEPs between the pairs BOY–SAVED and SAVED–THE cannot be explained. Therefore, a heterarchical model must provide still another feature, a relative weighting of the strengths of association represented by each of the connections on the graph.

(a)

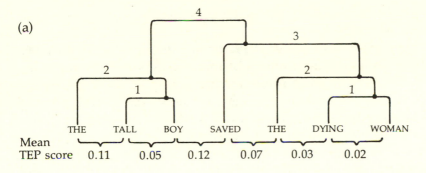

	THE	TALL	BOY	SAVED	THE	DYING	WOMAN
Mean TEP score	0.11	0.05	0.12	0.07	0.03	0.02	

(b)

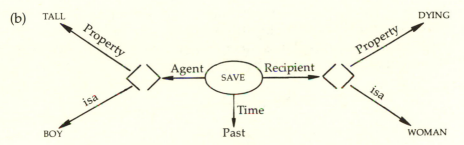

Figure 3.1. (a) Orrery diagram for one of the sentences used by N. F. Johnson (1965). (b) LNR case diagram for the sentence in N. F. Johnson's (1965) experiment.

Modulating the hierarchical structure: dependency and the work of Levelt

In contrast to the many psycholinguistic experiments on underlying structure that use more or less covert measures, W. J. M. Levelt developed a direct method of assessing the underlying structure of sentences. He gave people a string and asked them to estimate the relatedness of every possible pair of words in the string, instructing them to base their judgments on how the words are related in the sentence. Three methods are used: *triadic comparison*, where the subject decides which one of two words is more related to a third word; *dyadic comparison*, where the subject estimates the degree of relatedness, usually on a seven-point scale; and *free grouping*, where the subject arranges the words into related piles of any number of words each. The methods are listed in descending order of their usefulness in Levelt's work.

The results we review here use only the triadic and dyadic comparison methods.

In his earlier work, Levelt (1970) considered whether or not a hierarchical constituent model of underlying structure could account for the data from the relatedness judgments made by his subjects. For very simple strings such as KARLA RUNS FAST, the structure produced by a hierarchical clustering analysis (M. Johnson, 1967) of the relatedness data provides a good fit to the simple hierarchical structure shown in Figure 3.2(a). That is, subjects estimate RUNS and FAST to be closely associated with each other and less close to KARLA. However, "the constituent model predicts less well as the hierarchy becomes more complicated" (Levelt, 1974:39). And this difficulty still obtains when inferred underlying structures are used instead of those derived directly from surface constitutents of the string. For example, consider the string

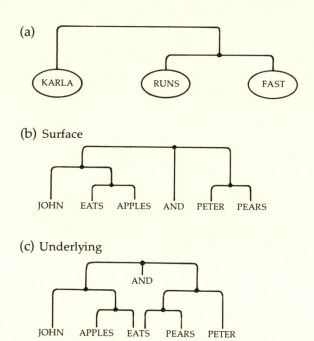

Figure 3.2. (a) Hierarchical structure for the simple string KARLA RUNS FAST (no dependency shown). (b) Surface structure and (c) underlying structure for the string JOHN EATS APPLES AND PETER PEARS (no dependency shown).

JOHN EATS APPLES AND PETER PEARS. In the relatedness judgments, PEARS was more related to EATS than to any other word in the string. An ordinary phrase structure constituent analysis would not reflect this high degree of relatedness – PEARS would be most closely joined with PETER. Figure 3.2(b) illustrates this structure.

But a hierarchical model does not have to use the order of the surface constituents to describe the underlying structure. In transformational theory, the underlying structure may have a different order from the surface structure. In the orrery model, the underlying structure has no order. For both models EATS PEARS forms a unit that in turn is connected to PETER. Figure 3.2(c) shows this structure. The second structure is much more in agreement with the relatedness judgments produced by Levelt's subjects. The finding that underlying structure rather than surface structure determines the psychological reality of a language string is cited by transformational psycholinguists as support for their theory (Fodor, Bever, and Garrett, 1974).

However, in his 1974 book, Levelt reports further experiments that cause him to reject the inferred transformational underlying structure version of the hierarchical constituent model. He writes:

> We may then conclude that the transformational extension of the constituent model must also be rejected. . . . The model is not capable of accounting for either the strong relation between the article and the corresponding noun, or the weak relation between the same article and the other words in the sentence. Yet this result is not surprising to the intuition. It shows that the relation between article and noun is asymmetric; the article is dependent on the noun, and the noun is the head of the noun phrase. A phrase structure or constituent model is not suited for the representation of such dependencies. [Levelt, 1974:50]

Levelt's move is to abandon the hierarchical model and adopt a dependency connectedness model. We can illustrate this with an example. Figure 3.3(a) is a matrix of relatedness judgments among the words of the string HE PUT HIS COAT ON (Levelt, 1974:56). Levelt suggests that these relatedness values can be portrayed in a connectedness graph with dependency values represented by the vertical distance separating any two words. This is illustrated in Figure 3.3(b) (Levelt, 1974:56). The relatedness of any two words on the graph is shown as the sum of the vertical

(a)

	HE	PUT	HIS	COAT	ON
HE	–	9	17	15	13
PUT		–	8	6	4
HIS			–	2	12
COAT				–	10
ON					–

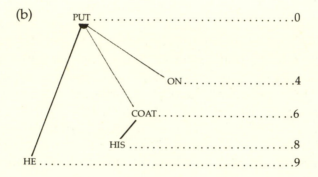

(b)

PUT 0

ON 4

COAT 6

HIS 8

HE 9

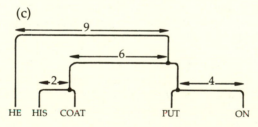

(c)

HE   HIS   COAT   PUT   ON

Figure 3.3. (a) Relatedness judgments for the string HE PUT HIS COAT ON. (b) Dependency connectedness graph for the string HE PUT HIS COAT ON. (c) Orrery diagram with dependency for the string HE PUT HIS COAT ON.

distances separating them on the graph. For example, in the matrix of Figure 3.3(a), HE and ON have a relatedness value of 13. On the graph this is represented as the sum of the vertical distance from HE to PUT (the only node in common between HE and ON) plus the distance from PUT to ON, or 9 + 4 = 13. The smaller the number, the greater the degree of relatedness.

Levelt's abandoning hierarchical structure in favor of a dependency connectedness graph has the disadvantage of making it difficult to invent a syntactic mechanism that can map the underlying structure onto string order and inflection. The advantages of a hierarchical syntax compared with one based on a connectedness graph are discussed in Appendix A, on computer simulation of syntax. On the other hand, if we are to take Levelt's experimental data seriously, dependency must be considered in any representation of underlying structure. The model we are proposing, the orrery, has the advantage of hierarchical structure and at the same time is able to portray dependency relations in a way consistent with Levelt's data. Figure 3.3(c) shows an orrery diagram for the string HE PUT HIS COAT ON. With the dependency feature, the relatedness values obtained by Levelt can be directly shown as the distance between terminal nodes on the diagram. For example, corresponding to the values in the matrix of Figure 3.3(a), PUT is 9 units from HE, while ON is 13 units from HE. It is the modulation of hierarchical scope by the dependency feature that permits a hierarchical structure to accommodate the lack of symmetry in constituent relatedness found by Levelt.

Left-to-right sequence in underlying conceptual structure

As we indicated in the preceding chapter, both standard and case versions of transformational theory consider the left-to-right order of the nodes in phrase markers to be crucial structural information. The order is used by the projection rules for·semantic representation. In contrast, the orrery and the Lindsay, Norman, and Rumelhart case models do not consider left-to-right (or any other) sequence to be part of the structural information. Of these two models, the orrery is hierarchical and the LNR case model is heterarchical. Earlier we presented some experimental evidence that favored hierarchical models over heterarchical models. In this section we are going to present some evidence suggesting that left-to-right sequence is absent in underlying structure.

The work of Levelt described in the preceding section presumed that sequence was unimportant. This presumption was in the nature of the experimental technique used. Subjects were asked to evaluate the relatedness of two words from a sentence either using a magnitude estimation scale or else they had to select which of two words was more related to a third. Levelt counterbalanced or randomly ordered the stimuli to be rated, thus obscuring any sequence effects. However, other experiments do provide a way of assessing the presence of sequential information in underlying structure.

Weisberg (1969) constructed a set of simple active-declarative (SAD) sentences from words that were not responses to each other in the free association studies by Cofer and Bruce (1965). One example was SLOW CHILDREN EAT COLD BREAD. Subjects memorized the SAD sentences or variants of the SAD form that had the same basic underlying structure. Later, each word in the sentence was used as a prompt in a word association task. For example, subjects were given CHILDREN and asked for the first word that came to mind.

The results of the experiment supported the hierarchical structure claim made earlier. Nearly always, the word that came to mind was in the same constituent as the prompt word. Thus SLOW and CHILDREN were associated with each other and so were COLD and BREAD. The results also supported the dependency claim. Subjects associated EAT both with COLD and BREAD but more strongly with BREAD, because that is the main component of the pair COLD BREAD. But important for the purposes of this section, the words that were members of the same constituent usually evoked each other with equal probability. Thus for example, BREAD evoked COLD as frequently as COLD evoked BREAD. If the members of a constituent were ordered from left to right in underlying structure, it would be likely that some asymmetry in performance would be found. The symmetry of many constituent associations found by Weisberg suggests that subjects are accessing structural information that is *not* ordered from left to right.[2]

Is the lean orrery model adequate as a representation of underlying structure?

With scope and dependency as the only features in its structure, the orrery carries less information than other models of underlying conceptual structure. On grounds of parsimony the orrery has an advantage, but only if it can be shown that the leaner representation can do the work of richer representations. In this section, we present an empirical argument in support of the adequacy of the orrery model.[3] In effect, we are going to demonstrate that scope and dependency alone are able to carry enough structural information to permit the encoding of relations of concepts. The argument depends upon a comparison of the lean orrery model to one whose structure is richly differentiated so that it is capable of carrying a great deal of information about relations of concepts. We will show that the added information of the rich model is redundant to scope and dependency. By showing that the lean model can do the same job as the rich model, we enable considerations of parsimony to favor the orrery.

Because it is clearly described and also well known to psychologists, the rich model we will use for the comparison is the case theory of Lindsay, Norman, and Rumelhart (Lindsay and Norman, 1972, 1977; Norman, Rumelhart, and the LNR Research Group, 1975; Rumelhart, Lindsay, and Norman, 1972). We will continue to refer to this model as the "LNR case model." The preceding chapter described the LNR model in enough detail to provide background for this discussion.

Recall from earlier discussions the role of underlying structure during language use: it is an information structure giving the relations of concepts that can be derived from a language string and that also can be used to derive a language string. If such an information structure were directly assessable, one could examine it for reliable correspondences with particular (unambiguous) language strings. But this is clearly impossible for human subjects, although such an examination might be accomplished for some computer simulations of language use.

This experiment simulates the use of underlying structure in language production by providing an external representation of each model for the subjects. Subjects are taught the conventions of each model. An orrery or case diagram is drawn up from a particular sentence and a subject tries to derive the original sentence from the diagram. If the structural features of the model are adequate to encode the relations of concepts expressed by the language string, the final sentence should be identical in meaning to the original.

It is a little unusual to use a representation of a psychological model to play the role of the cognitive structure being modeled. But this should not be disturbing. The experiment is one that tests the weak psychological reality of the models; in other words, it assesses the adequacy of the information contained in the model. It is not a test of the operations that must be performed to use this information. We have claimed that the orrery diagram is a graphic representation of the information structure that describes the relations of concepts expressed by a language string. Rumelhart, Lindsay, and Norman claim that the case diagram of the LNR model "allows the user to see the inter-relationships of the information structure more readily" (1972:201).

To outline the procedure: We compiled thirty sets of words containing from five to twelve lexemes and function words each. Each set was capable of being arranged to form at least five different sentences. The words representing lexemes were not ambiguous as to what concept they expressed. For example, LIGHT was not used because it could express "not heavy," "ignite," or "illumination." In order to make clear that lexemes rather than particular parts of speech were intended, some lexemes were written as sets of alternative inflected forms. Two examples of the word sets are:

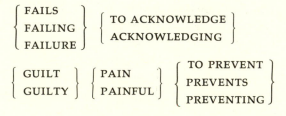

$$\left\{ \begin{array}{l} \text{FAILS} \\ \text{FAILING} \\ \text{FAILURE} \end{array} \right\} \quad \left\{ \begin{array}{l} \text{TO ACKNOWLEDGE} \\ \text{ACKNOWLEDGING} \end{array} \right\}$$

$$\left\{ \begin{array}{l} \text{GUILT} \\ \text{GUILTY} \end{array} \right\} \quad \left\{ \begin{array}{l} \text{PAIN} \\ \text{PAINFUL} \end{array} \right\} \quad \left\{ \begin{array}{l} \text{TO PREVENT} \\ \text{PREVENTS} \\ \text{PREVENTING} \end{array} \right\}$$

{MARY}   {BARNEY}   {SUPPER}

{FOR}   {TRUSTING}   {COOKS}

Each word in a set was written on a small card and the cards for each set were placed in an envelope in random order. Four control subjects treated the word sets as sentence anagrams. Their task was to generate six different sentences by arranging the words in strings. The order in which the sentences were generated was recorded. The second part of the control subjects' task was to rate the relative likelihood that each of the sentences they produced was the one that actually appeared in "a newspaper, book, or other source." They did this by distributing 100 percent of likelihood over the six sentences.

Two sentences with low probability of occurrence were chosen by the following method from each of the word groups, making a total of 60 sentences. High-likelihood sentences were eliminated until the total mean likelihood for the remaining sentences was under 50 percent. Then from the remaining sentences two were chosen that were not produced by more than two subjects, and were not the first or second ones produced by any subject. This gave us a set of sentences that could not be understood without using syntactic information. Lexical and pragmatic information alone were not adequate. The job now was to represent the syntactic information for each sentence according to the LNR case and orrery models.

Two experimenters independently drew orrery and LNR case diagrams for each of the sentences. For the few diagrams where they disagreed, a third experimenter arbitrated. The lexemes appeared in the diagrams in random spatial positions. This meant that the only way the diagrams could be decoded, i.e., translated into sentences, was by using the information about relations of concepts represented by scope and dependency for the orrery and case relation labels for the LNR model.

Eight experimental subjects were taught how to interpret LNR and orrery diagrams using programmed, self-paced training manuals based on examples that had been used in the literature to describe the two models. Of course none of the sentences used in the actual experiment appeared in the training manuals. The training included frequent testing and was designed to have the subjects "overlearn" the features of the models.

Next, the eight experimental subjects were given the task of decoding the orrery and LNR case diagrams into sentences. The orders of the diagram types and the individual sentences were counterbalanced. Two blind judges independently scored the sentences produced by the experimental subjects for similarity to the original sentences using a 0 to 4 rating scale: 0 = main and secondary idea(s) wrong; 1 = main idea wrong but secondary idea(s) correct; 2 = main idea correct but secondary or modifying idea(s) wrong; 3 = similar in meaning – emphasis or connotation different; 4 = identical, or essentially equivalent in meaning. The two judges agreed with a reliability of 0.73. They differed, although rarely by more than one point, on only 94 of the 480 sentences. For the disagreements, a third judge arbitrated the difference.

Subjects decoded the case and orrery diagrams with identical degrees of accuracy: 89 percent for each model. We can support our claim that performance on the two tests was the same by following the statistical procedures used to show that two tests (e.g., two versions of an IQ test) are parallel: The case and orrery tests could differ in any of three main ways. The mean scores across subjects could differ; the variances (a measure of variability) could differ; or the shape or profile of the scores could differ (Gullikson, 1950). A t test for matched samples yields $t = 0.74$ $(0.50 > p > .40)$ showing that there is no statistically significant difference in the means. The variances do not differ significantly because $F(7, 7) = 2.48$ $(p > 0.10)$. The similarity in the shape or profile of the distribution of scores across subjects can be assessed by a Pearson product-moment correlation coefficient. Since this statistic $= 0.80$, which is significant at $p < 0.02$, we can conclude that the profiles are highly similar. Since there were only eight subjects in the study, each statistic taken alone is not powerful, but the three tests taken together provide a greater confidence that there was no difference in decoding performance on the LNR case diagrams compared with the orrery diagrams.[4]

Most of the errors made by subjects were unsystematic, careless ones. Nevertheless, some general errors indicate possible weaknesses in each of the two models of underlying conceptual structure. For the LNR case model, some of the problems were the following: The scope of certain modifiers was not determinable from the heterarchical case diagram. For example, the sentence FIRST A PHOTOGRAPHED WOMAN RUINED THE CAMERA was rendered by some subjects as A PHOTOGRAPHED WOMAN FIRST RUINED THE CAMERA and by others as A PHOTOGRAPHED WOMAN RUINED THE CAMERA FIRST. The three sentences differ in implications at least. To the extent that these differences are important, the heterarchical structure of the LNR case model should be modified to accommodate them. The orrery, with its hierarchical structure, did not present any difficulty with this sentence type. In addition, consistent with the findings of Shafto (1973) and Bobrow (1970) discussed below, subjects had difficulties interpreting case relations other than agent, instrument, and object. This was especially true when there was no agent case present, for example in the diagram of the sentence THE WELFARE OF FUTURE CHILDREN DEPENDS ON THE COUNTRY. This is consistent with the results of a study by Braine and Wells (1978), whose subjects also had difficulty working with case categories in sentences that had no agent case. We discuss this study below.

The orrery displayed an inadequacy that seems to be intrinsic to its leanness. Figure 3.4 shows an orrery diagram that some subjects decoded into a sentence different from that which we used to generate the diagram. The problem is that the component LOSING BUSINESS is not distinguishable from BUSINESS LOSSES by scope and dependency alone. While it is true that there is not a

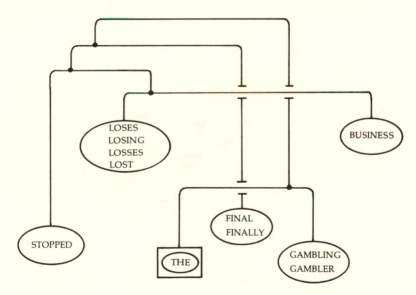

Figure 3.4. Orrery diagram for the sentence THE GAMBLER FINALLY STOPPED LOSING BUSINESS, which also encodes THE GAMBLER FINALLY STOPPED BUSINESS LOSSES.

great deal of difference in the meaning of the two phrases, there is a difference nonetheless. To overcome this inadequacy one might distinguish LOSSES from LOSING by claiming that they do not express the same concept. Such a distinction does not require that there be a systematic way of distinguishing all words that derive from the same root. For example, it need not be supposed that the language user marks both LOSING and GAMBLING by some one feature such as "activity." To suppose this would be to move in the direction of case theory. All that needs to be claimed now is that users of English distinguish LOSSES from LOSING, but not that there are distinguishing *general* feature(s) that differentiate other pairs of related concepts.

In summary, we can conclude from the results of this experiment that the orrery can encode information about concept relations using scope and dependency as adequately as the much richer LNR case model.

Experimental tests of case categories

In the preceding chapter, we directed a number of formal arguments against the case model. We argued that cases were too ill-defined to apply to more than a small subset of the concept relations that actually occur in natural language. In this section we are going to consider experiments that attempt to test the psychological reality of case categories. There are few experiments reviewed in this section because there are few in the literature. Convincing studies on the psychological reality of cognitive structures are difficult to do. But the recent popularity of case theory among psychologists is likely to have inspired many more experiments looking for evidence for case categories than have been reported.

Bobrow (1970) pitted case categories against an alternative model that characterizes concepts in a sentence in terms of a set of semantic features. Subjects were first exposed to one of three types of sentence lists. One kind of list contained pairs of sentences whose nouns were matched for case category but not for referent. For example, such a list might contain the following pair of sentences:

THE EPSOM SALT (instrument)
   LITTERED THE SHIP'S DECK (object)

THE TABLE SALT (instrument)
   COVERED THE OBSERVATION DECK (object)

Another list contained sentences whose nouns belonged to different cases as well as different referents. For example:

THE EPSOM SALT (instrument)
   LITTERED THE SHIP'S DECK (object)

THE OLD SALT (agent)
   CUT THE CARD DECK (object)

A control list contained sentences that were exact duplicates so that both case and referent were identical.

Bobrow supposed that either subjects learn case relations or they learn the meaning of the individual terms (but not both). He attributes to case proponents the argument that "people learn case grammar relationships when they study sentences instead of conceptual meaning of words" (1970:369). Subjects were prompted with the first noun in a sentence and were asked to recall the second noun. Bobrow's version of the case theory prediction is that subjects would remember sentences whose nouns belong to the same case category, even though their meanings differed (the first pair of examples in the preceding paragraph), just as well as the duplicated sentences of the control list. And of course each of these tasks would be easier than recalling the list where both case and meaning were different. Bobrow's alternative hypothesis was that the "same case–different referent" list would be more difficult for subjects than the list containing duplicated sentences. This alternative is indeed what happened.

Bobrow takes his results to argue against the psychological reality of case categories. However, we believe that Bobrow's pitting of case categories against word meaning is not fair to case theory. It is unlikely that case theory proponents would claim that case category alone plays a role in memory for sentences and word meaning does not. One might be able to draw a conclusion if the experiment had included a condition where subjects learned a list containing sentences that had different cases but the same referents. Such a list would contain pairs like the following:

THE EPSOM SALT (instrument)
LITTERED THE SHIP'S DECK (object)

THE EPSOM SALT (object)
WAS HIDDEN BY THE SHIP'S DECK (instrument)

If these were remembered as well as sentences that had the same case *and* same referent, one could conclude that case categories have no mnemonic value.

Kintsch (1972) developed a model for memory structure that is also based on case relations. He reports an experiment testing the psychological reality of case relations. In particular, his study was intended to test the psychological reality of the *case frame*, a way of characterizing verbs proposed by Fillmore. A case frame is a list of the case relations that a particular verb can have. For example, KILL has a case frame made up of agent, instrument, recipient (less commonly, object), location, and so on. This might be contrasted with the frame for TYPE, which would not have a recipient but would have an object instead. Kintsch gave subjects short sentences in which only a few of the possible case relations for the verb were made explicit, for example, THE SECRETARY TYPES. The subjects were asked to supply all the information implied by but not directly given in the sentence. In response to the example sentence above, subjects said that a typewriter, paper, verbal text, and a secretary's typing skill were implied. Kintsch analyzed the first three as location, instrument, and object. From this he concluded that people organize their knowledge of verbs in case category fashion. But this conclusion is not justified. What the results tell us is only that the subjects know that typing is done on paper, using a typewriter, and that a verbal text is the input and/or output of the process. This is the pragmatic knowledge that any theory would say is part of the meaning of the verb TYPE. It is case theory that imposes categorizations on the knowledge. And the three case categories given by Kintsch in this example are not even so clear-cut: Is the paper really the location of the typing and the verbal text the object (the thing affected)? Perhaps the most significant weakness in the case claim is that Kintsch was unable to classify the fourth piece of information provided by the subjects in terms of a case category – the fact that typing skill was involved, Kintsch called a *semantic implication*.

But it seems clear that all four of the implications drawn by the subjects are semantic implications; some of them just happen to be classifiable in terms of the categories specified by case theory. We can conclude from Kintsch's study that people do have access to the pragmatic information associated with verbs in context, but that this information is encoded in terms of case categories has not been demonstrated.

In the best-known paper on the psychological reality of case categories, Shafto (1973) reports two experiments. The first experiment used a concept-formation technique. Subjects were presented with a list of sentences. In each sentence one noun was underlined. They were told that the relationship of each underlined noun to the meaning of the sentence as a whole belonged to one of four categories. The categories were agent, experiencer, instrument, and object, although the subjects knew them only as A, B, C, and D. Shafto found that subjects could adequately learn to categorize the appropriate nouns as agents. The experiencer category was also learned although not so well as agent. However, subjects were poor at classifying nouns in the instrument and object categories. Subjects tended to use the features of animate-inanimate and active-passive to do their classifying. This was one of the reasons that subjects confounded the instrument and object cases. In Shafto's words, subjects "are unwilling to attribute active roles to non-living nouns, so that Instruments are displaced towards Objects along the active-passive dimension" (1973:555).

Shafto's rationale for the experiment is like an argument once used by Descartes: If subjects were able to classify nouns on the basis of case relations, that is, were able to recognize instances of case categories, then the case categories must correspond to "clear psychological relations" (Shafto, 1973:552). The experimental results showed that the category agent was an adequate basis for classification, experiencer somewhat less so, and instrument and object quite poor. When a putative category fails to serve as an adequate basis of classification, we can, on Shafto's argument, conclude that it is not a clear and distinct idea and thus has little psychological reality. Instrument and object would then have to be challenged as psychologically real and distinct cases on the basis of Shafto's experiment because they "encompass a variety of notionally distinct semantic relations" (p. 561). Furthermore, if a category turns out to be viable in a concept-formation task, this only means that it is a learnable category. This does not automatically justify the claim that it was a *preexisting* category in language cognition.

Shafto's second experiment follows the false recognition paradigm. Subjects were given a list of sentences containing a basic sentence form and three variant foils. For the basic sentence, THE GANGSTER (experiencer) OWNED THE CADILLAC (object), one foil had the nouns in the same case relationship as the basic sentence but in a different order: THE CADILLAC (object) BELONGED TO THE GANGSTER (experiencer). Another foil had the nouns in the same order but in a different case relation: THE GANGSTER (agent) WRECKED THE CADILLAC (object). The third type of foil had different order and different case relations: THE CADILLAC (instrument) APPROACHED THE GANGSTER (location). The foils appeared sometime later in the list than the base sentence. Subjects were asked whether they had seen each sentence before. Shafto's hypothesis was that if the case model were correct and people encoded sentences by their case relations, the case-congruent foil sentences should produce the greatest number of false positives. This is what happened. However, this does not mean that people encode sentences using case categories. The problem is that Shafto's case-congruent foil sentences had the same meaning as the base sentences. Even though he used a different verb, each foil sentence verb was the semantic complement of the verb in the basic sentence (OWNED/BELONGED (TO), CAUSE/RESULT (FROM), LOAN/BORROW, CONVINCE/BELIEVE). Therefore, the property of case congruence was confounded with meaning similarity. And every theory of language competence would claim that confusions must occur more frequently among semantically similar sentences.

A recent paper by Braine and Wells (1978) reports a series of concept-formation studies using children from three and a half to six years of age as subjects in order to eliminate the possibility that formal language training might contribute to knowledge of case categories. Braine and Wells trained children to place a small set of tokens on a picture that accompanied a sentence describing the event portrayed. Each token represented a particular case category. The task was to place each token on the object in the picture that filled the case category for the sentence. For example, in BIRD FLY IN CAGE and BOAT SAIL DOWN RIVER, children learned to place one particular token on the bird and the boat in the pictures, and another token on the cage and the river. The first token represented an actor case, which is a combination of agent and instrument; the second token represented location. Braine and Wells report some interesting results about the types of categories that are easiest for children to learn. Interestingly, the results depart from the system of categories proposed by any of the various case theories. Although children demonstrate that they can easily use an animate-inanimate distinction, they do not make this distinction for agent and instrument; they use the same token for anything, animate or inanimate, that does the action. Only when both agent and instrument are contained in the same sentence do they demonstrate the distinction. Even if one accepts case theory, this suggests that case categories cannot be notionally defined independent from one another, that they interact. Another finding from the Braine and Wells study is that determination of categories is not purely semantic, but depends on the syntactic form of the string. This is suggested by the children treating "subjects of predicate adjectives as a separate category, here called the Subject of Attribution, distinct from Actor, and functionally independent of objects of transitive verbs" (1978:100). Since case theory wishes its categories to be ontologic rather than syntactic, this may raise some problems for the theory.

The evidence presented by Braine and Wells, like that from other concept-formation studies, does not show that the categories were ones the subjects brought with them to the experiment rather than ones taught during the study. The whole argument hinges on the claim that subjects demonstrate they have learned the categories quickly. As Braine and Wells put it:

> The extremely rapid learning suggested that these meaning categories were ones that the children brought with them to the experiment and to which they assimilated the content of the training pictures and sentences. Thus, these results confirmed that the method might prove useful for exploring the nature and boundaries of children's case categories. [Braine and Wells, 1978:102]

The argument is not convincing. Children learn simple categorizing tasks very quickly, and the case categories used in the Braine and Wells study were simple and clear. This is supported by the fact that they used only instances of case categories that could be portrayed in simple one-frame picture form. There is no control concept with which to explicitly compare the speed of learning. In fact, however, there is one datum incidentally reported by Braine and Wells that suggests a noncase distinction was learned as rapidly as the case categories. In one experiment, they happened to use two different actor tokens in the training sessions, one token in strings of one form and another for a different form. Both tokens represented exactly the same case, actor. Case theory would predict that the two actor tokens would be used interchangeably when the opportunity arose. "We had expected that the children would confuse the two Actor tokens (but only put them on actors). . . . . However, contrary to our expectations, they almost always chose to use [the token for the form] that had been used . . . in the training" (Braine and Wells, 1978:104). That this incidental property was also learned during the training trials to a significant degree ($p < .01$) weakens the claim that the case categories must have been present in the children's cognitive structure before the training began.

A recent experiment (Robinson, 1979) does provide a comparison for how rapidly a subject can learn to use case categories. The rationale of the experiment is somewhat different from the training studies we have just reviewed. The subjects were to learn a miniature artificial syntax by arranging a set of words in a string to form a correct description of a picture of a simple event. The subject looked at the picture and tried to arrange the English words in conformity with the artificial syntax. The correct string was given after each attempt. The dependent measure was the number of trials the subject took to learn the syntax, using a criterion of four correct strings in a row. Two syntaxes were used, one fairly simple with all strings having the same structure; the other was more difficult with varying structure and length. A control group had only the pictures and word sets. A case experimental group was given cues to the conceptual structure according to case theory: each word was labeled as to its case category using nontechnical terms. These subjects received feedback as to the case frame of the sentences. An orrery experimental group received cues to the conceptual structure underlying the string by providing the scope relations of the set of words: A set of nested boxes was superimposed over the training strings.

A naive theory would predict that the control subjects would learn faster than either group of experimental subjects because the latter had more information to process. Case theory would predict that since discovering the case relations of a string is the heart of syntactic inference, providing the case frame explicitly should speed up the learning. Analogously, the orrery theory would predict that providing scope information explicitly would shortcut the syntactic inference required to learn the word-order code to conceptual relations.

Subjects in the scope-cue condition learned the syntaxes significantly faster than either the control subjects or the case-cue subjects. The case-cue subjects did learn significantly faster than the control subjects. There was no interaction between experimental treatment and syntax. This suggests that case category information may not play as important a role in syntax as scope information.

Our experiment was similar to that of Braine and Wells in that it required the subject to do a concept-formation task. In their study only case category concepts were involved. Their claim was that the rapid learning of the application of case concepts indicated that the subjects already had case categories in their cognitive structure. However, they did not provide any comparative basis for judging whether the time and exposure needed to apply the case category concepts was really too short to be explained without appeal to preexisting knowledge. In our experiment, case category concept formation was pitted against scope hierarchy concept formation. To hold the claim made by Braine and Wells, one then would have to hold that scope hierarchy distinctions were also present in the cognitive structure of language users, and to a greater degree than case-category concepts.

Future research on underlying structure: work in progress

One area of current interest is the exploration of how underlying conceptual structure mediates translation from one natural language to another. In Chapter 2 we considered the putative universality of various features of underlying conceptual structure. We argued against the universality of any small set of particular kinds of relations of concepts. At the same time, we suggested that scope and dependency were such general features that they would be present in all languages. We have begun to explore the problem of feature universality using a technique similar to that of the experiment reported in the preceding section.

One group of subjects takes a sentence in language A and portrays it either as a case diagram or an orrery diagram. We then randomly change the left-to-right order of the elements of the diagram, convert words to lexemes so that their syntactic role is not revealed, and then, using a dictionary, translate the words into language B. For case diagrams, the labels for the case relations are also translated. A second group of subjects, fluent in language B and trained in the interpretation of the diagrams, tries to derive the proper sentence from the diagram. Finally, a group of judges evaluates the fidelity of the two translation processes. A high-fidelity translation means that the model of underlying structure portrayed by the diagram is capable of carrying enough information to explain language processing. While our pilot study using English and French is too small for statistical conclusions, case and orrery diagrams appear to do the job equally well. We would like to try this experiment using a language such as Hopi or Nootka, where the syntax seems to depend on a set of ontological distinctions different from English.

A second study attempts to test the strong psychological reality of underlying conceptual structures. It is an attempt to use the speed of human language performance to evaluate models of underlying conceptual structure. The rationale is to use the relative complexity of a sentence according to a particular model of underlying structure as a predictor of the relative amount of time it takes to understand the sentence. This rationale has been used a great deal in experimental psycholinguistics, especially within transformational theory.

Fodor, Bever, and Garrett (1974) provide an excellent review along with a very pessimistic critique of research that tries to find experimental correlates between theoretically defined underlying complexity and sentence processing time. In essence, they argue that understanding a language string typically does not involve an orderly sequence of operations, each corresponding to one step in the theoretical model's process. Rather, sentence comprehension is characterized by analysis-by-synthesis, where semantic and syntactic redundancy are used to take shortcuts in ways that are difficult to specify. Further, it is difficult to estimate the number of such processes that are going on in parallel. Given these complications, Fodor, Bever, and Garrett conclude that actual measures of sentence comprehension time cannot be predicted from theoretical measures of the complexity of underlying structure.

The study we are working on avoids many of the criticisms presented by Fodor, Bever, and Garrett. We use materials we developed for some of the studies reported above. Recall that our experimental material consisted of lexemes with few or no inflection cues and functors, and that we used only strings derived from low-probability sentence anagrams. This means that semantic redundancy is completely or nearly eliminated. Therefore, it is impossible for the subject to correctly anticipate syntactic information from (lexical) semantic information. The subject is required to perform all or most of the parsing operations involved in understanding the sentence.

Another way our experiment is unique is that instead of using a purely theoretical measure of complexity, our measure of complexity is partly empirical. This is most easily described in the context of the experiment itself. Here is the rationale: Each model of underlying conceptual structure claims to represent the cognitive structure used in sentence comprehension. Proponents of both the LNR case model and the orrery model claim that the diagrams they use portray the essential features of the respective models. In this study we derive a measure of relative complexity by seeing how long it takes subjects to decode LNR case and orrery diagrams of the sentences used in the comprehension speed task. In effect, this is asking subjects to perform overtly on the cognitive structures that have been proposed as models of language performance.

Now it is clearly true that decoding an LNR case or orrery diagram must involve at least some psychological operations that differ from those involved in comprehending a sentence presented in conventional format. One task requires the perception of topologically portrayed relations and the other requires the perception of sequence and inflection cues. We could not expect subjects to perform the two different sets of operations with identical speed. This is true at least for the reason that subjects are highly practiced at perceiving syntactic information from ordinary sentences but only newly acquainted with the diagram decoding task. However, since each model claims that the information contained in the diagram is the information that needs to be extracted from the ordinary sentence and used in the parsing operation, we can expect there to be a relationship between the rank-order relative speed across sentences between the two tasks. That is, the faster sentences in the diagram decoding task should be the faster sentences in the ordinary comprehension task *if that form of diagram correctly represents the information needed to parse sentences.* Using diagrams for competing models, the experimental analysis can help us determine how well each model predicts the relative difficulty of parsing each of a set of sentences.

We are currently trying to determine good methods of measuring diagram decoding and sentence comprehension times. We have completed a pilot study requiring subjects to match the sentence to the best of four diagrams for one task and to the best of four paraphrases for the other. Unfortunately, the multiple choice situation proved too noisy for significant conclusions to be drawn.[5]

Summary

In the preceding chapter we introduced the orrery model of underlying conceptual structure and formally compared it to case and transformational models. In this chapter we have looked at some empirical arguments that bear on the models. First we considered the topological organization of the components of underlying structure and looked at some experiments suggesting that hierarchical rather than heterarchical organization better characterizes human language structure. This conclusion favors the orrery and transformational models and causes difficulties for the heterarchical LNR case model. Then we looked at evidence that underlying structure contains dependency information. This evidence favors the orrery over the transformational model. Next we reviewed some experimental evidence that the hierarchical organization of underlying structure does not contain information about left-to-right order. This again favors the orrery over the transformational model. Then we reported an experiment that suggests the lean orrery with only scope and dependency information carries enough information about conceptual structure to permit as complete language comprehension as the much richer LNR case model. Next we presented a brief critical review of the evidence for the psychological reality of case categories. We concluded that case categories have not received strong empirical support. The chapter closed with a sketch of projects we have begun to explore: the cross-language universality of case and orrery models, and the use of case and orrery diagrams to predict human parsing performance.

4

Syntax: background and current theories

In this chapter we will first discuss Chomsky's criteria for the adequacy of a theory of grammar and how they are related to (1) the use of computers in linguistic research, (2) the assumption of an ideal language user, (3) the role of linguistic universals in a theory, and (4) the connection between syntax and semantics. We will look at some of the ways to compare and evaluate theories of syntax. Then different accounts of syntax will be examined and compared. In the next chapter we will discuss our own model of syntactic operations and compare it with those discussed here.

Chomsky's criteria for an adequate theory

Noam Chomsky (1957) proposed three criteria that an adequate theory of grammar should satisfy. By grammar, he meant both syntax and morphophonemics, but we will be concerned only with syntax. Theories of syntax in their present stage of development are far from providing a complete account of all language; instead they propose programs or directions for research, setting out the kinds of rules that would be necessary for a complete account. No theory actually satisfies Chomsky's three criteria, but many justify their programs in terms of the likelihood of doing so. As we shall see, the interpretation of how the criteria are to be met differ from theory to theory.

The criteria are:

1. A theory of grammar should provide a set of rules that can generate all and only syntactically correct strings.

118

2. The rules should also generate correct structural descriptions for each grammatical string.
3. The theory should be formulated in terms of features universal to all languages.

Originally, Chomsky argued for *explanatory power* as a criterion of a theory:

> There are many facts about language and linguistic behavior that require explanation beyond the fact that such and such a string (which no one may ever have produced) is or is not a sentence. It is reasonable to expect grammars to provide explanations for some of these facts. [Chomsky, 1957:85]

Later, he identified the notion of explanatory power with a universal grammar:

> Universal grammar, then, constitutes an explanatory theory of a much deeper sort than particular grammar, although the particular grammar of a language can also be regarded as an explanatory theory. . . . To bring out this difference in depth of explanation, I have suggested . . . that the term "level of descriptive adequacy" might be used for the study of the relation between grammars and data and the term "level of explanatory adequacy" for the relation between a theory of universal grammar and these data. [Chomsky, 1972:27–28]

Generation of all-and-only grammatical strings

It has long been thought that the purpose of syntax should be to distinguish grammatical from ungrammatical strings. Chomsky's first criterion requires that this distinction be made by a limited set of rules that can be combined to generate strings automatically. As we discussed, using abbreviated Goodlish as an example in Chapter 1, the main argument for this is that people can produce novel grammatical strings and distinguish between grammatical and ungrammatical sequences that they have never had experience with before. Therefore, it seems reasonable to suppose that they do this, not by using something like a catalog of all grammatical strings, but by generating (and parsing) strings using some general principles. A catalog method is something like what people use to count from one to ten. The names of the numbers and their sequence have just been memorized. However, many people can also count indefinitely high, because in addition to the names of some numbers they have also learned principles for combining the names – principles that can be employed to generate or parse novel number names.

Now we could try to describe the principles used to generate number names in terms of a set of rules for combining number words. And Chomsky's first criterion could be applied to our rules for number names. If our rules generated names that were not well-formed names of numbers, such as THIRTY-ELEVEN, then something is wrong with our rules. And if our rules could not generate some number names, such as FIFTEEN HUNDRED, then our rules are inadequate.

Our ability to distinguish grammatical from ungrammatical strings involves many different properties of language strings. To a lay person, some properties of language strings appear to be paradigmatic distinguishers of grammaticality. For example, consider the properties that distinguish the correct from the incorrect in the following strings.

★I ARE AWAKE	I AM AWAKE
★I HAVE WENT	I HAVE GONE
★I EAT BEFORE I SLEPT	I ATE BEFORE I SLEPT

Properties such as noun-verb agreement, verb tense, pronoun and tense agreement across clauses may appear to describe differences that are more striking than many of the examples syntactic theories concentrate on. While the contrast between the correct and incorrect strings above may be very salient, there are syntactic distinctions that are more basic to our understanding of strings. We *can* interpret the sentences on the left correctly even though their forms are ungrammatical. But there are some ungrammatical strings we cannot interpret without ambiguity, if at all. For example: OR SMILE TALK DON'T, READ LEARN TO I, and WATERS JUMPS HIGH IT. Of central concern for theories of syntax are those properties of grammaticality that enable us to understand a string, to figure out how the concepts expressed by the lexemes are related. Unlike the job of the prescriptive grammarian, the important thing for a theory of syntax to explain is not why I HAVE GONE is correct and I HAVE WENT is incorrect, but how people can regularly and automatically produce one form rather than the other, whichever one it is.

Generation of strings by a computer

Let us now take a closer look at Chomsky's first criterion: A theory of syntax should provide a set of rules that generate all and only well-formed grammatical strings. In science, a common strategy is to isolate and delimit a target phenomenon in order to be sure that no unnoticed or ill-defined variables are at work. This is just what Chomsky did with syntax. One way to test whether a set of rules can generate correct strings and not generate incorrect ones is to program a computer with the rules and see what happens when the computer uses them to generate strings. This method has the added advantage of ensuring that only the specified rules are employed. If the rules were manipulated by humans, other, unknown, abilities, including prior knowledge of the difference between a grammatical and ungrammatical string, might be used unwittingly. The computer's output can be checked against a human language user's knowledge of correct strings. The random generation of strings by a computer is very unlike the production of strings by a language user. But the idea of a computer test is to isolate the grammatical mechanism from other cognitive abilities, not to replicate normal language use.

In addition, the particular rules responsible for failures and near-successes in a computer simulation can be illuminating. This way of testing how well a set of rules satisfies the first criterion has become so widely accepted that computer simulations are fairly standard (see Appendix A). However, such a test using syntactic rules without any other features of language to generate strings at random is, at best, only a check on one aspect of a theory: the extent to which it satisfies Chomsky's first criterion.

Correct structural descriptions

Chomsky's second criterion is that a linguistic theory should assign the correct structural descriptions to grammatical strings. That is, the rules of syntax must also provide information that is not in the string alone – how the terms go together. Using the number name example, the structural description might include how to group the terms in the name, for example in Roman numerals XXIX is to be read as XX(IX) and not as X(XI)X. The structural description might also include more about how the terms are combined, specifying, for example, that IX signifies "I less than, or before, X" and not "X more than, or after, I."

Notice that the structural description (representation of the combining principles) depends on the lexical information in the number names. That is, we need to know which symbols stand for smaller numbers than other symbols. A structural rule would use this information to specify how the symbol standing for the smaller number is to be combined with the larger one preceding or following it, for example, IV versus VI. One needs lexical information as well as the correct structural description for Roman numerals to understand what number is being expressed.

Ambiguity in structural descriptions

In the development of linguistic theory, ambiguous sentences have served as test cases for Chomsky's second criterion. Although a string may be ambiguous because it contains one or more ambiguous lexemes, the second criterion is concerned with strings that are ambiguous because we cannot tell how the concepts expressed by the lexemes go together. As we discussed in Chapter 2 the correctness of a theory's structural description is often demonstrated by its providing similar structures for strings expressing similar relations of concepts, and different structures for strings, or a single ambiguous string that express(es) different relations of concepts. For example, the string THE CANNIBAL ATE SOUP WITH A MISSIONARY can be interpreted with the missionary serving either as dining companion or main course. The syntactic structures corresponding to these interpretations can be shown easily by bracketing the constituents: either A CANNIBAL ATE [SOUP WITH A MISSIONARY] or A CANNIBAL [ATE SOUP] [WITH A MISSIONARY]. The second criterion requires that syntax provide a different structural description for every interpretation of a syntactically ambiguous sentence. This must be true even for strings where our pragmatic knowledge makes one interpretation so unlikely that it doesn't cross our mind. For example: MARIE ATE A HAMBURGER WITH JOHN. It is possible, although very unlikely, that someone with the name Marie is an anthropophagite with a large appetite.

Universal properties, essential properties, and acquisition

Chomsky's third criterion for an adequate theory of syntax is that it should be formulated in terms of features universal to all languages. The obvious thrust of the criterion is to require theories to be expressed in such a way as to cover more than a restricted domain. But Chomsky (1965:59) had something particular in mind for the third criterion: "Thus it may well be that the general features of language structure reflect, not so much the course of one's experience but rather the general character of one's capacity to acquire knowledge – in the traditional sense, one's innate ideas and innate principles." Just as it is an important universal fact about language that language users can generate and understand novel strings, so also is it an important fact that language users *acquire* the ability to do so. Thus the third criterion requires that theories of language be formulated so that it can be shown how the acquisition of language is possible. However, Chomsky's particular view of how language is acquired – that children have an innate language acquisition device which only needs to be "fine-tuned" to the grammatical patterns of a particular language – is not central to the criterion. Without subscribing to the nativist/rationalist doctrine, we can adopt a variant of the third criterion: An adequate linguistic theory should be formulated in terms of the properties that are *essential* to language. If properties are essential to language, they will be universal to all languages. By looking for essential properties rather than universal properties, one avoids the possibility of discovering properties that happen to be found in all languages either by accident or because of some other aspect of human or primate nature independent of language. Moreover, it should be possible to show how language can be acquired using the essential properties hypothesized.

Rules for an ideal language user

To apply the first criterion – generation of all and only grammatical strings – we need to have some idea of what counts as a grammatical string. This is not a trivial problem. We want to be able to account for what people actually say. But we don't want to force our account to handle all the *um*s and *er*s, false starts, interruptions, and sloppiness of actual speech. What we want are syntactic rules that describe the speech that might come from an ideal language user, someone who uses language without the random variations that occur in the speech of real people. The positing of an ideal language user is really no more than a heuristic device for explaining what part of language a theory of syntax is going to concentrate on.

Describing a theory of syntax in terms of an ideal language user is analogous to describing a theory of planetary motion in terms of point masses. Both theories employ abstractions that do not exist in the real world. Each makes a claim that certain properties of the real world are essential for the phenomenon being described: rules of syntax for language; position and mass for planetary motion. Neither claims that these are the only properties that can affect their respective phenomena.

Even within one dialect community, individuals will differ as to what they judge to be a correct string. Each person has a slightly different "idiolect" because each has had slightly different experiences with language and language changes. These idiolect differences could be handled by a syntactic theory as slight differences in the rules employed by different people. However, the test of a syntactic theory rests not on any particular rule it gives, but on its claim that rules of a particular sort, with particular sorts of properties, can serve as the basis for an explanation of syntax.

Not all unacceptable strings are ungrammatical

What is more of a problem for syntactic theories than the existence of idiolects is that, even when there is agreement that a string is incorrect, it is not always clear that it is incorrect or unacceptable because it is ungrammatical. Consider two clear cases first: Everyone might agree that SHE WITNESS THE IS is an unacceptable string and agree it is unacceptable because it is ungrammatical, the lexemes are not in any well-formed order. And everyone might agree that the insertion of the sentence SOIL EROSION IS NOT A SERIOUS PROBLEM IN ZAMBIA (not as an example) in the last paragraph of this chapter would be unacceptable, but that it would be unacceptable because of its inappropriate subject matter – it is semantically out of context, not ungrammatical. In between these two extremes are many cases where there is no easy agreement. The string may be unacceptable, but it is not clear whether it is because of the meaning, the context in which it appears, or syntax. The following strings are unacceptable to many people:

> THE CONCLUSION THAT PIGS CAN FLY REVEALED HIMSELF TO BE FALSE (Bach, 1974)
>
> THE WINDOW STRUCK (Fillmore, 1968)
>
> JOHN HAS MORE MONEY THAN HARRY IS TALL (Fodor, Bever, and Garrett, 1974)
>
> BE DIVISIBLE BY FIVE (Fodor, Bever, and Garrett, 1974)

In each case the question of whether the string is unacceptable because it is ungrammatical may involve more than the question of whether it falls under a particular rule of syntax. It usually involves a question of how semantics, the meaning, is related to syntax, the organization, of a string. It also may involve a question of what sorts of regularities in language are characterizable by automatic rules, rather than by less exact, heuristic strategies, and a question of what sort of rules a syntactic theory needs to have: For example, the first and third strings can be eliminated only as violations of rules that coordinate one part of a sentence with another, distant part.

Acceptability depends on more than syntax alone

We believe that the attempt to formulate rules to determine every aspect of acceptability is a mistake. The rules that eliminate many unacceptable strings would also eliminate some acceptable strings unless modified by an unlimited number of exceptions. Our view is shared by others, and we shall include their criticisms along with our own. We agree that a theory of syntax should be able to distinguish grammatical from ungrammatical strings and should assign more than one structure to most syntactically ambiguous strings. But just how much of ambiguity and acceptability is to be analyzed in terms of rules is highly disputable. Pragmatic information, our knowledge of the world, also contributes to determining the acceptability and ambiguity of strings. And there is no reason to suppose that the job can be done without this information. In fact, there is reason to believe that pragmatic information is necessary in many cases, for example, to handle pronoun agreement from paragraph to paragraph; to recognize that the string FRASER HAS MORE POWER THAN ALI IS FAST is acceptable, although the similar string JOHN HAS MORE MONEY THAN HARRY IS TALL might appear unacceptable; to realize that BE DIVISIBLE BY FIVE muttered by someone working on a problem in mod five arithmetic makes sense; and to understand stories or recounts of dreams in which stones can cough, windows strike, and cannibals named Marie do their thing at McDonald's.

Adding features to delimit acceptability

Some proponents of an autonomous role for syntax have argued that much of this pragmatic information could be coded in the syntactic theory in the form of features derived from the meaning of individual concepts. Each concept would be characterized in terms of a limited set of features available for use by syntax. The syntactic mechanism would contain restrictions on which categories of morphemes, as described by the features, could occur together. For example, a typical feature is *gender*. With all nouns and pronouns marked as to their gender, a syntactic rule could enforce the agreement of pronouns, thus preventing one of the examples above: THE CONCLUSION THAT PIGS CAN FLY REVEALED HIMSELF TO BE FALSE. Other restriction rules would also prevent THE CONCLUSION from being combined with RAN INDOORS DURING THE WINTER, FED ON PLANKTON AND OTHER SMALL SEA CREATURES if the verbs and their modifiers were coded only to accept [+ human] or [+ animate] subjects. However, the kind of coding that would eliminate the above combinations and still permit the acceptable THE CONCLUSION RAN IN HER HEAD DURING

THE INTERMISSION; THE CONCLUSION FED ON SUSPICION AND RUMOR would have to introduce additional features to make a distinction between running indoors and running in someone's head, between feeding on plankton and feeding on rumor. Once these additional features are accepted by the theory, new sentences would require still more features, since the world does not provide the language user with a limited set of properties and relations to talk about, nor prearranged categories of what sort of concepts can go together.

Could features work to determine acceptability?

The question here is one of feasibility. Adherents of this view are proposing a direction for research, not offering a finished theory. So it is not a question of whether the theory does what it claims but whether it is likely that there could be a finished theory that does what is claimed. They suppose that there are a limited set of features that can encode concepts and be operated on by syntactic rules, so that all ambiguous strings will have more than one description and only acceptable sentences can be generated.

Bolinger (1965) argued convincingly that the number of such features would have to be unmanageably large. Rather than having a limited set of features for classifying all concepts, he argued that the number of features would have to increase with each variation in meaning among concepts in order to make correct distinctions for judging acceptability and resolving ambiguity.

Another problem with this proposal for incorporating semantic features in syntax is that it ignores an important aspect of language. Language is constantly changing. There are new ways of saying old things and new things being said about relations of concepts that have not been seen as related before. If a preestablished set of rules was totally responsible for determining which concepts could and could not be related, then it would be hard to understand novel and deviant strings that violated the syntactic/semantic classification rules. And yet people do understand novel and deviant strings quite readily. One conclusion of a large empirical study of how people interpret difficult and deviant strings (Gleitman and Gleitman, 1970:159–160) is: "The ordinary speaker apparently rejects an utterance just in the limiting case in which the sequence has no semblance of structure. . . . Typically, the listener will assume that whatever is said has meaning."

Some theorists (e.g., Katz, 1964; Ziff, 1964) who believe that the syntactic mechanism does contain category restrictions that rule out deviant strings, then account for the ready interpretation (and less common production) of deviant strings by postulating a supplementary mechanism that "relaxes" the category restrictions. Reviewing these proposals, Gleitman and Gleitman conclude:

> But no one has commented usefully on just what these rules are to be, how to write them, and particularly how to limit them. Therefore, we have to conclude that no one has developed a theory to account for the comprehensibility of deviant sentences. Semi-grammatical sentences are systematic deformations of grammatical sentences and somehow the speaker-listener knows how to undo these deformations in very many instances. [1970:163–164]

What syntax need not do

Our position is that the acceptability of strings is governed in many cases by the nature of the concepts expressed and the situation in which they are expressed. And where semantic and pragmatic information processing can determine ambiguity or acceptability, it is unnecessary to require syntax to do the same job. We believe much of semantic and pragmatic information processing that determines the acceptability of strings will not be amenable to characterizations in terms of explicit procedures and automatic rules. This position, however, is independent of our model for syntax, which tries to describe only the minimal and essential aspects of syntax. A set of categorization rules and semantic markers could be added to our theory as easily as to any other theory, were such entities found to be convincing.

We believe there are some aspects of language processing that can be formulated in terms of explicit procedures and automatic rules. But we do not think that all language processing can be characterized in such terms. For some operations, there are strategies and heuristics that may guide, but do not alone determine the path of, the processing. There is good reason to believe that the order of lexemes and the occurrence of inflections and function terms are, for the most part, processed automatically by language users. A theory of syntax is an explanation of this automatic process. Linguists have wanted their theories of syntax to be as powerful as possible. So it is tempting to describe a theory as a program that could by itself (eventually) provide rules for resolving all ambiguities and generating all and only acceptable strings. But as Bolinger and others have pointed out, such rules, if they existed, would be burdened with an enormous system of fine syntactic and semantic classifications and would be inconsistent with the language user's ability to interpret and express novel relations that violate the rules.

Instead, we suggest that syntax does not have to do its job in isolation; for example, syntactic structures need not resolve all ambiguities. Ambiguities are recognized because the language user knows that the concepts expressed can be related in more than one way. Syntax cannot distinguish all the possible ways concepts can be related. Fortunately, it does not have to. The language user can employ pragmatic information.

As for judgments of acceptability: When pragmatic information processing can determine unacceptability, syntactic criteria of acceptability are redundant.[1] When pragmatic information cannot rule out the conceptual relations expressed in an unacceptable string, then it must be syntax that determines the unacceptability. In between these extremes, how much does the syntactic mechanism do in determining acceptability? That is hard to answer. Perhaps the earlier example *I EAT BEFORE I SLEPT is anomalous because the different tenses of EAT and SLEPT conflict with the meaning of BEFORE. If such distinctions can be completely accounted for by pragmatic and lexical information (in this case, that things in the present do not occur before things in the past), then we would not have to invoke syntactic rules to make the distinction. We do not expect there to be a rigid boundary between the contributions of syntax and semantic/pragmatic information processing. For syntax and pragmatic information processing to overlap would provide a measure of redundant control, insuring adequate language performance where neither by itself could effect reliable distinctions.

The fuzzy borders of the realm of syntax

Let us look more closely at some problems of defining an exclusive realm for syntax. Most people would agree that a syntactic mechanism should be able to generate the following strings:

THE SMALL BIRD	THE OLD BIRD
THE OLD HOUSE	THE SMALL BIRD HOUSE
THE OLD HOUSE BIRD	THE BIRD THAT IS SMALL
THE BIRD HOUSE THAT IS OLD	THE SMALL HOUSE

and many other strings using the same lexemes.

The criterion that an adequate theory be able to generate all and only grammatical strings requires that a syntactic mechanism not be indiscriminate in its generative capacities. It should not also generate strings that are clearly ungrammatical, for example:

★SMALL BIRD THE   ★THAT THE IS HOUSE OLD

Sometimes it is not clear whether a string is grammatical. Consider, for example:

HOUSE SMALL BIRD   THE FATHER HOUSE

Other strings with the same grammatical categories, noun-adjective-noun and article-noun-noun, are acceptable:

MILE HIGH GIANT   THE BIRD HOUSE

In order to treat the first two as ungrammatical and the second two as grammatical, the syntax could classify MILE as a different sort of noun than HOUSE, for example. If MILE belonged to the category noun$_1$ and HOUSE to the category noun$_2$, then the rule system could allow strings of the form noun$_1$-adjective-noun and not allow strings of the form noun$_2$-adjective-noun. A distinction could also be made between HIGH and SMALL, or FATHER and BIRD. Of course such a distinction would have to permit distinctions between acceptable and unacceptable strings of other sorts as well.

Such classifications would increase the complexity of the rule system. Since this distinction can be, and is, made on pragmatic grounds, we would argue that there is no reason for linguistic rules to duplicate the distinction. In other words, English-language users do not produce strings like THE FATHER HOUSE (or HOUSE SMALL BIRD), not because their rule system is organized to make such strings impossible to generate, but because they do not conceive of any sensible relation between the concepts expressed by FATHER and HOUSE under ordinary circumstances.

For the string, THE FATHER HOUSE, English-language users, if pressed as in the Gleitmans' study, would try to imagine some relationship between the concepts expressed by FATHER and HOUSE: the original house, the house where the father lives, a house where fathers go, and so on. And if any such connection of concepts appears appropriate, the expression THE FATHER HOUSE would be readily employed.

In discussing syntactic models, we will frequently provide examples of the sorts of strings they can generate and the sorts they cannot. We do not intend our illustrations about what is and what is not grammatical to be definitive. Situational and individual differences affect such decisions. Different language users may appear to be using different rules. In some cases the language users making the judgments of acceptability are the very ones who argue for particular theories of syntax. We need to consider this problem of possible bias directly.

Comparing syntactic theories

Chomsky's criteria serve as standards by which a theory of syntax can measure itself: Does it provide rules that automatically generate all and only grammatical strings, with their structures, from basic properties that characterize all languages? However, Chomsky's criteria are difficult to apply when actually comparing theories, for what distinguishes one theory from another is very likely to depend on differences in what each judges to be a correct structure, a linguistic universal, or even a well-formed string. Theorists who believe there are rules that will distinguish any unacceptable string from acceptable ones and that will provide more than one structure for any ambiguous string, will classify each unacceptable string as ungrammatical and each nonlexical ambiguity as a grammatical ambiguity. Further, a commitment to a particular theory, as in any other field, may lead the language scientist to look at the data in a different way, for example, considering a string that others would find acceptable or only mildly awkward to be ungrammatical. As Greene (1972:9) comments on decisions about grammaticality: "These intuitions can vary widely, from the judgment in 1957 that 'colourless green ideas sleep furiously' is grammatical, to the judgment in 1971 that 'even John came but then maybe no one else did' is ungrammatical."

In our discussion of syntactic theories, we will see that they consider different phenomena in need of explanation and employ different properties in their explanations. Within a theory also there may be wide disagreement about particular rules, the phenomena that are part of syntax, and restrictions on what constitutes a legitimate answer. In what follows we will discuss some of the most prominent theories. Our discussion will not be exhaustive. We will omit some theories whose principles are very different from our model, e.g., categorial grammars (Adjukiewicz, 1935). Nor will our discussion be comprehensive for the theories we consider. We try to be sympathetic to the best in each theory and to discuss aspects of the theories that are representative and the focus of critical interest. While the version of transformational grammar we present is now being disputed and revised, there are many linguists who still accept it, and it is the version being presented in most current texts – if only because it is more worked out than its offshoots (see, for example, Akmajian, Demers, and Harnish, 1979).

Constituent analysis: bracketing, tree graphs, and phrase structure rules

The problem for any theory of syntax is to explain how relations of concepts are expressed by relations of lexemes. Frequently we can indicate something about the relations of lexemes by showing how elements in a string are grouped together using brackets[2] around the terms that belong together: *immediate constituent analysis*. For example, the constituent structure of THE HOUSE IS SMALL would be shown by ([THE] [HOUSE]) ([IS] [SMALL]).

Although the nested brackets are imposed on the linear sequence of a string, they indicate hierarchical organization and should not be mistaken for a system that merely relates single adjacent elements. A pair of brackets is to be read as connecting all enclosed symbols as a unit to all the symbols contained in the adjacent pair of brackets. In the previous example, THE and HOUSE

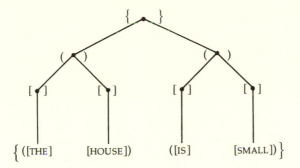

Figure 4.1. Tree graph representation equivalent to nested bracket notation for the string THE HOUSE IS SMALL.

as a unit are connected to IS and SMALL as a unit. The subunit HOUSE is not more directly connected to IS than to SMALL even though HOUSE and IS are adjacent in the string THE HOUSE IS SMALL.

The hierarchical nature of the nested bracket notation can be more easily seen when it is converted into a tree graph as described in Chapter 1. Figure 4.1 illustrates the equivalence of nested brackets and a tree graph for the string THE HOUSE IS SMALL. The nonterminal nodes of the tree are marked to indicate the particular set of brackets that each is equivalent to.

The immediate constituent analysis of THE HOUSE IS SMALL, as shown by the bracket notation or the tree representation, is straightforward. One unit is formed by THE and HOUSE, and another by IS and SMALL. The two units might be described in syntactic terms as subject and predicate, but this is not essential. However, the analysis of immediate constituents may be more complicated. The sources of these complications have played important roles in the development of language theories.

One problem involves syntactic ambiguity. For example, the appropriate constituent analysis for the string WHEN EATING FISH DO NOT LAUGH can only be determined by the context – whether it is about the behavior of the fish or advice on how to avoid choking when eating seafood. If the first, then EATING and FISH are not grouped together; if the second, they are.

Another problem in constituent analysis occurs when parts of the string that should be grouped together as one constituent are

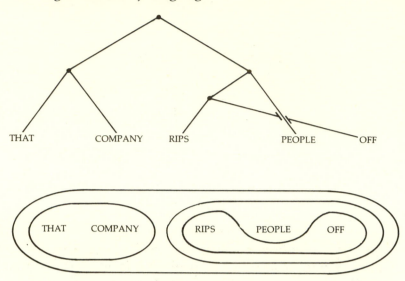

Figure 4.2. Two unconventional but simple ways to portray an analysis of discontinuous constituents.

separated by one or more words that do not belong to that constituent: the problem of *discontinuous constituents.* For example, in the string THAT COMPANY RIPS PEOPLE OFF, RIPS and OFF should be grouped together as a unit to be joined with PEOPLE. This grouping is impossible for the standard bracket notation or the ordinary tree graph to portray. This impossibility has taken on great importance in language theory. As we will discuss, it is the basis for one of the major arguments favoring transformational grammar over immediate constituent grammars. There *are* simple, but unconventional, ways of portraying an analysis of strings with discontinuous constituents (see Figure 4.2). However, the problem for a theory of syntax adopting such a representation is how to come up with a set of rules that will parse and generate strings with discontinuous constituents into and from the proper structural description. The grouping portrayed by bracketing or the sharing of nodes on a tree graph gives information about the structure of individual strings but tells relatively little about how the structure of one string is related to that of another. For example, bracketing or trees by themselves cannot tell us that THE SMALL HOUSE, THE CAT, IT, and JAMIE could each be substituted for THE HOUSE in the string THE HOUSE IS SMALL to produce a different well-formed string. Nor could it tell us that the above phrases cannot be substituted for IS SMALL in the same string. Something more than mere grouping is needed; we need to categorize the groups in such a way that terms that are substitutable for each other belong to the same category. To keep track of categories, we must also label them.

Labeling the categories is the equivalent of labeling the nodes of the tree graph or labeling the sets of nested brackets. The information carried by the labels accounts for more of the regularities of language than a representation of grouping alone. It shows that some words or phrases can be substituted for some others to yield well-formed strings. The substitutability of syntactic units is indicated by their sharing the same category label. Although traditionally the categories are labeled with the terms of classic grammar, other terms, such as numbers, can and are sometimes used instead. Figure 4.3(a) shows a tree diagram with labeled nodes and a sample of labeled syntactic units that may be substituted in the original string to yield a new well-formed string.

Labeling each node according to its syntactic category is important for describing the regularities of structure that characterize the strings of a language. These regularities, as we indicated in Chapter 1 with the comparison between Goodlish and Badlish, are crucial to understanding how language users are able to produce and understand new strings. They allow the properties of syntactic units to be generalized across the members of a category. The regularities are usually described in terms of production, or rewrite rules. Because these rules describe the grouping of constituent phrases in strings, they are also called *phrase structure rules*. Each rule describes how a particular node is related to the nodes immediately below it. Figure 4.3(b) lists the production rules corresponding to the tree graph in Figure 4.3(a).

Although formally equivalent to the tree graph or labeled bracket representations, the set of rewrite rules has important advantages. By breaking up the information contained in the structure into small independent chunks, it is very easy to analyze the similarities across different strings as the sharing of production rules. For example, the string THE CAT LOOKS LONELY shares with the string THE HOUSE IS SMALL all of the production rules in the

(a)

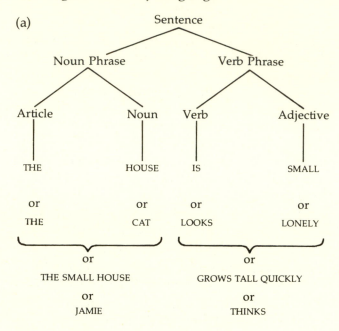

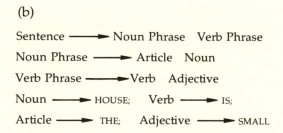

(b)

Sentence ——→ Noun Phrase   Verb Phrase

Noun Phrase ——→ Article   Noun

Verb Phrase ——→ Verb   Adjective

Noun ——→ HOUSE;   Verb ——→ IS;

Article ——→ THE;   Adjective ——→ SMALL

Figure 4.3. (a) Tree graph of THE HOUSE IS SMALL. (b) Production rules corresponding to the tree graph.

first three rows of Figure 4.3(b). The two strings differ only in the production rules that control the lexical items, for example NOUN → HOUSE in one case and NOUN → CAT in the other.

The phrase structure tree compared with the orrery

For simple strings, a phrase structure tree graph looks somewhat like an ordered orrery diagram with the arms bent in a different way. However, there is an important difference between the rep-

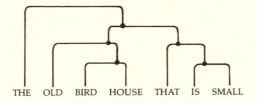

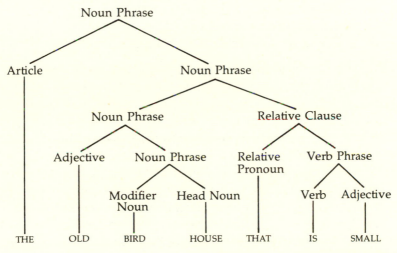

Figure 4.4. Orrery and phrase structure tree for the string THE OLD BIRD HOUSE THAT IS SMALL.

resentations. The orrery indicates dependency relations in the structure, while the phrase structure tree does not. Figure 4.4 compares the two representations. Indicating the dependency relations by marking the main component of each constituent unit enables the structure to encode differences between phrases such as VISITING PROFESSORS (meaning peripatetic scholars) and VISITING PROFESSORS (meaning the paying of social calls on faculty members). The inability to structurally portray differences such as these is a commonly mentioned shortcoming of phrase structure grammars.

A phrase structure grammar could try to overcome this deficiency by adding a set of rules that would determine dependency relations from the labels of the nodes. For example, a noun could be listed as the main component of a noun phrase, a verb as the main component of a verb phrase. In the noun phrase THE SMALL HOUSE, HOUSE is the noun and hence the main component. However, such rule systems to derive dependency relations from node labels do not yet exist and may be difficult to formulate. The traditional category labels do not lend themselves to a systematic ranking of dependency relations.

Phrase structure grammar criticized by transformational theory: examples of phrase structure constructions

Transformational theory objects to phrase structure grammar on two main grounds: (1) its rules are too numerous and too complex and (2) it ignores important syntactic generalizations and distinctions. These arguments can be illustrated using three types of English constructions: *phrasal verbs* (forms containing more than one word), different *sentence modes* expressing similar relations of concepts (interrogative, negative, etc.), and different *sentence forms* expressing the same idea (paraphrases). Other constructions have been used to illustrate inadequacies in phrase structure grammar, but the arguments on these are similar to the ones we present here. Readers who are familiar with the arguments on the inadequacies of phrase structure grammars, or who are willing to accept that such grammars are inadequate, may prefer to skim the following section.

Phrasal verbs

In what follows we will present an example of each construction; the phrase structure rule required by that construction; and an explanation. We will give simplified rules for verb phrases that do not treat subject-verb agreement and list only one verb modifier, an optional adverb.

1. *Modal auxiliaries:* THE HOUSE WILL CREAK
   S→NP Predicate Phrase; PredP→M VP
   M→WILL, CAN, MAY, SHALL, MUST

We cannot use a rule such as VP→M VP because it could be applied more than once in a sentence to allow ⋆THE HOUSE WILL

CAN CREAK. And we cannot make M optional because it is needed for negation.

2. *Negation:* THE HOUSE WILL NOT CREAK

Add an optional Neg to the PredP rule: PredP→M (Neg) VP

Neg→NOT

If M were optional, the rules could generate ⋆THE HOUSE NOT CREAK.

3. *Progressive tense:* THE HOUSE IS CREAKING

VP→BE V +ING (Adv)

With S→NP VP, this rule generates THE HOUSE IS CREAKING, and with S→NP PredP and PredP→M VP, it generates THE HOUSE WILL BE CREAKING.

4. *Perfect tense:* THE HOUSE HAS CREAKED

VP → HAVE V + ED (Adv)

Note that all the separate VP rules carry the same modifiers.

5. *Perfect progressive:* THE HOUSE HAS BEEN CREAKING

VP→HAVE BE +EN V +ING (Adv)

The rules for perfect and for progressive cannot be combined, so each requires an independent rule.

6. *Passive:* THE HOUSE IS CRACKED

VP→IS V +ED (Adv)

The verb CREAK does not take the passive. The string ⋆THE HOUSE IS CREAKED is unacceptable. To handle this syntactically, the rules must assign CREAK to a different category than CRACK, i.e., formalize the difference between transitive and intransitive verbs. More will be said about the relation of active and passive sentences below.

7. *Perfect passive:* THE HOUSE HAS BEEN CRACKED

VP→HAVE BE +EN V +ED (Adv)

8. *Progressive passive:* THE HOUSE IS BEING CRACKED

VP→BE BE +ING V +ED (Adv)

9. *Perfect progressive passive:* THE HOUSE HAS BEEN BEING CRACKED

VP→HAVE BE +EN BE +ING V +ED (Adv).

Phrase structure grammar, as we have shown above, needs to add a new rule for each of the different sentence forms. However, each one of the rules is just a different combination of basic verb parts. Table 4.1 lists the verb parts needed for each of the basic

Table 4.1. *Phrasal verb forms as combinations of verb form parts*

Modal	WILL					
Perfect		HAVE	{ED, EN}			
Progressive			BE	ING		
Passive				BE	{ED, EN}	
Verb					CRACK	
Modifiers						OPEN
Sentence	WILL	HAVE	BE +EN	BE +ING	CRACK +ED	OPEN

forms of sentence construction. The suffix that belongs with an auxiliary always appears attached to the next verb part. The table gives the perfect progressive passive form as an example, showing how it combines elements from the table.

Since phrase structure grammar has no provision for inserting elements of one rule in between the elements of another, it cannot take advantage of the way complex verb forms can be constructed from simple components. Although this lack of economy has been the target of criticism, transformational theory has raised a stronger objection: The separate rules for each phrasal verb form treat each construction independently from the others. Thus phrase structure rules fail to show the relationships across these several forms. The difficulty is multiplied when we consider sentence modes, such as yes-no questions, and negation.

Sentence modes

1. *Modal auxiliary questions:* WILL THE HOUSE CREAK? WILL THE HOUSE HAVE CREAKED?

   Q→M NP VP?

Combined with the verb phrase rules given under "Phrasal verbs," all the verb forms with modal auxiliaries can be produced in a question form. However, there are also questions that do not begin with modal auxiliaries.

2. *Questions without modal auxiliaries:*

   IS THE HOUSE CREAKING?

   Q→BE NP V +ING (Adv)?

   HAS THE HOUSE CREAKED?

   Q→HAVE NP V +ED (Adv)?

HAS THE HOUSE BEEN CREAKING?
Q→HAVE NP BE +EN V +ING (Adv)?

IS THE HOUSE CRACKED?
Q→BE NP V +ED (Adv)?

HAS THE HOUSE BEEN CRACKED?
Q→HAVE NP BE +EN V +ED (Adv)?

IS THE HOUSE BEING CRACKED?
Q→BE NP BE +ING V +ED (Adv)?

HAS THE HOUSE BEEN BEING CRACKED?
Q→HAVE NP BE +EN BE +ING V +ED (Adv)?

Phrase structure grammar needs all these separate rules even though all the question forms are constructed on the same principle: The first auxiliary of the verb appears to the left of the noun phrase. Given the regularity across the question forms, plus their relationship to declarative forms, transformational theorists argue that it would be better to have a single rule that incorporates both regularities: To form a question, move the first auxiliary in the declarative form to the left of the main noun phrase.

Of course, such a rule is not a phrase structure rule. In fact, it is a very different sort of rule. It requires a standard initial order for questions that is unlike the order in which they finally appear, then a rearrangement of that order during which the categories (main noun phrase) and order (*first* auxiliary) are kept track of.

3. *Negation with modal auxiliary:* THE HOUSE WILL NOT CREAK
   PredP→M (Neg) VP
4. *Negation without modal auxiliary:*
   THE HOUSE IS NOT CREAKING
   Neg VP→BE Neg V +ING (Adv)

   THE HOUSE HAS NOT CREAKED
   Neg VP→HAVE Neg V +ED (Adv)

   THE HOUSE HAS NOT BEEN CREAKING
   Neg VP→HAVE Neg BE +EN V +ING (Adv)

   THE HOUSE HAS NOT BEEN CRACKED
   Neg VP→HAVE Neg BE +EN V +ED (Adv)

HAS NOT THE HOUSE CREAKED?
Q→HAVE Neg NP V +ED (Adv)?

IS NOT THE HOUSE CREAKING?
Q→BE Neg NP V + ING (Adv)?

HAS THE HOUSE NOT CREAKED?
Q→HAVE NP Neg V +ED (Adv)?

IS THE HOUSE NOT CREAKING?
Q→BE NP Neg V +ING (Adv)?

The new symbol, Neg VP, has to be introduced to prevent negative verb phrases from being used with PredP → M (Neg) VP.
Otherwise sentences such as: ★THE HOUSE WILL NOT HAVE NOT
BEEN NOT CREAKING would be permitted. However, if one does
not wish to rule out the multiple negatives by syntactic rules, the
Neg VP symbol is not needed. But this does not obviate the additional rules that are required.

Phrasal verbs are not limited to the main verb phrase of a sentence. Other clauses and phrases take restricted subsets of the
forms allowed main verbs. Infinitive phrases can take phrasal
verbs without modal auxiliaries, noun agreement, and tenses:

TO EAT	but not ★ TO ATE
TO BE EATEN	★ TO EATS
TO BE EATING	★ TO HAS EATEN
TO HAVE BEEN EATEN	★ TO CAN EAT
TO HAVE BEEN EATING	
TO BE BEING EATEN	
TO NOT BE EATEN	

In addition, all the usual verb modifiers can accompany infinitive
verbs.

Verb phrases that act as subjects, verb complements, and dependent clauses can be formed from that part of a phrasal verb
which occurs after the BE of the progressive BE V +ING auxiliary.

WAITING
BEING WATCHED } IS A STRAIN
BEING CAREFUL

WAITING,
BEING WATCHED, } THEY LEFT THE HOUSE
BEING CAREFUL,

THE DOG SAW THEM $\begin{cases} \text{WAITING} \\ \text{BEING WATCHED} \\ \text{BEING CAREFUL} \end{cases}$

In other words, they are formed by adding +ING to a simple verb, to the auxiliary of a passive, or to the copula of a predicate adjective or predicate nominative (IS CAREFUL, IS THE ROYAL FAMILY). Dependent clauses can also be formed by adding +ING to a more complex phrasal verb provided that there is no tense, agreement, or modal auxiliary (the same restrictions as on infinitives).

$\left.\begin{array}{l} \text{HAVING WATCHED ALL DAY,} \\ \text{HAVING BEEN WATCHED ALL DAY,} \\ \text{AFTER HAVING WATCHED ALL DAY,} \end{array}\right\}$ THEY LEFT THE HOUSE

Probably even:

> HAVING BEEN WATCHING ALL DAY, THEY WERE TIRED

but not:

> ★HAVING WATCHED IS A STRAIN (acceptable to some speakers)
>
> ★THE DOG SAW THEM HAVING WATCHED
>
> ★HAVING WATCHING THEY LEFT THE HOUSE
>
> ★THE DOG SAW THEM BE WAITING

Each of these participial +ING phrases can, in other constructions, take all the verb complements of a main verb, including other participial phrases:

> SUSAN WAS INTERESTED IN WATCHING THEM BEING CAREFUL

Sentence forms

It is easy to overlook the great variety of ways there are for saying approximately the same thing. Here are some sentences that express similar relations:

> THE TRUCKS ARE CRACKING THE HOUSE
>
> WHAT THE TRUCKS ARE CRACKING IS THE HOUSE
>
> IT IS THE TRUCKS THAT ARE CRACKING THE HOUSE
>
> IT IS THE HOUSE THAT THE TRUCKS ARE CRACKING
>
> THE HOUSE IS BEING CRACKED BY THE TRUCKS
>
> IT IS THE HOUSE THAT IS BEING CRACKED BY THE TRUCKS
>
> IT IS THE TRUCKS THAT THE HOUSE IS BEING CRACKED BY

And here are some ways of questioning those relations:

> ARE THE TRUCKS CRACKING THE HOUSE?
> IS WHAT THE TRUCKS ARE CRACKING THE HOUSE?
> IS IT THE HOUSE THAT THE TRUCKS ARE CRACKING?

Plus the tag questions:

> THE TRUCKS ARE CRACKING THE HOUSE, AREN'T THEY?
> WHAT THE TRUCKS ARE CRACKING IS THE HOUSE, ISN'T IT?

And here are some ways of denying those relations:

> THE TRUCKS ARE NOT CRACKING THE HOUSE
> WHAT THE TRUCKS ARE CRACKING IS NOT THE HOUSE
> WHAT THE TRUCKS ARE NOT CRACKING IS THE HOUSE
> IT IS NOT THE TRUCKS THAT ARE CRACKING THE HOUSE
> IT IS THE TRUCKS THAT ARE NOT CRACKING THE HOUSE

If we combine questioning and denial, then there are about seventy sentences that involve the same relations among THE TRUCKS, CRACKING, and THE HOUSE. Even though the individual sentences are in different modes and emphasize different concepts, they still share the same core set of relations among concepts. Phrase structure grammar would require different rules for each of these seventy sentence types.

Phrase structure grammar criticized by transformational theory: the arguments

Transformational theorists criticize phrase structure grammars because:

1. They are uneconomical. Too many rules are needed to account for a variety of related structures that could be generated by many fewer rules of a different sort.
2. They cannot portray the systematic relations across different grammatical forms.
3. They cannot portray the correct constituent relations among discontinuous constituents, since their only way of showing that terms belong to the same constituent is to show them as products of the same rewrite rule.

The variation in phrasal verbs and their parts makes an impressive case for treating the parts of phrasal verbs as separate elements that are added, deleted, and arranged for each of the different constructions. The regularity of the restrictions on which parts of verbs can occur in infinitive and participial phrases, and the ordering of auxiliary verb parts in phrasal verbs, questions, and negation are not explainable in terms of pragmatic or lexical information processing. These regularities are syntactic and ought to be accounted for by a syntactic theory. Phrase structure grammar can only accommodate these regularities as the products of several independent and unrelated rules. The alternative is to treat the parts of rules as components that may be added, deleted, and rearranged for each of the different constructions. However, the operations of addition, deletion, and rearrangement are beyond the capabilities of phrase structure grammar.

Phrase structuralists would rejoin that the regularities across the different forms could be the result of parallel relations across sets of separate rules. There are not so many extra that they would make the cognitive burden too large. After all, we really have no idea *how* much information is too much for a human to process. Of course, *some* people, they would admit, may have developed an automatic procedure for constructing a question, for example, by moving the main auxiliary to the front of the corresponding declarative string, but we should not change drastically the kind of rules used in syntax in order to accommodate strategies that are supplemental and perhaps uncommon. Very articulate people may have generalizations and shortcuts for forming complex strings, and even paragraphs. Some novelists seem even to have a formula for writing entire books. But a theory of syntax is supposed to explain what is necessary for coordinating relations of lexemes with relations of concepts, not what is possible. That is how the phrase structure grammarian would reply.

Ignoring the regularities that occur across so many different kinds of constructions also makes it difficult for the phrase structure grammarian to account for the evolution of language. If the individual rules for each separate construction were truly independent from each other, it is surprising, at least, that they all developed the same way. The phrase structure grammarian might counter that this is an example of convergent evolution – analogous structures arising independently in response to a general "linguistic selection pressure." But this is just moving the generality one step outside the set of rules.

Phrase structure adherents would challenge the portrayal of regularities of syntax that require other than local rules. Supposing there are global rules that use information about other parts of the tree structure (for example, determining which terms are part of the noun phrase, which is the first auxiliary) is supposing too much about language processing. What is the mechanism that looks at the tree structure as a whole, that for example recognizes a noun phrase, determines the first auxiliary (rather than an adverb) of the verb phrase? Is there a little linguist inside the head of each language user in order to do all these things? Phrase structuralists would thus challenge claims for the existence of a further set of special rules that delete, substitute, and move elements around: Prove that such rules are necessary to describe the way people actually do language.

This raises an important point. Syntactic rules are theoretical entities whose purpose is to describe some syntactic regularities of language. It is only this ability that allows them any status at all. Phrase structure rules have no special status in linguistic theory. If there are syntactic properties that phrase structure rules do not characterize, there should be no hesitation in adopting rules that do capture the regularities. The question then is not whether there should be rules that show such regularities to be related, but what sort of rules these should be, and how plausible is their explanation of the regularities.

Not only do phrase structure rules show some regularities uneconomically and fail to show others at all, but the relations shown may be incorrect. For example, the scope relations given for one mode of a sentence are not consistent with the scope relations for another mode. Consider the two mode variants THE HOUSE IS CREAKING and IS THE HOUSE CREAKING? It appears that the IS of the first string is the same IS found in the second string, only its position is different in the two modes. The IS belongs to the verb phrase regardless of the mode of the sentence. However, because phrase structure rules do not have any provision for portraying discontinuous constituents, they portray the IS as part of the verb phrase only in the first string, but not in the second. Figure 4.5 illustrates the different hierarchical relations assigned to IS in the two strings.

The criticisms of phrase structure grammars can be at least partially avoided by beefing up the rules with new devices. The devices that have been suggested sacrifice the elegance of in-

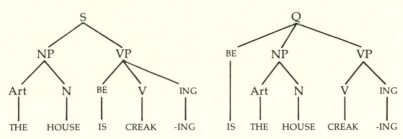

Figure 4.5. Difference in scope of IS for two mode variants.

dependent, locally effective rules (see Chapters 1 and 5). One device is *context sensitivity*. It enables a given rule to produce one set of terms in the context of (i.e., in the same string as) another particular type of rule or term and to produce still a different set of terms in a different context. For example, without context-sensitive rules there would have to be a separate phrase structure rule for every combination of gender, number, and negation in a tag question to coordinate the pronoun of the tag with the main noun and add negation in the tag if it is not in the main verb. The context-sensitive rule would contain the following kind of information: Where the noun is masculine singular, insert HE in the tag; where the main phrase does not contain a negative, insert a negative in the tag; and so on. For example, THE STALLION RAN, DIDN'T HE? Phrase structure rules could also be supplemented with a device to show the relatedness among the parts of discontinuous constituents. This would mean providing syntactic rules to perform operations such as those shown in Figure 4.2 for the string THAT COMPANY RIPS PEOPLE OFF.

In the linguistic debate between transformational theory and phrase structure grammar the latter is generally seen as the loser. The inadequacies of phrase structure grammar are more serious than the difficulties of introducing the global rules of transformational grammar. In Chapter 5 we present a theory that has the simplicity of local rules and at the same time offers the parsimony and representational advantages of transformational systems.

In the following section we examine transformational theory and how it overcomes the objections it leveled at phrase structure grammars. This will not be a comprehensive presentation of the theory and all its recent variants. For more complete explanations, we refer readers to the sources cited in the following section. For our purposes we hope merely to be able to show the kinds of explanations and rules given by transformational grammars. Again, this section may be skimmed or skipped by those who are either familiar with or uninterested in transformational theory.

Transformational grammar

The central idea in transformational theory is that strings are generated, not by a single stage of operations, but by several stages, each characterized by a different kind of operation. First an underlying syntactic structure is generated. Called a *base,* this consists of a phrase marker, which is similar to the syntactic diagram used by phrase structure grammar, with the morphemes and some of the syntactic elements further specified by sets of *features.* Then the terminal elements of the phrase marker are mutated by a set of transformation rules. These rules perform operations like reordering, deleting, and adding morphemes. The transformation rules themselves are under the control of still other rules. The result is the sequence of morphemes in a well-formed language string. In the following subsections, we will sketch the main properties of each of these components of transformational theory and then discuss briefly some variations on the theory.

Features

Features classify morphemes and syntactic elements of the base structure. A morpheme or syntactic element can be classified positively for a feature F [+F], negatively [−F], or not at all.

Specifying features is a way of making grammatical distinctions without providing additional rewrite rules. For example, the following nouns will have, in addition to [+N], the features:

HOUSE	[+common, −animate, +count, . . .]
MINISTER	[+human, +common, +count, . . .]
ETHEL	[−common, +human, −masculine, . . .]
ICE	[−count, +concrete, . . .]
PSYCHOLOGY	[+abstract, . . .]

Although the names of the features sometimes look like semantic categories, the criteria for assignment of features are claimed to be syntactic, for example, [−masculine] does not directly represent the sex of the referent of a noun, but the linguistic gender for purposes of agreement, as in FRANCE, SHE. . . .[3]

Features can give the syntactic categories of morphemes [+N]: finer syntactic distinctions [+count]; the names of transformation rules that can (or cannot) be applied to them [+passive] (in one version). In addition, features can classify a morpheme in terms of the syntactic types that can occur as its complementary constituents. Thus a morpheme that can occur to the right of a constituent with the feature [+F] would have the feature [+ [+F]———].[4] For example, in addition to [+V], the verb CRACK would have the positively marked features:

[+ ——— NP (PrepP)]

THE BURGLARS CRACK THE DOOR WITH THE CROWBAR

[+ ——— #]

THE DOOR CRACKED (# indicates a stop)

[+ ——— (PrepP)]

IT CRACKED IN THE RAIN; THE MINISTER CRACKED UP
   THE CAR

[+ ——— LIKE predicate nominative]

IT CRACKED LIKE AN EGG

[+ ——— manner adverbial]

IT CRACKED SLOWLY

The differences between contexts where CRACK can appear and those where the verb CREAK can appear are reflected by the differences in their features. In order to prevent THE BURGLARS CREAK THE DOOR from being generated, CREAK would not have the first of the above features. The negatively marked features for CRACK would include:

[− [+abstract] ——— [+abstract]]

This rules out: PSYCHOLOGY CRACKS VIRTUE

[− [+animate] ———]

This rules out: ETHEL CRACKS

[− [+NP] ——— [+abstract]]
This rules out any NP in contexts such as———
CRACKS VIRTUE

Base structure

The base structure is the first stage of generative syntactic processing. It consists of hierarchical phrase markers with morphemes and features. In the base phrase markers, complementary constituents are always adjacent: They are connected to (dominated by) the same node. Thus units that are in each other's scope are portrayed as connected together, avoiding the problem of discontinuous constituents. There is one basic form and order of morphemes for the base phrase markers. Complex sentences are represented in terms of phrase markers for individual simple sentences, conjoined or embedded. Thus only a relatively small set of phrase structure rules are needed to construct the base.

As we discussed in Chapter 2, it is commonly (but not universally) held by transformational theorists that the base structure is the part of syntax that is closest to the idea expressed by the language string. From the information in the base, projection rules would determine the idea expressed by the string. In language production, the base is operated on by transformation rules to produce the surface structure phrase marker. As the next section details, transformation rules may take the immediate constituents of the base and combine them with other elements, delete, substitute or move elements and combine phrase markers, and coordinate a change in one part of a string with a change in another part. Thus it is possible for complementary constituents, which are adjacent in the base, to be discontinuous in the surface phrase marker. The transformation rules are not supposed to affect the meaning, but merely operate on the form of the base.

Believing the base to be the syntactic stage closest to semantic interpretation and believing that there is a one-to-one correspondence between base structure and meaning, transformational theorists attributed the following properties to the base: (1) there should be similar base structures for language strings that express similar relations of concepts; (2) there should be more than one base structure for structurally ambiguous language strings; (3) because they have meaning, all lexemes should be added in the base; (4) features and categories that are supposed to characterize syntactic properties may describe semantic properties as well (for example, [+animate], [+concrete], time adverbial, place adverbial).[5]

There are recent arguments that many of the semantic properties once attributed to the base are more appropriately handled by operations upon the surface structure (e.g., Jackendoff, 1972). These newer arguments diminish the significance of the base structure and reduce the appeal of the transformational model.[6] But even if the base is no longer seen as exerting full control over the semantic interpretation, it is still held that "initial phrase markers generated by the base have significant and revealing syntactic properties" (Chomsky, 1975:82). Brame (1976), Bresnan (1978), and others have argued against the existence of several central transformation rules. They propose that many regularities across different grammatical forms, once thought to be produced by identical or similar base structures, have base structures closer to their surface structures. However, they still explain the regularities across different grammatical forms in terms of rules that change or restrict order, rather than as structural similarities. And these new rules are still global with respect to the elements (noun phrase, verb, etc.) they operate on.

Transformation rules

Transformation rules convert base phrase markers into intermediate phrase markers and finally into surface phrase markers. Each transformation rule can be described in terms of the kind of structure it operates on (*structural index*), the kind of change it makes (*structural change*), and special conditions on its application. Table 4.2 lists the operations transformation rules can perform.

Illustrating transformation rules with phrasal verbs

To see how transformation rules work, let us look again at phrasal verbs. Since the formulation of both base and transfor-

Table 4.2. *The five basic operations transformation rules can perform*

Operation	Structural index	Structural change
Deletion	S / A B̲ C	S / A C
Substitution	S / A B C̲	S / A B D̲
Sister adjoin	S / A B C	S / A B C Q̲
Chomsky adjoin	S / A B C	S / A B C / C Q̲
Feature change	[+F̲₁] A B C	[+F̲₂] A B C

mation rules is still subject to debate, the rules used here are only intended to illustrate the general principles of the theory.

As we saw in the discussion of phrase structure grammar, the several components of phrasal verbs can be arranged in several different orders, each corresponding to a particular grammatical form. But since transformational theory represents all variants in the base by a standard order plus mode and tense markers, the number of base rules needed is minimal.

$$S \rightarrow NP \quad PredP$$
$$PredP \rightarrow Mode\ VP$$
$$Mode \rightarrow (Neg)\ Aux$$
$$Aux \rightarrow Tense\ (M)\ (Perfect)\ (Progressive)$$
$$Tense \rightarrow [\pm past]$$
$$Perfect \rightarrow \text{HAVE} + \{\text{EN, ED}\}$$
$$Progressive \rightarrow \text{BE} + \text{ING}$$
$$VP \rightarrow V\ (NP)\ (NP)\ (Manner\ Adv),\ldots$$

These rules have the proper consitituent relations and they do not need to duplicate parts of rules over and over as did phrase structure grammar.

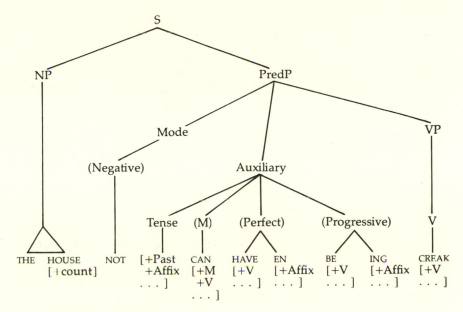

Figure 4.6. Base structure for the string THE HOUSE COULD NOT HAVE
BEEN CREAKING.

To the base structure, morphemes with their appropriate features are added. The feature [+V] is assigned to HAVE, BE, modal
auxiliaries (M), and the verb; the feature [+affix] is assigned to
+ING, + {EN, ED}, and tense elements. To illustrate, the base
structure for the string THE HOUSE COULD NOT HAVE BEEN CREAK-
ING is shown in Figure 4.6. Now, transformation rules are applied to get the terms in the proper order. First, we can apply a
rule called *affix shift*. Here is its formal description followed by
the application of the rule to our example in Figure 4.6.

        Structural index: x [+affix][+V]   Y
        Structural change: x   [+V][+affix] Y
        Condition: obligatory

When we apply this transformation rule to the elements in the
base structure in Figure 4.6,

     NOT   +past   CAN   HAVE   EN   BE   ING   CREAK

the result of moving the affixes as shown by the arrows is

     NOT   CAN   +past   HAVE   BE   EN   CREAK   ING
which becomes:

NOT   COULD[7]   HAVE   BEEN   CREAKING

Now we need to move the NOT to a position after the first auxiliary. This can be done with a transformation rule called *negative place.* This rule too is formally described in terms of a structural index, structural change, and conditions of application, but for simplicity we just illustrate its operation on the form that resulted from the application of the previous transformation:

COULD   NOT   HAVE   BEEN   CREAKING

which is the correct form for the surface string.

With these two transformation rules, in addition to the base rules, simple declarative sentences with any combination of modal auxiliary, negation, progressive, and perfect tenses can be generated from the same basic structure. Compared to the phrase structure grammar presented earlier, this represents an enormous economy of rules. Moreover the similarity across variations in form is reflected in the similarity of the rules used to produce the forms.

In addition there are transformation rules that move the auxiliary and the negative for yes-no questions; rules to insert DO when there is no auxiliary present for negation and question forms, as in THE HOUSE DOES NOT CREAK or DOES THE HOUSE CREAK? rules to convert embedded sentences into infinitive phrases, verb complements, dependent clauses, and subjects of sentences, and that replace the tense, modal auxiliary, and subject agreement of the Aux node with TO or +ING, as in THEY WANT (THE HOUSE CREAKS) → THEY WANT THE HOUSE TO CREAK; or (THE HOUSE'S CREAKING) BOTHERED THEM, THE HOUSE STARTED (CREAKING IN THE WIND), THEY HEARD (THE HOUSE CREAKING).

The passive

As discussed in the preceding section, the passive is a phrasal verb form that can be combined with other forms:

Passive: IS RESCUED
Passive progressive: IS BEING RESCUED
Passive perfect progressive: HAS BEEN BEING RESCUED
Passive perfect: HAS BEEN RESCUED

But there are other regularities in the passive besides its surface form and the way it can be combined with other phrasal verb forms. First, there is the obvious relation between the active and passive forms of sentences:

THE DOG RESCUED THE TOY

THE TOY WAS RESCUED BY THE DOG

in which the active form, NP1 . . . V + past . . . NP2, expresses the same relations as the passive form, NP2 . . . BE + past V + {EN, ED} . . . BY NP1. These relations of sentence types are paralleled by relations of certain noun phrases:

THE DOG'S RESCUE OF THE TOY

THE RESCUE OF THE TOY BY THE DOG

If these pairs of strings express the same relations, transformational theory holds that the deep structure for the two forms should be similar.

In one version of transformational theory (Chomsky, 1957), active and passive sentences and noun phrases that express similar relations were all assigned the same base structure. The phrase marker of the base was that of a sentence in the active form. Transformation rules were applied to change this form into the passive or to convert the sentence into a noun phrase. Ambiguous noun phrases, such as THE RESCUE OF THE DOG, have two possible base structures and transformational histories: (Unspecified subject) RESCUE THE DOG versus THE DOG RESCUE (unspecified object). The relationship across the meanings of the different strings was explained as their sharing of the same base structure. In this version of the theory, transformation rules contributed to meaning by, for example, converting the base into a question. The base structure was not given a special role in relation to the semantic component; it contained only phrase structure rules, no features.

In a later version (Chomsky, 1965), the base included morphemes with features. Transformation rules were restricted so that they could not change meaning. The base structures of active and passive forms differed because the BY of the passive appeared in the base along with a "marker" that indicated the passive transformation rule should be applied. The base phrase structure for the passive string THE TOY WAS RESCUED BY THE DOG is shown in Figure 4.7.

The presence of the passive marker requires that the passive transformation be applied. The phrase marker for the active form

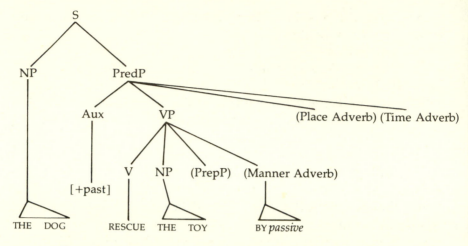

Figure 4.7. Base for a passive sentence according to Chomsky (1965).

does not have this element. This version no longer portrays the similarity of the active and passive forms in terms of identical base structures, although the structural relationship between the noun phrases is essentially the same. The whole phrase marker would be dominated by an NP in order for THE RESCUE OF THE TOY BY THE DOG to be produced through the application of transformation rules.

Versions of transformational grammar since 1965

The relationship and functions of transformation rules, base structure, and surface structure are still very much disputed. The questions of which regularities of language can be characterized by syntactic rules, how to handle exceptions to the regularities, and what sort of rules there should be, are much debated within transformational theory. One trend has been toward a richer base representation and an increase in the power of transformation rules. Another trend has been toward a leaner base component and a decrease in the use of transformation rules.

Richer representations

By 1965 transformational theory had already encoded semantic distinctions in the syntactic rules. For example, the BY of a passive was assigned a different place in the base than the BY of a time adverbial (HER DEATH WAS MOURNED BY PASTEUR versus THE PASTURE WAS FLOODED BY MORNING). About this time, linguists tried to account for other sorts of relations that could be expressed by different syntactic forms. The branch of transformational theory known as *generative semantics* wanted to explain the similarities in the relations expressed by, for example (Lakoff, 1968):

> I USED THE KNIFE TO CUT THE SANDWICH
>
> THE KNIFE CUT THE SANDWICH
>
> I CUT THE SANDWICH WITH THE KNIFE

In each string, KNIFE, SANDWICH, and CUT are related to each other in the same way, although their syntactic roles according to the standard version of transformational theory are very different from one string to another. Generative semantics proposed using more semantic information in underlying structure to explain the similarity of the three strings. For these examples, the underlying structures would be based on a phrase marker of I CAUSED THE SANDWICH TO BE CUT WITH THE KNIFE.

Adding still further to the semantic richness was a synthesis of case theory with transformational theory. Stockwell, Schachter, and Partee (1969) proposed that the phrase markers of underlying structure contain nodes bearing the names of the appropriate case categories (see Chapter 2). Thus, for each of the above examples, KNIFE would be governed by an *instrument* node and SANDWICH by a *neutral* node (equivalent to the *object* case in the LNR system discussed in Chapter 2).

In this case/transformational theory, the underlying representation is ordered. However, the order is different from standard transformational theory, and no subject or object appears in the underlying structures. The base structures for passive and active forms are the same (and are similar to related noun phrases) but neither passive nor active is the source of the other. The use of cases allows a greater variety of language strings expressing similar relations of concepts to be assigned similar underlying structures. Cases also allow finer distinctions among relations of concepts to be made than was possible in Chomsky's 1965 version of transformational theory. For example, THE BIRD OPENS THE DOOR and THE KEY OPENS THE DOOR can be assigned structurally dif-

ferent underlying phrase markers because BIRD is governed by an
agent node and KEY by an *instrument* node.

Chomsky (1970:9) allowed that case distinctions could play a
role in semantic interpretation but argued that pairs of sentences
like the example above should be given structurally identical
syntactic bases. However, he claimed the difference between
transitive and intransitive forms of the same verb, for example,
THE BIRD BROKE THE WINDOW versus THE WINDOW BROKE, should
be distinguished in underlying structure. Chomsky (1970:32)
suggested that "an intransitive with the feature [+cause] becomes transitive and that its selectional features are systematically revised so that the former subject becomes the object."

Leaner representations

In 1970 Chomsky proposed that sentences and related noun
phrases have different underlying representations. For example,
the relations among DOG, RESCUE, and TOY are the same in both of
the following:

THE DOG'S RESCUE OF THE TOY

THE DOG RESCUES THE TOY

Earlier it had been assumed that they both had the base structure
of a SAD sentence to which different transformation rules had
been applied. However, irregularities in the way noun phrases
could be produced by transforming SAD sentence bases would
require numerous and specialized transformation rules. Consider the variety in the way nouns are formed from corresponding verbs:

Verb	Noun
RESCUE	RESCUE
DESTROY	DESTRUCTION
EMPLOY	EMPLOYMENT
DENY	DENIAL

In addition, there are other unsystematic syntactic differences,
such as whether the noun form will be a count or mass noun.
Chomsky concluded that such noun phrases should not be analyzed as products of transformation rules operating on SAD sentence base structures. Therefore, the similarity between a SAD
sentence and the corresponding noun phrase was no longer at-

tributed to their sharing the same or even similar base structures. Thus, in THE DOG'S RESCUE OF THE TOY, DOG was no longer considered the underlying subject of RESCUE, nor TOY the underlying object. Instead, the similarity between the two forms was attributed to their sharing the same lexeme (RESCUE) and to similarity rather than identity in parts of their underlying structures.

Chomsky proposed new base structure rules that portrayed the similarity between noun phrases and corresponding sentences as similarity in the *topology* of the underlying structures. This replaced the previous representation of semantic similarity in terms of similarity in node labels or the sharing of large portions of the underlying phrase marker tree.

Chomsky's new modification devalues the role of node labels and transformations in the representation of similarity across different grammatical forms. The role of the topology of the phrase marker tree, that is, the scope relations, is greatly increased. Furthermore, the categories proposed in the new version's base structure emphasize, although informally, the dependency relations and minimize the number and importance of syntactic categories. There are nouns, verbs, sentences, complements, along with a convention of writing bars above the letter symbols such that N is the main constituent of an $\bar{N}$, which in turn is the main constituent of $\bar{\bar{N}}$, and similarly for Vs. New production rules for the base include:

$$\underline{S} \rightarrow \bar{\bar{N}}\ \bar{\bar{V}}$$
$$\bar{\bar{N}} \rightarrow \text{Specifier-of-}\bar{N}\ \bar{N} \qquad \bar{\bar{V}} \rightarrow \text{Specifier-of-}\bar{V}\ \bar{V}$$
$$\bar{N} \rightarrow \text{N Complement} \qquad \bar{V} \rightarrow \text{V Complement}$$

Specifiers-of-$\bar{N}$ include articles, possessives (e.g., THE DOG'S); specifiers-of-$\bar{V}$ include tense and auxiliaries. A noun complement could be a prepositional phrase (e.g., OF THE TOY); a verb complement could be a noun phrase, an $\bar{\bar{N}}$ (e.g., THE TOY).

Another move toward leanness has been the use of surface structure in semantic interpretation. For example, sometimes the active and passive forms do not express the same relations. Consider:

1a. EVERYONE LOVES SOMEONE
1b. SOMEONE IS LOVED BY EVERYONE
2a. THE DOG HASN'T SEEN MANY HORSES
2b. MANY HORSES HAVEN'T BEEN SEEN BY THE DOG

3a. DOGS USUALLY DIG HOLES
3b. HOLES ARE USUALLY DUG BY DOGS

The most likely interpretation of 1a is that everyone loves someone or other (perhaps only themselves). The most likely interpretation of 1b is that there is one person whom everyone loves. In
order to avoid taking examples of this sort as counterevidence to
the putative regularity between passive and active forms, these
examples have been treated as special cases. Their special status
is attributed to their use of quantifiers (SOME, MANY, ALL), either
explicitly or implicitly by the use of general terms in the subject
position (e.g., DOGS, HOLES) and negation, which are interpreted
from the surface structure (Jackendoff, 1972; Chomsky, 1975). In
1975 Chomsky proposed that all semantic interpretation could be
done from surface structure with the addition of "traces" indicating where elements had been moved by transformation rules.
This again decreases the importance of the base.

Recently Bresnan, Brame, and others have gone farther in this
direction. Bresnan (1978), when summarizing other research,
concludes (1) that the relation between pronouns and their referents should not be specified by rules of grammar at all, making
within sentence connections governed by the same semantic and
pragmatic considerations as cross sentence connections; (2) that
all "function-dependent" (that is, relating subject and object)
relations be taken care of by lexical rules rather than transformation rules. For example, the relation between active and passive
forms – once central in the arguments for the existence of transformation rules – is shown by lexical rules similar to Chomsky's
(1965) strict subcategorization rules (Bresnan's "syntactic contexts") and selectional restriction rules (Bresnan's "functional
structures") (see note 4). Bresnan gives the following list in illustration:

Syntactic contexts	Functional structures
V, [———]	NP1 SLEEP
V, [——— NP]	NP1 HIT NP2
V, [——— NP],	NP1 EAT NP2
[———]	($\exists y$) NP1 EAT y

This list explains the relation of SLEEP, HIT, and EAT to direct objects: EAT can take an object, SLEEP cannot, and HIT must (for most
speakers). As Bresnan (1978:14) says: "As nontransformational

relations are factored out of the transformational component, the transformational complexity of sentences is reduced, deep structures more closely resemble surface structures, and the grammar becomes more easily realized within an adequate model of language use."

The foundation for Bresnan's proposal is the arguments presented by Brame (1976) that many central transformation rules are not well justified. Although Brame's proposed solution differs from Bresnan's, they both, as do other transformationalists, assume that the similarity among different grammatical forms must be specified by the rules themselves.

The different versions of transformational grammar not only have different transformation rules, they also have different base categories, different orderings for the components of the base, and different features for the morphemes and syntactic elements. As well as differences in accounting for the passive-active relation and other regularities of language not discussed here, there are differences in (1) how to represent similarities in syntactic relations (by the same base, by a base phrase marker with the same topology, by the same node labels); (2) which regularities in language have to be explained (subject/object relations, agent/instrument differences, and the like); (3) how the base structure is related to the semantic interpretation; (4) whether all lexemes are entered before transformation rules apply; (5) how many similarities and differences in relations of lexemes are to be explained in terms of similarities and differences in base structures.

What all the versions of transformational grammar have in common is: (1) an ordered base structure portrayed by rules of the phrase structure type; (2) transformation rules that convert the order of the base structure to the order of the surface structure; and for most versions (3) a lexicon whose entries are marked for features that restrict the contexts in which they can appear.

Control of transformation rules

In principle, a transformation rule can convert any arrangement of elements into any other arrangement. The power of transformation rules is both an advantage and a source of embarrassment

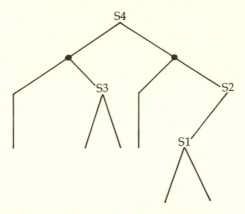

Figure 4.8. Partial base structure tree with embedded sentences.

for transformational theory. To preserve the advantages and avoid the embarrassments, linguists have specified a number of restrictions on the kinds of changes a transformational rule is permitted to make:

1. Only the five types of changes listed in Table 4.3 should be permitted. However, even these minimal types are disputed; some theorists are critical of the feature-change principle or of having both sister adjoin and Chomsky adjoin principles in the same system (e.g., Stockwell, Schachter, and Partee, 1969).
2. Transformation rules should introduce no meaning changes.
3. Transformation rules should not add structure (Chomsky adjoin is a small exception).
4. Transformation rules should be as simple and as few as possible. This applies both to the formulation of individual rules and to the set of rules as a whole. This restriction is taken very seriously and plays a key role in arguments for extrinsic constraints on transformation rules, and in recent arguments for lexical and surface interpretation rules to replace transformation rules.

The number and/or complexity of transformation rules can be reduced if the rules are extrinsically ordered, that is, if the sequence in which they are applied is controlled.[8] For example, greater simplicity is achieved if the transformation rules are restricted to apply first to the most deeply embedded sentence in an underlying phrase marker, then to the next most deeply embedded, and so on in repeated cycles through the tree. In terms of Figure 4.8, all the transformation rules apply in order first only to

S1, then they apply to either S2 or S3 (in this case it makes no difference), and finally they go through their ordered cycle again for S4. However, ordered cyclically applied transformation rules are not adequate to produce correct grammatical strings of all types. Various suggestions have been made to solve problems with the application of transformation rules.

One suggestion is that some transformation rules not be applied until the last cycle. These last-cycle-only rules are to be ordered along with other transformation rules but not used on the other cycles. Then there must be something that detects when the last cycle is occurring, thereby permitting these last-cycle-only rules to apply. It has also been suggested that there should be precyclic rules – rules that operate on the full base structure before any cyclic rules are applied (Lakoff, 1970). In addition, there seems to be a need for restrictions on the kinds of movements transformation rules can permit in order to prevent the generation of certain ungrammatical sentences (Ross, 1967).

Another suggestion is for a new type of transformation rule. Transformation rules are global with respect to the parts of a phrase marker they involve (see Chomsky, 1965:99, 215) but local with respect to the sequence of transformation rules in the derivation from base to surface structure.[9] Each transformation rule operates only on a single phrase marker, either an initial phrase marker of the base structure or the product of another transformation rule. A transformation rule does not use global information about which transformation rules have already been applied, or about previous phrase markers earlier in the cycle. Lakoff (1970) suggested that some transformation rules would have to use information from more than one stage in the transformational derivation. For example, to account for the verb agreement in:

THERE WERE BELIEVED TO BE TWO UNICORNS IN THE GARDEN
THERE WAS BELIEVED TO BE A UNICORN IN THE GARDEN
[Bach, 1974:234]

there would have to be a rule that says in effect: "The verb that at *this* point of the derivation has THERE as its subject must agree with the NP that *was* the subject of the relevant embedded sentence at an earlier point of the derivation" (Bach, 1974:235).

Chomsky (1973) suggested that a principle of "subjacency" be

imposed on transformation rules: A rule can only move something in an embedded sentence to the next level of embedding.
For example, in Figure 4.8 no transformation rule in the first cycle
could move anything from S1 to any part of the structure that was
not in S2. On the next cycle, something could be moved from S2
to S4.

Emonds (1976:1) has argued that restrictions on transformation
rules "are not ad hoc specifications on the individual rules but,
rather, reflections of some deeper grammatical principles." He
proposes limiting transformation rules to three exclusive types:
(1) those that apply to the whole sentence structure and change
that structure (for example, to make questions); (2) those that
apply to adjacent elements under certain conditions (such as interchanging object NP and verb particle); and (3) those that apply
to embedded sentences or other syntactic elements resulting in a
type of structure that is determined by the base rules (such as
moving the subject NP to the object of a preposition for the passive). One also needs restrictions on permissible base structures,
since they are not determined by surface structure but only by
the transformation rules one wants to use.

Theoretical evaluation

Transformation rules were developed in order to account for the
regularities of language strings and to explain how different
strings could express the same relations and how ambiguous
strings could express more than one relation of concepts by the
same surface structure. Transformation rules reorganize language elements in order to show how paraphrases are derived
from a common structure and how two different structures could
both give rise to the same ambiguous string.

Since transformation rules are in principle of unlimited power
– that is, they could make any string out of any underlying structure – restrictions have been suggested to avoid the embarrassments of too much theoretical power. With these restrictions,
transformational theorists are developing a set of rules that can
describe the regularities of a growing subset of English syntax.

Chomsky (1964, 1975) assumes that the nature of the restrictions on transformation rules is related to the innate organization

of the human mind. However, it is also possible to take the restrictions as evidence that the system of transformation rules used to convert underlying structures to language strings is inadequately formulated or wrongly conceived.

The positing of rules and metarules in order to explain the regularities of language is fine – laws, mechanisms, and boundary conditions are common entities in science. But for a theoretical entity to be valuable in an explanation it should have certain properties. For example, it should not be too powerful; that is, it should not equally well explain regularities that do *not* occur as well as those that do. It should not require ad hoc mechanisms to work properly or to restrict the overgenerality of a too-powerful principle. On these criteria, transformation rules with their systems of restrictions appear to have shortcomings. Theoretical entities should also be justified in as many different ways as possible. This criterion is taken very seriously by language theorists. For example, Stockwell, Schachter, and Partee (1969) were concerned to justify the introduction of case nodes not only to explain the case relations posed by Fillmore but also to show the relationship between the SAD sentence and related noun phrase forms. However, this criterion by itself may not be so very discriminating; language is such a complex phenomenon that it is not unlikely a rule can be invented that will affect more than one aspect of the language. What would be most helpful would be independent evidence for the existence of transformation rules in the behavior of language users. Unfortunately for the theory, such evidence has been sought vigorously, and only very weak support for the existence of psychological operations analogous to transformation rules has developed (Fodor, Bever, and Garrett, 1974, Chapter 5).

What has maintained the preeminence of transformational theory has been the lack of a competitive theory. There have been no alternative theories with the ability to describe as many of the syntactic regularities as can transformational theory. In the next chapter, we introduce an alternative theory with the descriptive power of transformational theory and without the complex mechanics of transformation rules and metarules to control the transformation rules.

Transformational grammar and its goal of explaining the regularities of language in a way that was cognitively plausible gave us a generation of exciting research. It is the result of this research that has led to recent calls for changes in the theory – away from the use of transformation rules, away from attempts to provide rules for every aspect of language, and away from the hypothesis of a deep structure that is different from surface structure. We welcome these trends and see them as moving the theory from within in a direction that will eventually converge with the model we are proposing.

5

The syntax crystal model

In the preceding chapter, we described the role of syntax in language processing and the criteria to be met by an adequate theory of syntax. Then we introduced phrase structure grammar and discussed its inadequacies from the point of view of transformational theory. The syntactic mechanisms of transformational theory were then described.

Transformational theory incorporates a large number of different global operations, from the transformation rules themselves to the metarules that in turn control their application. As we discussed in Chapter 1, global operations are less satisfactory in a model than local rules. Global operations are usually expressed in general terms; to actually use them, a further set of procedures must be specified.

In a cognitive model, a global operation is an incomplete explanation. It does not explain *how* the disparate parts controlled by the global operation are recognized and operated on; it only states that they are. A model of a cognitive process that invokes complex global operations presupposes additional cognitive processes for the model to work. Such a model, in effect, requires a homunculus, a little person inside, who performs the additional operations that are needed to explain the cognitive processes. The model still has to explain how the homunculus operates. Explanation by homunculus is open to the kind of criticism that Miller, Galanter, and Pribram (1960) directed at Tolman's (1948) explanation of navigation behavior that posited a "map control room in the brain" and left unexplained the details of how the maps were drawn and used. To adopt their phrasing, the problem with complex global operations in a model of language is that

167

they "leap over the gap from knowledge to [utterance] by inferring cognitive organization from [language] behavior, but that still leaves outstanding the question of the language user's ability to leap it" (Miller, Galanter, and Pribram, 1960:9). Many transformational theorists recognize the disadvantages of relying on global operations in the theory. This is indicated by their reluctance to accept global metatransformation rules, and/or the reluctance to add case category distinctions to deep structure.

In this chapter we introduce a new model of syntax whose aim is to minimize the use of global operations and emphasize the use of local rules. As a cognitive model, it is more explicit about what may be the operations bridging the gap between knowledge and language behaviors such as parsing, generating, and the acquisition of syntax.

In the linguistics literature, a theory of syntax claims to be superior when it can explain more grammatical constructions and regularities than competing theories. Unlike other theories, our main claim is not that our model explains grammatical constructions and regularities that other theories do not. In fact we rely heavily on the research of the past twenty years in discovering regularities of syntax. Our model is not unique in what it explains so much as how it is explained. Behind the explanatory metaphor we employ is the motivation to present the model in mechanically clear terms and show how it can reduce the regularities of syntax to properties on a smaller level.

To achieve these goals we introduce a new theoretical construct, the syntactic *module,* which reduces ordinary syntactic rules to independent, component parts. Roughly, each module corresponds to an element of a rewrite rule. So, for example, corresponding to the rule "noun phrase→determiner + noun" will be a module for determiner and a module for noun. Each module represents a local operation based on a small amount of scope and dependency information. Modules connect together to form the syntactic structures. The connections are governed by the local rules of the modules plus a few simple global operations.

Reducing syntactic rules to modules allows for a more complete explanation of syntax. Not only does our model describe *what* procedures are necessary but specifies *how* the procedures might operate – in effect, offering an explanation for the homunculi remaining in other models. Reducing syntactic rules to modules follows a standard procedure in science: Theoretical constructs are introduced to explain a phenomenon whose only description is at a global level. The gene was introduced to explain the partially independent assortment of hereditary traits; the neutrino to explain the conservation of energy, momentum, and spin during beta decay of an atomic nucleus; the TOTE unit to explain adaptive behavior. This does not mean that we expect there to be a physiological entity corresponding to a module, but we do suggest that the module might correspond to a *functional* unit in the cognitive organization of the language user.

In addition to introducing a smaller unit of analysis, our model makes structural distinctions unlike those of other theories. Every model of syntax must have enough resolving power to distinguish between language strings that are structurally distinct. Most theories do this by relying on distinctions made using information in node labels. Instead, our model introduces dependency as a feature. This enables it to make many more structural distinctions topologically, that is, by the shape rather than the labels of the structure. Therefore, specific information from the particular rules (modules) that comprise a structure is not usually needed to convert a syntactic structure to a semantic representation. A further difference, related to the absence of an important role for node labels, is that our model does not require the assumption that all language productions are based on covert complete sentences.

In what follows, we will first explain the rules of our syntactic mechanism and their relationship to the orrery model of underlying conceptual structure. Then we will show how the model can be used to parse and generate language strings, to show similarities across paraphrases, and to resolve syntactic ambiguities. Then we will describe the formal properties of the syntactic mechanism, their mathematical antecedents, and distinguish their essential features from those of heuristic convenience. Alternative methods of displaying the rules, including computer implementation, are described here and in Appendix A. We also suggest how the model can be applied to languages like Latin, which use inflection encoding instead of sequence encoding.

We next apply the rules of our model to the syntactic construc-

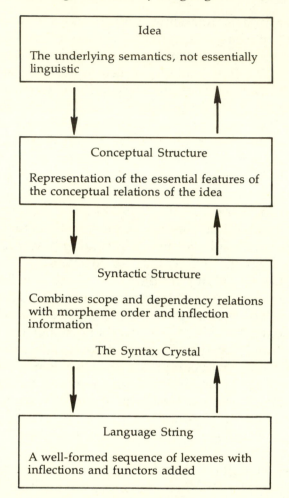

Figure 5.1. Overview of language generating and understanding.

tions used to illustrate the power of transformational theory in the preceding chapter. We demonstrate how each of these historically important tests of a syntactic theory is passed by our model. In Appendix B, additional constructions are presented.

To get our bearings, let us look again at the diagram of the four parts of language processing, repeated here as Figure 5.1. In Chapter 2 we looked into the contents of the second box, the conceptual structure underlying sentences and other language strings. We examined various models of conceptual structure and discussed their adequacy as a means of conveying the contents of the first box – the idea to be expressed in a language string. In Chapter 1 we looked into the fourth box, arguing for the existence of hierarchical structures governing language strings. Now we want to look into the third box, which mediates between the language string and the conceptual structure. This is syntax, the encoding of relations of concepts by sequences of lexemes with functors and inflections added.

In Chapter 2 we argued that the orrery model, whose only features are scope and dependency, is a plausible representation of the information in the second box. In Chapter 3 it was demonstrated that, with pragmatic and lexical information, the orrery model provides sufficient information about conceptual structure to reliably encode an idea. We now need a mechanism to convert orrery relations into a language string to express the idea represented by the orrery.

The syntax crystal is our model for such a mechanism. It correlates information about the scope and dependency relations of concepts given by the orrery model with information about lexeme sequence and the occurrence of functors and inflections found in language strings. It combines the two types of information so that either type of information may be used to gain access to the other.

Syntactic rules: the modules of the syntax crystal

The syntactic mechanism is called the syntax crystal by analogy to molecular crystallization. Each syntactic rule is portrayed in the form of a rectangular module with a *connection code* on at least one of its edges. Two modules may be connected if their apposing edges bear matching codes. Assembling a set of modules under the restrictions of the connection codes results in a "crystal" structure that places morphemes in the proper sequence and adds inflections and functors. The geometry of the connected modules enables them to portray conceptual relations in terms of the scope and dependency features of the orrery.

Modules may be classified into two general types. One type contains information that actually appears in a language string, the basic units of surface syntactic analysis: *morphemes*. There are two types of morphemes: lexical morphemes and grammatical morphemes. Lexical morphemes are what we have been calling lexemes; they express concepts. An example of a grammatical morpheme is the 'S that attaches to nouns to mark the possessive. Sometimes it is not clear whether a morpheme is grammatical or lexical, but the modules do not need to make this distinction.[1]

The second type of syntax crystal module contains only information that does not appear in the surface form of a language string. These are called *structure modules* because they combine to form the underlying structure of a language string. Each syntax crystal module represents a syntactic rule *type* with an unlimited number of *tokens* of each type available. In other words, even if we have used a module in one place in the structure of a particular string, we can use duplicates of it in other places as many times as we need to. For example, the morpheme THE may appear more than once in a given string.

The basic operations of syntax crystal modules

The function of any syntactic mechanism is to map the underlying structure, from which meaning is derived, onto the surface form of the language string and vice versa. For our model, the orrery structure's scope and dependency features must be mapped onto the proper sequence of morphemes. Consider a simple orrery connecting together the elements A, B, and C such that A and B form a unit which in turn is connected to element C. Of the unit A and B, let B be the main component with respect to the connection to element C. As Chapter 2 indicated, orrery relations by themselves tell nothing about the sequence in which the elements are expressed in a language string. For an orrery of three elements, six different permutations of the sequence are possible. Figure 5.2 illustrates in the left column how the same orrery may have these six different arrangements.

With ten different structure modules, these six different permutations of sequence can be constructed so that each exhibits the same scope and dependency relation. This is shown on the right side of Figure 5.2. The orrery relations appear on the completed crystals by tracing through the connection codes.

The structure of crystals 1 and 2 is straightforward. Each mod-

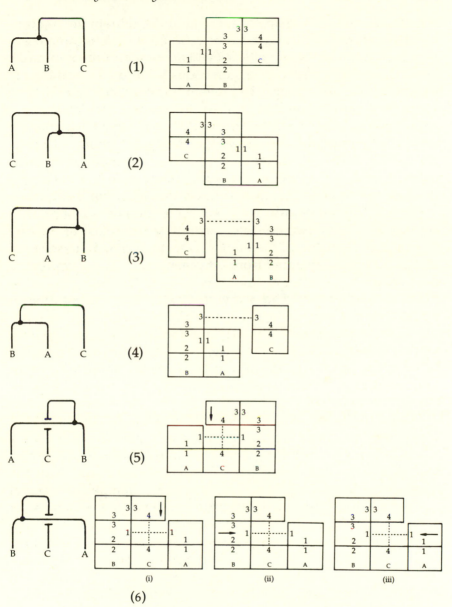

Figure 5.2. The six arrangements of one orrery (where C connects to A and B as a unit above B, the main concept).

ule directly adjoins the one or more modules with matching connection codes. No edge with a connection code is left unmatched. But direct adjoinment of modules will not work for the remaining crystals: Modules with connection codes 1–1 and 4–C would be in conflict for the same space. To prevent this conflict, crystals 3 and 4 employ a convention that requires the modules which are connected higher up on a column to yield position to any module which is connected lower down on the same column. That is, lower modules have *positional priority*. Thus the modules in the C column move out of the way for the modules in the A column because the latter are connected lower down on the B column.

Crystals 5 and 6 require an exception to the positional priority convention. These two crystals illustrate the problem of the discontinuous constituent: Element A is in the immediate scope of element B but is separated from B by element C. The exception to the positional priority convention is indicated by an arrow on the module requiring it. The arrow indicates that the module to which it points preempts positional priority over any other module.[2] Thus, in crystals 5 and 6(i), the modules in the A column were required to move to allow the C module positional priority. With this principle, the syntax crystal is able to handle discontinuous constituents, unlike phrase structure and categorial grammars.

The positional priority convention is a global procedure. However, both the way it is specified and the operations it demands are much simpler than the global rules of transformational grammar. A transformation rule must distinguish particular syntactic elements in particular syntactic contexts and then perform global movement, insertion, deletion, or feature-change operations. In contrast, the positional priority convention requires that *any* (nonarrowed) module yield position to *any* other module that interferes with the first module's bottom code connection. This can be translated into a simple recursive procedure: (1) attempt to complete bottom code connection; (2a) if no positional conflict, proceed; (2b) if positional conflict, move one space horizontally and go to step 1. Transformation rules and their metarules are much more difficult to translate into step-by-step procedures. As we argued earlier, models of cognitive processes should minimize the number and complexity of global procedures.

As described in Chapter 2, orreries contain only the names of

the concepts expressed by a string, possibly some mode indicators (e.g., "Past"), and the connections among them in terms of
scope and dependency. The left-to-right order of the elements is
not constrained. On the other hand, a syntax crystal for a language string must have its terminal modules in the proper
sequence. Syntax crystals also contain inflections and functors
that do not appear in a representation of underlying conceptual
structure. These grammatical morphemes are assigned scope and
dependency to indicate which of the lexical morphemes they
operate on. Therefore, an orrery derived from parsing will be
somewhat different from an orrery for generating a string.

The syntax crystal is not a finite-state Markov process

In 1957 Chomsky argued that it was impossible to generate all the
sentences of a natural language by a "finite state Markov process." Since then, his and similar arguments have been assumed
to invalidate all attempts to explain syntax on "associationist
principles" (Katz, 1964, for example). Chomsky's argument is
directed against associationist principles that apply to linear
word-word associations. We have also argued that such connections would be inadequate (see Chapter 1). But in order to show
that these arguments do not apply to the connections made by
the syntax crystal, we will summarize them and show that the
syntax crystal can meet the objections.

Chomsky gave three examples of artificial languages with just
two elements, A and B. In one language the A's are always followed by an equal number of B's. So, AB, AABB, and AAAABBBB are
typical strings in that language. In another language, the strings
are symmetric around the center, so AA, BAAB, and AABBAA are in
that language. And in the third, each series of A's and B's is duplicated so that AABAAB, BABA, and AABAAABA are strings. No finite
number of word-word associations would be able to generate the
strings of these miniature languages. To the extent that natural
languages have the generative power of these miniature languages, permitting repetition of elements and phrase types in expansions, they demonstrate that syntax must include more information than just which elements follow which other elements.

Using syntax crystal modules, we will show that it is possible

to produce strings of the symmetric language by simple associative connections between modules. But the association is not the
chainlike linear sort from element to element that is criticized in
the above argument. The associative connection is a kind of connection that can be used over again in the same string and connects elements in the string to each other indirectly through a hierarchical connection.

Just a few module types will produce the symmetric language.
We start with two uncoded lexeme modules in Figure 5.3(a). We
add codes and connect them via structure modules to produce AA
and BB in 5.3(b). To one of each pair of structure modules (we will
choose the left ones), we add optional top codes (3, 4) and add
these new modules in 5.3(d). Now with these ten modules and
the positional priority rule, any string in this language can be
generated, for example, AABBBBAA in 5.3(e). These modules provide dependency information making the left element of each
symmetric pair the main constituent. They also provide scope information, connecting each inside symmetric pair as a unit to the
next outer pair. An orrery for the above structure is shown in Figure 5.3(c). The first of the artificial languages is even easier to
generate using syntax crystal modules. The basic construction is
shown in Figure 5.3(f). The third language requires different
modules for each subseries so that AAB would be followed only
by AAB, for example. Since in natural language coordinate constructions are formed from a limited number of syntactic types,
there would be no need to have rules for every possible string,
just rules for the different major syntactic categories.

Assembling the modules of the syntax crystal

Instead of the abstract examples shown in Figure 5.3, let us now
consider how the syntax crystal might apply to a real language
string. We will use the modules shown in Figure 5.4(a). For con-

Figure 5.3. (a) Uncoded lexeme modules. (b) Lexeme modules attached
to structure modules to form AA and BB. (c) Orrery for AABBBBAA. (d)
Structure modules that attach to coded lexeme modules of (b). (e)
Structure and module types for symmetric language. (f) Modules for
"equal number of B's follow A's" language.

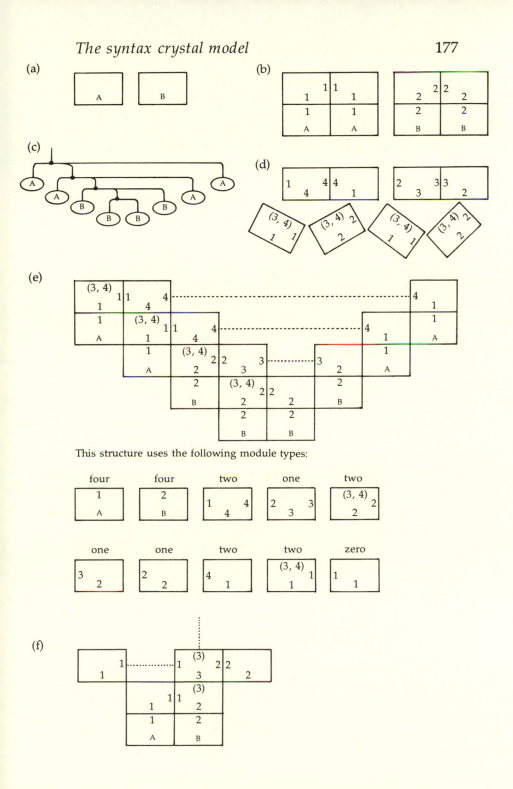

This structure uses the following module types:

venience, the connections codes are letter-number combinations; the code N2, 4 stands for "N2 or N4"; N1, 8–12 stands for "N1, N8, N9, N10, N11, or N12". Later in the chapter we explain further the notation of the codes; here we only need the principle that matching codes allow apposing modules to be connected. Figure 5.4 shows several orreries and corresponding crystals for combining BIRD, HOUSE, and THE.

The positional priority principle requires the A1–A1 structure module to move left along the path shown by the row of dots. Thus the A1–A1 module yields to the N5–N5 module in Figure 5.4(b). The N5–N5 module has positional priority because it is connected lower down on the column of modules above HOUSE. This does not mean that the connection between the A1 codes is any weaker than the connection between N5 codes; it does not matter how far apart connected modules are. In Figure 5.4(d) the A1–A1 module is connected higher on to the BIRD column than the O1–O1 module, so the O1 connection has positional priority.

The morpheme sequence in the language string is read along the bottom of each column of modules from left to right. In Figure 5.4(b) and 5.4(c), no inflections or functors need to be added. Using the structure modules in Figure 5.4(a), there are four ways that THE, BIRD, and HOUSE can be connected – the three portrayed in Figure 5.4(b,c,d), plus THE HOUSE's BIRD. Of the possible strings composed of these morphemes, all and only the grammatically correct ones can be generated with syntax crystal modules.

In Figure 5.4(b), BIRD and HOUSE are connected together as a unit and THE is connected to their connection from the top. This portrays the scope relations of the conceptual structure: BIRD and HOUSE are in each other's scope, and the scope of THE is the pair BIRD and HOUSE. The dependency relations are determined by which column has connection codes on its top, plus the fact that THE is connected to the modules comprising the BIRD–HOUSE connection through the HOUSE column. In Figure 5.4(c), THE is connected to the modules that comprise the BIRD–HOUSE connection on top of the BIRD column, showing that BIRD is the main constituent. In Figure 5.4(d), the scope of THE is smaller; this time only BIRD is in its scope. The main constituent of THE BIRD is BIRD, and therefore the connection to HOUSE, via the possessive morpheme, 'S, is made to the BIRD column.

(a)

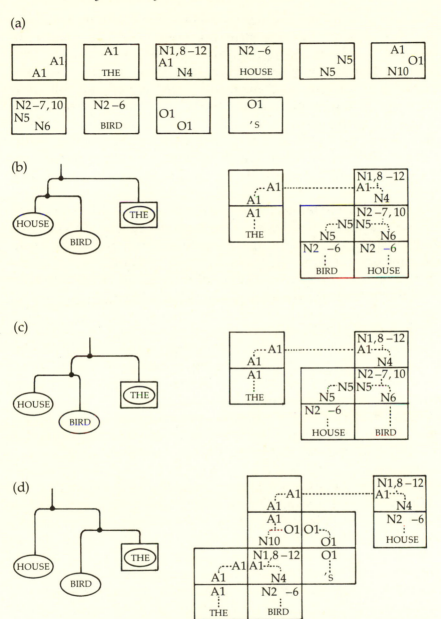

Figure 5.4. (a) Some typical syntax crystal modules. (b–d) Orreries and crystals for combining BIRD, HOUSE, and THE in different scope and dependency relations.

If one looks at the structure modules at the top of each connection, one can see that the structure module for the main morpheme has codes on its top, permitting other connections to it. In Figure 5.4(d), the only codes on the top of the structure modules connecting THE and BIRD are in the BIRD column, and the only codes on the top of the structure modules connecting THE BIRD to 'S also are in the BIRD COLUMN. But the codes on top of the modules connecting THE BIRD'S to HOUSE are on the top of the HOUSE column. The main constituent of THE BIRD'S HOUSE is HOUSE, and the other constituents are the subordinate, or the dependent, ones.

Appendix B contains a set of syntax crystal modules arranged in four stages of complexity. The modules can be photocopied and cut apart. By assembling the modules according to their connection codes and the positional priority conventions, the reader will be able to construct a sample of interesting English strings. Additional instructions are given in the appendix. We encourage the reader to do this.

Like other models of syntax, the syntax crystal offers only an idealized version of language processing. These idealized versions make very few claims about the actual parsing, generating, or acquisition processes that may employ a variety of strategies and be related to other cognitive processing. Here we are interested in describing the essential properties of language processing. Appendix A goes beyond this goal and relates the model to what is known about human parsing strategies.

The syntax crystal model can be operated as a random string-generating mechanism for testing its ability to generate any and only grammatical strings. The model can be worked by hand or in computer simulation to see how well it can produce syntactically acceptable strings. However, string production usually involves syntactic encoding for some purpose other than demonstrating an ability to generate grammatical strings. The syntactic mechanism is used to express ideas and to interpret strings: in our terms, to map the orrery relations onto a language string and to extract the orrery relations from the sequence, inflection, and functor information in a language string. So that is what we shall discuss now.

Generating a string from an orrery: expressing an idea

In terms of the orrery and syntax crystal models the process of *generating* a language string to express an idea would go like this: First, the idea is represented as an orrery. This contains information about the scope and dependency of the conceptual relations, but no sequence information is present at this stage. Suppose the idea is that which we would express as THE BIRD HOUSE. The orrery for the idea is shown on the top left of Figure 5.4(b). The left-to-right sequence is arbitrary.

To express the idea, the language user employs the syntactic knowledge embodied in the modules of Figure 5.4(a). Lexical morpheme modules representing the basic concepts are selected. (This does not mean that all lexeme selection is done before the syntactic mechanism is used.) Then those structure modules are chosen to connect the morpheme modules together that preserve the scope and dependency portrayed by the topology of the orrery branches. The morphemes BIRD and HOUSE must be connected as a unit so that they can connect to THE through the main morpheme, HOUSE. As one can see from the examples in Figure 5.4, BIRD, HOUSE, and THE can be connected through syntax crystal modules in several different ways. The modules that portray the correct orrery relations (traceable through the dotted lines shown on the modules) will give the correct order: THE BIRD HOUSE.

In a phrase we usually know what the main term is because we know how the phrase can combine with other morphemes and phrases. This knowledge is represented in the syntax crystal by the unconnected codes on the modules. The morpheme whose column contains unconnected codes on the top is the main morpheme.

Suppose the dependency relations were different and BIRD was the main morpheme, as in the orrery of Figure 5.4(c). The only way to portray these orrery relations with syntax crystal modules is to change the order of the morphemes, as in the second crystal of the figure.

Suppose we want the scope of THE to be different, as in the orrery of Figure 5.4(d). Although HOUSE is the main morpheme, the scope of THE is BIRD. There is no way to do this in English without adding other morphemes. In Figure 5.4(d) we have added the possessive morpheme 'S to produce this structure.

In each case, the crystal that corresponds to an orrery maintains the same topological scope and dependency relations as the orrery, but the information on the structure modules causes the morphemes to appear in the correct left-to-right sequence.

Parsing: extracting scope and dependency relations from a string

The other process that employs the syntactic mechanism is parsing. The language user confronts a string of morphemes and wishes to extract from it an idea. Concepts can be associated with lexical morphemes but the relation among the concepts must also be extracted. In our view, the language user needs to extract scope and dependency information, that is, to construct an orrery using data from the surface string. The syntax crystal mechanism performs the task as follows: First, the incoming string is represented in morpheme modules[3] with the sequence preserved (this does not mean that the whole string must be represented before parsing begins). Consider THE BIRD HOUSE as the incoming string.

The goal is to have all of the morpheme modules connected together into one structure without changing the left-to-right sequence. In other words, no connection codes must be left unmatched. Structure modules are selected to make these connections. With those available in Figure 5.4(a), there is only one set of structure modules that can do this and only one structure that can possibly result, the one shown in Figure 5.4(b). The scope and dependency relations may be read off as the "skeleton" of the crystal. If the connection among lexical morphemes in the resulting orrery structure is the same as the one from which the string was generated, the message carried by the string has been successfully communicated.

The examples of generating and parsing we have just presented are extremely simple and the syntactic knowledge represented by the small set of modules very elementary. As a result, the procedures for assembling a crystal structure subject to orrery constraints while generating, and to morpheme sequence constraints for parsing, were very easy to do. However, as we discussed in Chapter 1, global constraints on local operations are often difficult to specify in a precise and efficient way. A primitive procedure of exhaustively trying to fit structure modules at random will work eventually. But this method of parsing a complex string using a more complete set of modules might involve a lot of wasteful backtracking. Heuristic procedures can be used to make the process more efficient. We describe some parsing heuristics in Appendix A.

Fortunately, except for deciphering material like Lewis Carroll's (1872) poetry, natural language users do not need to perform syntactic analyses in isolation. The goal of parsing is to arrive at an orrery structure that represents the conceptual relations underlying the string. Along with a lexical analysis to find out the concepts expressed by the string, pragmatic information and primitive syntax offer powerful clues to conceptual structure. For a recent review of how these information sources aid parsing, see Clark and Clark (1977:72–79).

Representing ambiguous strings and paraphrases

Natural languages do not always map ideas onto morpheme strings in an unambiguous one-to-one fashion. It frequently happens that a given string can represent more than one idea. Sometimes this happens because a morpheme is ambiguous. Sometimes it happens because the string can be parsed into more than one sort of structure. As we discussed in the preceding chapter, syntactically ambiguous strings have been used as diagnostic tools for models of syntax. If a model cannot provide more than one structural description for a syntactically ambiguous string, it fails Chomsky's second criterion for an adequate theory. In terms of the syntax crystal, this criterion requires that if a string can express two (or more) ideas with distinct orrery representations, then it must be parsable into distinct crystals, one for each orrery. This leaves open the possibility that a string may express more than one idea whose orrery relations do not differ. Some structures may be ambiguous, just as some words are.

Here is an example: SMALL BIRD HOUSE. This can express two different ideas. It can mean "a house for small birds" or it can mean "a small house for birds." Figure 5.5(a) shows the orreries for the two interpretations along with the crystals for two different structures that use the same morpheme sequence (and the same modules). Not only may one string express more than one relation of concepts, but one relation of concepts may be expressed by more than one string. For example, THE HOUSE THAT IS SMALL is an alternative expression (paraphrase) for THE SMALL HOUSE. There may be stylistic differences between the two expressions, but they are close to synonymous. Figure 5.5(b) illustrates the crystal structure for THE HOUSE THAT IS SMALL along with the orrery derived from the crystal.

Comparing the crystals and orreries of Figure 5.5(b), we can see that the relations among HOUSE, SMALL, and THE are basically the same: In both, HOUSE and SMALL form a unit that is then joined to THE. In the right crystal the connection between HOUSE and SMALL is more direct than that in the left one because the latter connection is mediated by the modules controlling the morphemes THAT and IS. The crystals of both paraphrases have similar scope and dependency relations among HOUSE, SMALL, and THE. In other words, the similarity across the paraphrases is shown by the similarity in the *topology* of the syntactic structure: The basic features of the connections remain the same even though the parts of one crystal may be rotated and/or stretched with respect to the other.

It is not important that the modules which mediate the connections themselves be similar across the two paraphrases; were it not for reasons of economy, an entirely different set of modules might be used for the second paraphrase. This is consistent with our basic working principle – only the scope and dependency relations are needed for syntax; the details of the syntactic mechanism, the codes and their configuration, only serve to coordinate scope and dependency with morpheme sequence. Now we shall take a closer look at the connection codes.

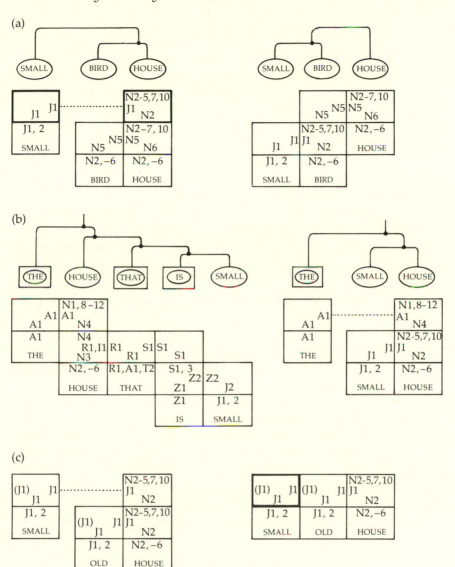

Figure 5.5. (a) Orreries and crystals for the ambiguous string SMALL BIRD HOUSE. (b) Orreries and crystals for connecting SMALL and HOUSE. (c) Hierarchical and heterarchical recursive structures for SMALL OLD HOUSE.

What the codes on the modules represent

Each code represents one-half of an abstract, mediated association. It is one piece of the underlying structure of sentences. No connection represented by the codes is ever expressed by a language user nor is it ever perceived directly. It represents part of the inferred hierarchical structure of language strings we argued for in Chapter 1. Like the syntactic rules of any linguistic theory, the codes, their arrangements on the modules, and their potential matching to those of other modules is an attempt to account for certain regularities of natural language strings. Further, as a model for performance, the codes are intended to suggest how language use can be described in terms that can be extended to cognitive mechanisms. Breaking down syntactic knowledge into the smaller units of connection codes rather than the larger units of production rules will enable us to present a procedure for syntax acquisition without assuming an innate, specifically linguistic acquisition device (see Chapter 6).

The connection codes coordinate scope and dependency information with sequence, functor, and inflection information in a language string. As abstract mediators, the letters and numerals used for the codes are intrinsically arbitrary. The only important thing is that the same letter + numeral combination is the same connection code; a different letter + numeral combination is a different connection, thus code: $B3 = B3 \neq B4 \neq C4 = C4$. How this sameness and difference are represented is not of theoretical importance. However, we are going to use codes to remind us of the grammatical categories we are familiar with: N for noun, V for verb, J for adjective, and so on. For example, modules with J codes build the part of underlying structure that connects adjectives to the things they modify. We use numerals after the letter codes to distinguish more finely among modules that participate in the same sort of syntactic operation. It is important to emphasize that this is done just for the convenience of our seeing what is going on and for comparing the syntax crystal structures with those of other linguistic theories. There is no claim that a language user, in being able to make a connection represented by a J code, need have any idea that there is a category of adjectives. Also, the fact that connection codes J1 and J3 share the same capi-

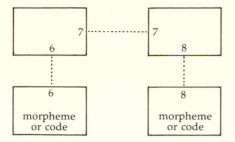

Figure 5.6. A single hierarchical connection between modules.

tal letter is only for convenience in discussing the theory. It should not be taken as a prima facie indication that, for example, J1 is more psychologically similar to J2 than is N3.

The codes on the modules are entered during the acquisition process. Originally, the modules are empty. The quantity of information portrayed by connection codes increases during the learning process. So also does the reliability of syntactic information processing. A more complete representation of syntactic information would have each connection code weighted as to its probability of effecting a connection, representing the relative strength of a piece of syntactic knowledge. However, in what follows, we are going to continue to represent the connection codes as simple "on-off" associations. Two modules either can, or cannot, be connected to each other.

The connection codes and their arrangements on the modules are intended to suggest something about the cognitive operations performed by language users when they generate and parse strings. However, we do not suppose that every operation of the model has a direct counterpart in the cognitive operations. For example, the syntax crystal models each hierarchical connection as a relation among four modules with three pairs of connected edges. This is illustrated by Figure 5.6. This does not mean that three cognitive operations are claimed necessarily to be involved. It is likely that some operations that occur together repeatedly or happen to articulate well together may become integrated into a single functional unit. In terms of the syntax crystal, two or more modules might become integrated into a single more or less stable unit, analogous to a chemical radical. If two or more morpheme modules are involved, this might represent a frozen form or such stuff as clichés are made on.

If two or more modules are used only together and never separately, we could represent them as collapsed into a single module. Figure 5.7(a) illustrates how two modules that are always used with their edges connected are replaced by a single module that functions equivalently. The replacement in Figure 5.7(a) also changes the dependency relations, as shown by the accompanying orreries. The process could also be reversed to make finer distinctions.

Representing modules economically

In Chapter 1 we described how syntactic rules are made more economical by combining the information from a number of simple rules into one, more complex rule. The syntax crystal can also be made more economical by collapsing several modules into a single module. For any syntactic system, the economy is achieved using the logical connectives we described in Chapter 1. Figure 5.7(b) illustrates a sample of the ways that one module can replace a number of other modules. Recall that an element in parentheses is optional; that elements separated by commas indicate that one only is selected; that square brackets constrain the choice of elements such that choosing the nth element in one set of brackets requires that the nth element in the other set of brackets also be chosen; and that $\emptyset$ stands for the null element.

Recursion in syntax crystal modules

In Chapter 1 we described recursion as a property of rule systems that permits the same kind of element to be introduced over and over again. The property of recursion allows there to be an unlimited number of strings in any language and allows the production of a string of unlimited length. The essence of recursion is that an element generates, either directly or indirectly, an opportunity for itself to be generated again. In a production rule system, $S \rightarrow X\ S$ is an example of a simple recursive rule. In the syntax crystal model, recursion is permitted anytime a module can be connected to another of the identical type. This will occur

(a)

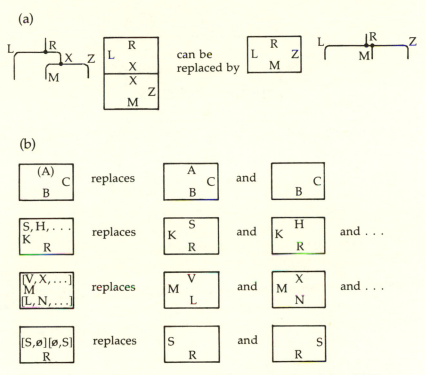

(b)

Figure 5.7. (a) Collapsing two constantly associated modules. (b) How modules are collapsed for economical representation.

when a module has the same connection code on opposite edges. As in production rule systems, indirect recursion may also occur, where one module connects to a different module (or set of modules) that in turn can connect to one of the first type.

In English, an arbitrarily large number of adjectives may modify a noun. As we discussed in Chapter 2, such modifiers may be arranged hierarchically or heterarchically depending on the particular relation of concepts. Figure 5.5(c) illustrates how these two types of constructions can be generated by module recursion in the vertical and horizontal directions, respectively. In contrast, only one article (or other determiner), and, for some speakers, only one relative clause, are permitted each noun phrase. In these constructions, the modules that govern their connections do not have any of the same codes on opposite edges and hence cannot be recursively repeated.

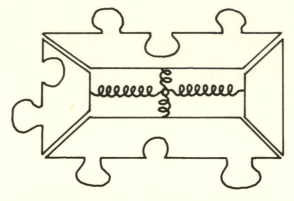

Figure 5.8. An alternative form for a syntax crystal module.

Alternative representations for the syntax crystal model

We have presented our syntactic rules in terms of rectangular modules that assemble under the control of connection codes on their edges. We selected this form for a number of heuristic reasons:

1. As will be discussed in the next section, a matrix of modules is the traditional and clearest way of representing the mathematical properties of the model.
2. The analogy with molecular crystallization is suggestive.
3. The geometry of the configuration of connection codes allows dependency to be mapped directly.
4. As the reader who used the modules in Appendix B has discovered, the modules can be assembled and manipulated by hand far more quickly and easily than writing out and rewriting the syntactic rules of any other system.

However, we do not mean to imply that there is anything sacred about the representation, or that the formal properties of the model depend on the crystal metaphor. For example, instead of connection codes, we might adopt the jigsaw-puzzle metaphor used by molecular biologists to explain the assembly of genetic material. Figure 5.8 illustrates such a module with geometric connection codes and springs to allow the unit to stretch to conform to the positional priority principle.

Although the modules are two-dimensional rectangles that assemble on a plane, there is no reason, other than the simplicity of presentation, that they must be two dimensional. There is certainly no psychological reason for limiting a language model to only two dimensions. Work on the cognitive psychology of semantics has shown that many representations of the psychological relatedness of concepts require three or more dimensions to be adequately portrayed. However, for the convenience of presenting the model on paper and comparing it with other linguistic theories, we will stick with two dimensions.

Syntax crystal modules can also be simulated on a computer. This allows more constructions to be tested in a shorter time than is possible by hand. It also tests whether the rules described have been specified clearly and precisely enough to be used in a program. In Appendix A a computer simulation of the syntax crystal is described.

Up to this point, we have presented the syntax crystal modules in their geometric form. The syntactic information is carried not only by the set of connection codes, but also in the geometric relationship of the codes to each other. It is the geometry that allows the system to carry dependency as well as scope information. However, syntactic models are traditionally presented in terms of production rules. In order to make it easier to compare syntax crystal modules with the rules of other models, it would be helpful to be able to translate them into a comparable form. Another advantage of the rule system is that it is a familiar format for a digital computer. By entering a set of rules in a computer with a program for combining them, the computer can parse and generate strings with no human intervention.

If we translate the modules in Figure 5.9(a) into the equivalent production rule of the ordinary kind (see Chapter 1), A → B D, we would lose the information that D is the dependent constituent and that B is connected to D through side code C. We can show dependency by underlining the main constituent and scope by using braces. Thus: A → { B D}. As long as the two modules are connected, the side code C has no way of affecting the pair's connection to other modules, so we do not need to include it as an element in the rule. However, the advantage of the syntax crystal depends on the independence of the modules. Therefore, we need a notation for single modules.

Modules of the general form in Figure 5.9(b) are translated as

(a)

$A \rightarrow \{\underline{B}\ \ D\}$

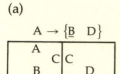

(b)

$A \rightarrow \{D/\underline{B}\backslash C\}$

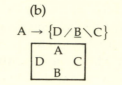

(c)

$D/B\backslash C$

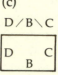

(d)

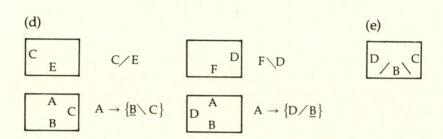

C/E   F\D

$A \rightarrow \{\underline{B}\backslash C\}$ $A \rightarrow \{D/\underline{B}\}$

(e)

(f)

The rule for the left one is: $A \rightarrow \{D/\underline{B}\backslash C\}$

The rule for the right one is: $\underline{ C/E }$

Combined, we get: $A \rightarrow \{D/\underline{B}\quad\ \ E\}$

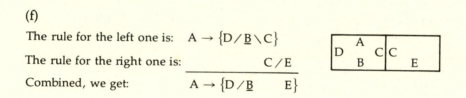

(g)

$A \rightarrow \{D/\underline{B}\ \ E\}$

$\underline{ F\backslash D }$

$A \rightarrow \{F\ \ \underline{B}\ \ E\}$

(h)

$A \rightarrow \{D/\underline{B}\}$

$\underline{ B \rightarrow \{\underline{K}\backslash H\} }$

$A \rightarrow \{D/\quad\ \ \{\underline{K}\backslash H\}\}$

(i)

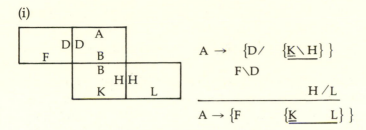

$$A \rightarrow \quad \{D/ \quad \{\underline{K}\backslash H\}\}$$
$$F\backslash D$$

$$\underline{\hspace{4cm}}\quad H/L$$

$$A \rightarrow \{F \qquad \{\underline{K} \qquad L\}\}$$

Figure 5.9. (a–e) Modules and corresponding production rules. (f–i) Combining modules and production rules.

$A \rightarrow \{D/\underline{B}\backslash C\}$. $\underline{B}$ is the main constituent with respect to A, since it is directly below it in the same "column." A module of the form in Figure 5.9(c) does not have the "A →" portion of the rule above. Its rule is $D/B\backslash C$. In this case, B is not under-lined because it is not the main constituent of anything that con-nects to it from the top. Note that the directionality of the arrow is not significant; syntax crystal modules can connect from the bot-tom up as well as from the top down, or side to side. The arrows are used in the rules for easier comparison with the rules of tradi-tional theories. Originally, production rules for syntactic struc-tures were written to produce the structures from the top down.

There are four other types of modules. They are in Figure 5.9(d) with their rule versions. The bottom code is always "under" the slash (that is, the top of the slash points toward the bottom code as if it were the denominator of a fraction written on a single line or as if it were sheltered by a lean-to). The side code "above" the slash is on the side it would appear on the module. Another way of looking at it is that the slash appears as if it were drawn to sep-arate the codes as they appear on the module in Figure 5.9(e).

The production rules can be combined by an arithmetic opera-tion that describes the combining of the corresponding modules. For example, two of the modules illustrated in Figure 5.9 com-bine as in Figure 5.9(f). The right side-code C in the first rule combines with the left side-code C in the second rule to cancel out. In other words, matching side-codes with opposite slashes combine and cancel out to represent a connection of modules. Once joined, the codes are not accessible to further connections. The combination of rules describes the pair of modules joined together: Top code A connects directly to left side-code D and bottom code B (the main constituent code), and through a side code to bottom code E (dependent constituent) on the right of a second module.

The connections can be compounded just like the connections among the modules. We can take the result of the operation performed in Figure 5.9(f) and add to it F$\setminus$D. We get A $\to$ {F $\underline{B}$ E}, which describes the three modules joined together in Figure 5.9(g). Modules can be joined at top and bottom edges as well as along the sides. This is how it works in the notation: A $\to$ {D$\diagup$$\underline{B}$} plus B $\to$ {$\underline{K}$$\setminus$H} yields A $\to$ {D$\diagup$ {$\underline{K}$$\setminus$H}} This is shown in Figure 5.9(h). If we then add F$\setminus$D we get A $\to$ {F {$\underline{K}$$\setminus$H}}, and if we now add H$\diagup$L we get A $\to$ {F { $\underline{K}$ L }}. This is shown in Figure 5.9(i).

The combining of rules for two modules is like the operation of production rules described in Chapter 1. An element on the right of the arrow of the first rule is further specified (rewritten) as another element or set of elements. The element to be further specified also appears in the second rule. The remaining elements of the second rule give the further specification of the element. By carrying down the braces, we can maintain the scope information in the rules. A single rule representing a set of joined modules has as its elements only the connection codes that are still available. The codes participating in joined edges are not represented.

The production rules may be used for generating and parsing in the same way the modules are used. An array of rules combines scope, dependency, and morpheme sequence information as does an array of modules forming a crystal. We can demonstrate the similarity by showing how an array of rules constructs the string THE HOUSE THAT IS SMALL, which is shown in crystal form in Figure 5.5(b). Each rule will be written on a separate line. The rules will be spread out to make room for elements of rules below them. To save space, elements to the left of an arrow will be written over in the left margin with their products taking their place under the preceding rule. For example:

A $\to$ {Q/$\underline{W}$}   instead of: A $\to$ {Q/$\underline{W}$}
 _   W $\to$ {$\underline{R}$$\setminus$N}   W $\to$ {$\underline{R}$ N}

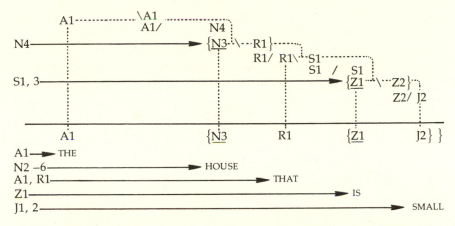

Figure 5.10. Array of production rules corresponding to the modules in Figure 5.5(b) for THE HOUSE THAT IS SMALL.

The array of rules is shown in Figure 5.10. The striped bars show how the orrery relations of scope and dependency are carried by the array of rules.

Beneath the rules for structure modules, we "sum them up" so that the elements representing joined edges drop out leaving only the elements that connect directly to morphemes. The braces are carried down and the products of any element that has been further specified are included within the braces. The summed formula shows the scope relations in the string by the nested braces. By carrying down the underline marker for major constituents, the dependency relations are also portrayed.

The rules have the other properties of modules: Morphemes with the same rule elements are interchangeable – for example, SMALL and OLD. The rules, like the modules, do not need any additional rules to control the order in which they are combined. The assembly of a rule array can be started with any rule, or even more than one rule at the same time. Rules representing modules that are exceptions to the positional priority rule have the arrow written after the bottom code, for example G1/ G1↓. The arrow is carried down when the rule is summed. However, when the rules are summed, scope information about the arrowed element may sometimes *not* be carried by the nested braces.

The importance of being able to translate the information contained in the syntax crystal modules into a production rule system or a computer program is to demonstrate that the principles of operation are not essentially bound to the physical model. Thus, in proposing the syntax crystal as a model of human natural language performance, we are making no claim about the specific set of properties of rectangular modules with coded edges.

The formal properties of syntax crystal's local rules

The syntax crystal is named by analogy to molecular crystallization because it shows how the global structures of an unlimited number of different strings can grow from the self-constrained accretion of small units of a relatively few types. The analogy is faithful in two other important ways. First, crystallization of the syntactic structures of a sentence is shown to be an automatic process. All the information needed is accounted for. No external guiding agency is required to link up the molecular units of the model. Second, the growth of the crystal may be constrained in general ways just as the general form of a chemical crystal may be constrained by placing its matrix solution in containers of various shapes. The analogy to the constraining container is the orrery – the syntax crystal shows how it is possible to grow the structure of a sentence and the proper linear order of its words from the nonordered scope and dependency constraints of the underlying conceptual structure.

Formally, the syntax crystal can be described as a cellular automaton (von Neumann, 1966): It is a system composed of subunits, or modules, that join together to produce coherent structures. The modules are of a restricted number of types, although there may be an unlimited number of tokens of each type. Although a general principle of assembly may be used, all the information to determine the form of the structure must be contained within the modules they join together to produce the structure. In other words, no global blueprint for the structure is used or exists in any one place. The information is distributed among the several modules. The information contained in each module tells only what other module, or modules, it can connect itself to and the geometry or direction of the bond. In terms of our discussion in Chapter 1, the syntax crystal is a device that achieves a globally coherent pattern by the combined effects of several local operations.

Coordinating nonadjacent elements by local rules

Karl Lashley (1951) argued that coordination among nonadjacent parts must be considered by any explanation of complex behavior. Lashley and, even earlier, Wundt (1901) suggested that disparate pieces of linguistic behavior – e.g., words at the beginning and end of an utterance – were joined together by an abstract hierarchical mediating structure. This structure rather than the intervening pieces of behavior (i.e., the words in between) coordinated the disparate parts. The rule systems of the syntax crystal, and other generative grammars, are representations of this structure. In the syntax crystal, coordination of disparate pieces of language can be traced through the connections of structure modules.

Information to coordinate two nonadjacent morphemes must be carried through the structure to the sites of the morphemes. For the syntax crystal, all the intervening structure modules between the sites of the morphemes must carry the information that coordinates them. The same is true for intervening rules in other models of syntax. Coordination of this sort is required for many types of agreement. For example, in the sentence THE GIRLS WHO HAVE BROUGHT THEIR DOG RUN DOWN THE STREET, the plural form of the verb RUN is coordinated with the choice of the plural morpheme attached to the noun GIRL. For number agreement, the intervening modules (or rules) for plurals and the intervening modules for singulars mediate many of the same sorts of constructions: For example, plural and mass nouns as well as singular count nouns, can connect to adjectives, modifier nouns, relative clauses, prepositional phrases, and others. To account for agreement through the structure requires alternative forms of rules for these connections. Figure 5.11(a) illustrates how the intervening modules might carry the information. In this figure, LEFT$_i$ is a form that agrees with RIGHT$_i$. This form has in common with other forms that it can take a morpheme whose module has

(a)

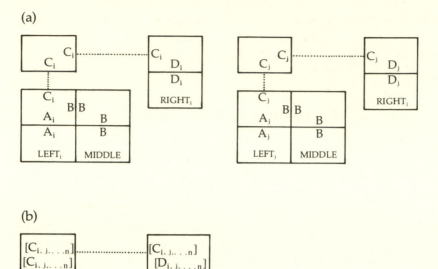

(b)

Figure 5.11. (a) How intervening modules coordinate nonadjacent elements. (b) Coordinating *n* pairs of nonadjacent elements using only one set of modules.

a B code, such as MIDDLE. For another form, say LEFT$_j$, which must be connected to RIGHT$_j$, all the modules with "i" subscripts must be changed to modules that can coordinate LEFT$_j$ with RIGHT$_j$. The more connections LEFT$_j$ has in common with LEFT$_i$, and the more RIGHT$_i$ has in common with RIGHT$_j$, the more sets of modules must be added to produce agreement. And the more forms there are that must agree, the more sets of modules there must be. Thus, in order to handle agreement through the structure, the complexity of any syntactic model must be considerably increased. As described earlier, most linguistic theories try to reduce the number of rules by combining them through logical notation. Figure 5.11(b) shows how the number of structure modules can be reduced by making individual modules more complex. Using the notation described in Chapter 1, the square brackets indicate an ordered constraint on the choice of connection codes on one edge by what has been selected at another edge. For example, if, A_k is selected from the left brackets, then C_k must be selected at the next connection, D_k at the next.

There is another way to economize on the amount of information required to coordinate nonadjacent morphemes. Instead of effecting the agreement of nonadjacent morphemes through the hierarchical structure, we can postulate that they are connected by some procedures outside the hierarchical structure. This outside procedure selects a morpheme at one site to correspond to the morpheme that appears at the other coordinated site. Because the selection at one site depends on what is at another site in the same string, the outside procedure is said to provide *context sensitivity*.

The rule systems that use context sensitivity appear to be much simpler because they do not have to carry information through the hierarchical structure. However, they do have to go back and operate on this structure. Consider how such a system would handle THE GIRLS WHO HAVE BROUGHT THEIR DOG RUN DOWN THE STREET. The rule that selects RUN instead of RUNS is: Select VERB + s in a context where preceded by a singular NOUN PHRASE; Select VERB $+\emptyset$ in a context where preceded by a plural NOUN PHRASE (Lyons, 1968:245). In order to determine whether the noun phrase THE GIRLS WHO HAVE BROUGHT THEIR DOG is singular or plural, one has to identify the main noun. And identifying the main noun can only be done syntactically by examining the hierarchical structure of the phrase.

The formulation of context-sensitive rules has been done only in terms of global operations. No attention has been paid to how the noun phrase is identified, nor how the hierarchical structure is used to identify whether the noun phrase is singular or plural.[4]

The syntax crystal model describes only grammatical relations that might be completely determined through the hierarchical structure. We argued earlier that many of the relations which have been attributed to syntactic rules can be explained better as the result of pragmatic information: Recently, others have argued that many of the relations previously attributed to the hierarchical structure, including transformation processes, are better attributed, either wholly or in part, to the surface structure (Jackendoff, 1972; Chomsky, 1975) or to lexical rules (Chomsky, 1972; Bresnan, 1978). We would agree that surface structure as well as pragmatic information contribute to syntactic processing, either in concert with the hierarchical structure or sometimes alone. Our immediate goal has been to describe the hierarchical structure. We have not yet investigated the details of how it might work in conjunction with other aspects of the string.

Inflected languages and local rules

There are some languages, such as Latin, that do not use sequence to carry syntactic information. Instead, they rely on inflections to indicate the relations of concepts described by a well-formed set of morphemes. We want to show that the syntax crystal can go from an orrery to a string of an inflected language as well as to the string of a language that employs sequential encoding. Figure 5.12(a) shows an orrery and a crystal for the idea expressed in English as THE DOG LOVES THE GIRL. The stem of each noun, CAN- and PUELL-, have added to them the nominative inflection (+IS) and the accusative inflection (+AM) respectively. The Latin sentence is, then; CANIS AMAT PUELLAM.

A language in which syntax is expressed by inflections rather than order would not use a positional priority rule for causing morphemes connected higher up on a column to appear farther away. Only the structure modules that connect to inflections need to be ordered so that inflections appear with their lexemes. These modules are portrayed with an arrow which indicates that modules connected lower down in the structure must move out of their way.

Notice that the modules with brackets on opposite sides use the logical notation described earlier to allow one module type to connect only to one side or the other. Such connection codes allow any structure grown on the right of a module with brackets to also be grown on the left (but not on both sides). This permits the morphemes of a Latin string to appear in any order. Of course, the inflections that appear at the ends of morpheme stems are not attached this way. The modules shown in the figure may be assembled to produce six different sequences of the three morphemes. Except for stylistic differences, they are semantically equivalent.

(a)

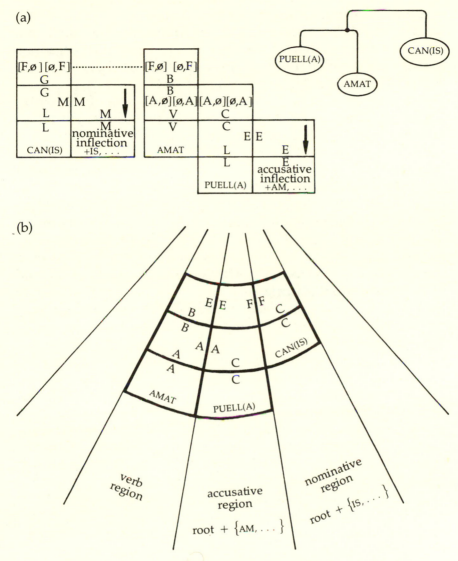

(b)

Figure 5.12. (a) Orrery and crystal of the Latin for THE DOG LOVES THE GIRL. (b) Abstract syntax crystal that maps an orrery onto an inflection space for the Latin sentence CANIS AMAT PUELLAM.

Although a Latin crystal does not arrange the morphemes in a fixed sequence, each assembly of the crystal produces some particular sequence or other. This is reasonable given that speaking, hearing, signing, and writing are necessarily sequential activities. However, this is not a necessary feature of syntax or of the model. (McNeill [personal communication] has suggested that some analyses of syntax might even be extended to an organism with a large number of organs of communication that could emit all the lexemes of a sentence simultaneously.)

Using a more abstract formulation, the principle of the syntax crystal could be extended to describe a sequence-free model for inflected languages. Representing sequential positions in a string by the order of the morphemes in a crystal (as for English) is a mapping convention – the space is used to represent sequence. A different interpretation could be assigned to the crystal space.[5] We might divide the space in which a crystal is assembled into sector-shaped regions. Each region would represent one type of syntactic form that can appear in a Latin string. Figure 5.12(b) shows a portion of such an *inflection space* with three of the regions labeled: verb region, accusative region, and nominative region. Associated with each of these regions would be a particular type of inflection. For example, the accusative is marked by the suffixes +AM and +UM for the first and second declensions.

When parsing strings, the lexical morpheme modules are placed in the regions corresponding to the inflection that accompanies them. Without moving the modules out of the regions, structure modules are applied. A crystal results, giving the scope and dependency relations among the morphemes. Such a crystal is shown in Figure 5.12(b). During string generating, the structure modules, assembled under the topological constraints of the orrery, will force the (uninflected) lexeme modules to lie in the appropriate region of inflection space. The sentence is emitted by applying to each lexeme the inflection corresponding to the region in which it has been placed. The lexemes with their inflections may be emitted without regard to sequence.

How the syntax crystal
handles English constructions

In Chapter 4 we described a sample of the constructions of English grammar that have played important roles in the justification of syntactic theories. For each of these constructions, transformational theory was shown to be superior to phrase structure grammar for its ability to portray the similarities and differences that characterize the regularities of English.

However, transformational theory achieved these advantages at the cost of introducing a great number of global operations – the transformation rules themselves, or in recent variants, extensive use of global lexical restrictions, and the metarules that control transformation rules. As we pointed out earlier, a syntactic theory which relies on global operations that have no obvious or plausible translation into local operations is deficient both as a complete explanation and in its ability to relate to theories on other levels of analysis. We are now going to demonstrate that the syntax crystal model can also generate these several forms of English strings and do it with the correct syntactic structures, i.e., portray scope correctly and indicate similarities and differences across the forms. To the extent that the properties of other syntactic theories can be reduced to scope and dependency relations, they are compatible with the syntax crystal. If the regularities treated by transformational or case theories can be handled by the local rules of the syntax crystal, the rules of those theories will have been reduced to a form more accessible to psychological explanation. Where other theories require properties that cannot be translated into syntax crystal properties, there exists a theoretical difference. Some of the differences with transformational grammar are described at the end of this chapter.

The number of different constructions that have been treated in transformational accounts is legion. In this chapter we treat only a tiny fraction of them, the ones that have figured most prominently in the literature comparing one theory with another. In Appendix B a number of additional constructions are demonstrated with syntax crystal modules. However, we are not claiming that the syntactic rules currently employed are complete, nor even that the syntax crystal is currently as powerful as transformational grammar. What we hope to demonstrate is that the syntax crystal model represents a serious alternative to transformational theories.

The following illustrations use modules with connection codes that correspond roughly to the abbreviations of traditional grammatical categories: V for verb, for example. Sometimes modules have been collapsed as described earlier and sometimes not, depending on the ease of illustration. These conveniences do not represent a claim about the nature of psychological operations. Whether syntactic performance depends upon fewer, more complex operations or upon more numerous, simpler operations is an empirical question and is likely to be a difficult one to answer. Readers who are willing to accept on faith that the syntax crystal model can handle the several forms of English may skim the following sections.

Phrasal verbs

Recall from the preceding chapter that complex verb forms can be analyzed in terms of component parts (see Table 5.1). Phrase structure grammars handle each of the several constructions involving these parts by a separate, independent rule. Transformational theory, to portray the relationship across the several forms, posits a single base structure with a standard order of components and a set of transformation rules that shift them to the correct positions.

The syntax crystal also takes advantage of the fact that the several phrasal verb constructions employ subsets of the same set of components. Unlike transformational theory, separate global rules are not required to order the components. The modules that connect the main noun phrase to a simple verb phrase are shown in Figure 5.13(a). The optional T3 code allows the sentence to be embedded in a THAT clause, as is demonstrated in Appendix B.

To add a modal auxiliary to this basic form, we insert between the above modules the additional ones shown in Figure 5.13(b).

Table 5.1. *Parts of complex verbs*

1. Modal auxiliary	WILL			
2. Perfect		HAVE +EN, +ED		
3. Progressive			BE +ING	
4. Passive				BE +EN, +ED
5. Verb (and modifiers)				WATCH

The new modules are shown in bold outline. Because, in formal English at least, DO does not connect to phrasal verbs, a different module (without code S1) is required to connect it: THEY MIGHT BE WAITING but not *THEY DO BE WAITING. (Dialects that accept both forms do not require a different module for DO.) The modal auxiliary DO with its connecting module is shown in the right side of the figure.

To construct the perfect tense form, the modules controlling the modal have to be replaceable by those controlling HAVE, the verb, and the perfect tense inflections. These are shown in Figure 5.13(c). In the figure, connection path I between modules allows the modal form to be combined with the verb phrase as in the previous figure, 5.13(b). The connection path labeled II allows the perfect tense form without the modal, and connections I and III together combine the modal with the perfect tense.

To this we can add modules for the progressive tense form and for the passive tense. These are shown in Figure 5.13(d). The modules for the several components can be combined to yield any of the well-formed constructions of English that they control

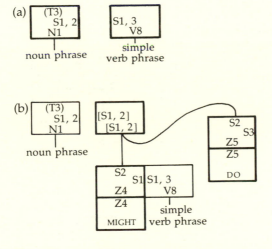

Figure 5.13. (a) Modules that connect main NP to main VP. (b) Modules for noun phrase, two different modal auxiliaries, and a verb phrase. *Continued on the next page.*

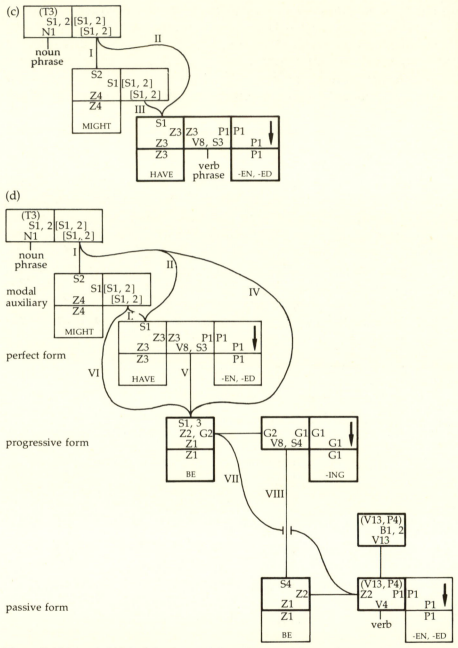

Figure 5.13 (*cont.*). (c) Modules for modal auxiliary and the perfect tense.
(d) Modules for NP (Aux) (Perfect) (Progressive) Passive VP.

and no illegitimate forms. The connection codes and their geometry on the modules force the components to go in the correct left-to-right order and prevent any connections that would result in an improper string. By connecting the modules along the pathways shown in the figure, any of the allowable combinations of verb parts can be obtained. Connecting along path I brings in the modal; paths II and III bring in the perfect form; paths IV, V, and VI bring in the progressive form; paths VII and VIII bring in the passive form.

Infinitives

Infinitive phrases are parts of verb phrases that take all possible verb complements, including other infinitives.

> I WANTED TO WATCH THE DOG EATING BREAKFAST SLOWLY
> I INTENDED TO ASK YOU TO WAIT FOR THE OTHERS

Infinitive phrases do not take noun agreement, tense, or modal auxiliaries.

> ★ I WANTED TO WATCHED
> ★ I WANTED TO CAN WATCH

However, other phrasal verb forms are acceptable.

> I WANTED TO BE WATCHED
> I WANTED TO HAVE BEEN WATCHING (connections I–VI in
> Figure 5.14 effect these constructions)

In addition to complementing verb phrases, infinitive phrases can

1. Complement noun phrases: THE HOUSE TO BUY, THE HORSE TO BE WATCHING TOMORROW (Figure 5.14, path VII)
2. Complement question adverbs: HOW TO EAT, WHETHER TO KEEP HOPING (Figure 5.14, path IX).
3. Connect to noun phrases as part of an object of the verb phrase to form a sentoid: I WANTED (MY SISTER TO EAT) (Figure 5.14, path X) as distinct from I WANTED THE PIZZA TO EAT HERE, THE KID WANTS A HOT DOG TO EAT (Figure 5.14, path VIII).
4. Can take the place of noun phrases: TO ERR IS HUMAN.

These modules are duplicated in Appendix B, where the reader may try various connections.

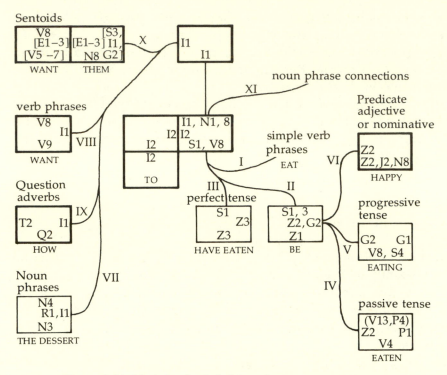

Figure 5.14. Modules for infinitive phrases.

Passive

In order to show the similarity across corresponding active and passive forms, the syntax crystal must provide the same scope and dependency relations, relative to the rest of the structure, for each of the following pairs: (1) subject of the active form and object of the preposition BY in the passive form; (2) object of the active form and subject of the passive form. Thus we need modules that will connect the subject noun phrase of the passive to the bottom of the verb column and the BY prepositional phrase to the top of the verb column. In addition, verbs that take particles in the active form must connect to the particles in the passive as well. For example: THE DOG LOOKED AT TV and TV WAS LOOKED AT BY THE DOG. Note that either the direct or indirect object in the active form can be the subject in the passive form: THE DOG GAVE THE BIRD THE KEY may be paraphrased as either THE KEY WAS

GIVEN TO THE BIRD BY THE DOG or THE BIRD WAS GIVEN THE KEY BY THE DOG. (Unlike case grammarians, we will continue to treat the prepositions, except for the passive BY, as lexical morphemes, not to be controlled by syntactic rules. We believe, however, that many prepositions are in fact determined by a combination of syntactic and semantic information.)

Figure 5.15(b) introduces some of the modules for the passive.

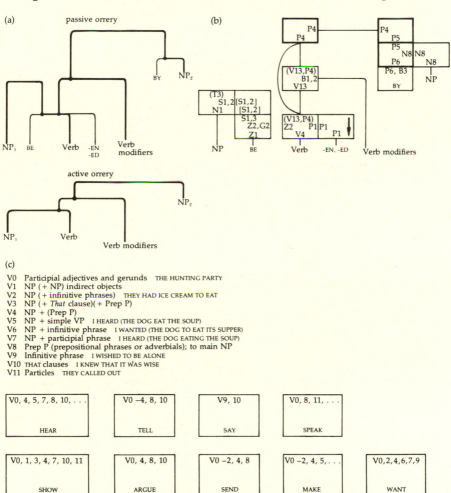

(c)

V0   Participial adjectives and gerunds   THE HUNTING PARTY
V1   NP (+ NP) indirect objects
V2   NP (+ infinitive phrases)   THEY HAD ICE CREAM TO EAT
V3   NP (+ *That* clause)(+ Prep P)
V4   NP + (Prep P)
V5   NP + simple VP   I HEARD (THE DOG EAT THE SOUP)
V6   NP + infinitive phrase   I WANTED (THE DOG TO EAT ITS SUPPER)
V7   NP + participial phrase   I HEARD (THE DOG EATING THE SOUP)
V8   Prep P (prepositional phrases or adverbials); to main NP
V9   Infinitive phrase   I WISHED TO BE ALONE
V10   THAT clauses   I KNEW THAT IT WAS WISE
V11   Particles   THEY CALLED OUT

Figure 5.15. (a) Similar relations in passive and active orreries. (b) Some modules for the passive form. (c) Some verb modules and the kinds of modifiers their codes connect to (V0–V11). *Continued.*

(d)

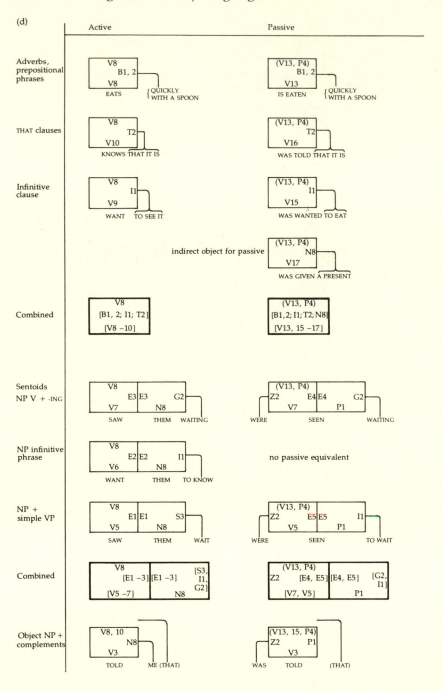

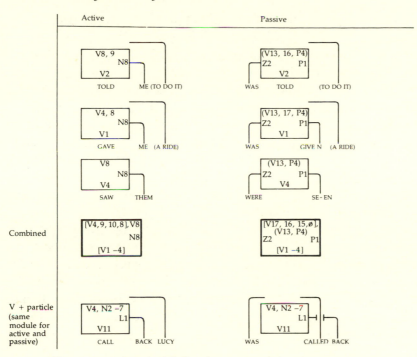

Figure 5.15 (*cont.*). (d) Combining modules that connect active or passive verbs to complements.

The same modules for the verb column can be inserted between the top and bottom modules for the passive form. The subject noun phrase connects at the *bottom* of the verb column through modules that have been used in other constructions. The optional P4 code *atop* the passive module (Z2/V4\P1) connects to the BY prepositional phrase. This permits the scope and dependency relations of the noun phrases in the passive to correspond to the scope and dependency relations of the noun phrases in the active.

Different verbs take different kinds of complements. Although in some cases differences in the complements may be attributed to differences in meaning (see, for example, the discussion on PERSUADE, which operates on sentient beings, and EXPECT, which can apply to events, in Appendix B), in other cases these complements appear to be purely syntactic matters. Figure 5.15(c) gives a sample of verb modules and an explanation of what their codes connect to in the active form.

In order to permit the same sort of connections in the passive form, new modules must be used and new codes must be assigned for verb complements. Now, it is true that global rules might be able to avoid this duplication. If global rules turn out to be a more accurate representation of a language user's knowledge, the local rules given here have at least provided a description of the information needed for the global rules to operate on. Note that a global rule that simply converted the active to the passive would ignore some active forms that do not have the same passive complements (for example, I WANTED THEM TO KNOW ABOUT IT but not ★ THEY WERE WANTED TO KNOW ABOUT IT BY ME; I RESEMBLE MY SISTER but not ★ MY SISTER IS RESEMBLED BY ME; I SAW THEM WAIT FOR THE LIGHT and THEY WERE SEEN TO WAIT FOR THE LIGHT). Figure 5.15(d) shows the corresponding active and passive complement modules for the verb column. It also combines similar modules into a single module with ordered connection codes.

Nominalizations related to the passive and active forms

In transformational grammar, the "subject" of a sentence is defined as the main, or first, noun phrase of the deep structure and the "object" the main noun phrase of the verb phrase. In order to avoid confusing this use of "subject" and "object" with that of other grammars, we can call the relation of the transformational subject to the rest of the sentence a type 1 relation and that of the transformational object a type 2 relation. Transformational grammar points out that the following groups of sentences all express a type 1 relation to I (ME) and a type 2 relation to THE DOG.

I SAW THE DOG EATING

THE DOG WAS SEEN EATING BY ME

I GAVE UP THE DOG

THE DOG WAS GIVEN UP BY ME

I GAVE MY COUSIN THE DOG

THE DOG WAS GIVEN (TO) MY COUSIN BY ME

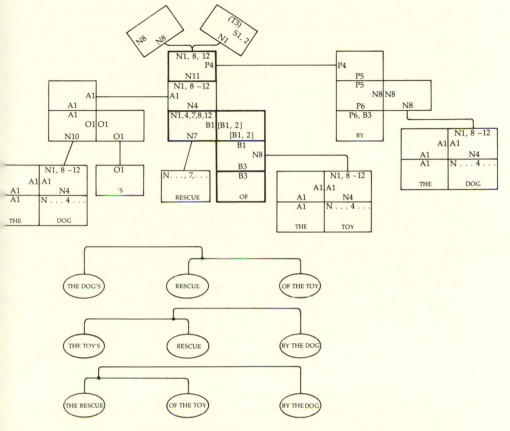

Figure 5.16. Modules for type 1 and type 2 relations in nominals.

The syntax crystal modules illustrated in Figure 5.15(d) can combine to show a type 1 relation with I (ME) and a type 2 relation with THE DOG. However, these relations are not defined in terms of the order in which they occur but in terms of their scope and dependency relations to the other morphemes in the string.

Similar scope and dependency relations will occur with modules for noun phrases that express similar relations. Remember, corresponding to THE DOG RESCUES THE TOY and THE TOY WAS RESCUED BY THE DOG are the nominals THE DOG'S RESCUE OF THE TOY and THE RESCUE OF THE TOY BY THE DOG. Modules for such nominals are given in Figure 5.16.

The orreries for the nominals in Figure 5.16 are topologically the same, and the same (except for placement of function terms) as those for the sentences: THE DOG RESCUES THE TOY and THE TOY WAS RESCUED BY THE DOG.

If the modules for TOY, DOG, and RESCUE have the *same* top codes, there could be combinations that would be hard to understand: THE RESCUE'S DOG, THE TOY BY THE RESCUE. If these were eliminated syntactically by using different top codes, they would be ruled out rather than treated as combinations that are well formed syntactically but semantically anomalous. Earlier, we argued against treating such distinctions syntactically. However, it is clear that the syntax crystal could follow other theories by making additional distinctions in the module codes so that, say, only abstract nouns can take BY prepositional phrase modifiers of the sort shown above. Further specialization of prepositions could also be attained.

The syntax crystal does not predict that a particular kind of modifier will involve a type 1 or a type 2 relation. Thus THE DOG'S RESCUE is ambiguous, i.e., the DOG may be either rescuer or rescuee. However, further specification can determine whether a type 1 or type 2 relation is expressed by these phrases. Thus in THE DOG'S RESCUE OF THE BOY, THE DOG has a type 1 relation, and in THE DOG'S RESCUE BY THE BOY, THE DOG has a type 2 relation.

Questions

Recall from the preceding chapter that for questions, as for phrasal verbs, phrase structure grammars require a number of independent rules, and transformational grammars posit a base structure different from the surface structure plus transformation rules to convert the base to the surface.

For the syntax crystal, ȳes-no questions can be formed using the modules in Figure 5.17(a). These can be connected to the auxiliary modules shown earlier in Figure 5.13 and again in 5.17(b). The optional Q2 on the left of one question module allows question adverbs to be connected. As long as the optional Q2 and the optional T3 (which serves to embed the sentence in a higher sentence) have not been connected, the yes-no question modules and the declarative sentence modules will be interchangeable. Thus it does not take a totally new set of rules to make the ques-

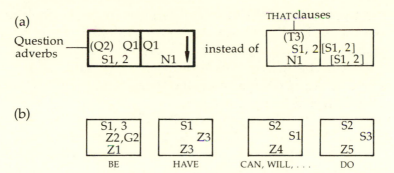

Figure 5.17. (a) Modules for yes-no questions. (b) Verb auxiliary modules.

tion form of various sentence types. Nor does it require the assumption that one form is basic and the other is derived from that form.

The arrow on the question module ensures that the noun phrase column will occur between the question auxiliary and the rest of the verb phrase. See Figure 5.18 for an example. Connections for the interrogative form are labeled I; those for the de-

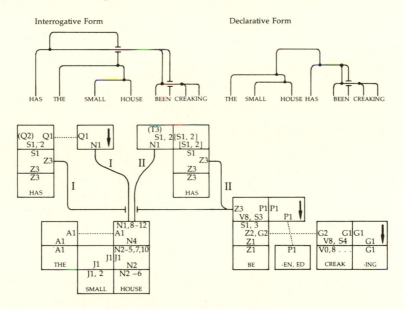

Figure 5.18. Modules for declarative and interrogative forms. Part of the crystal is the same for both forms.

clarative form labeled II. The differences between the interrogative and declarative crystals is that two modules are in a different position and two other modules are new. All the rest of both crystals is the same. Thus different modes with the same basic relations are shown to correspond and the syntactic rules are not multiplied beyond necessity.

We do not have to suppose that a language user generates a question by using cognitive operations analogous to moving two rules and changing two others in the declarative form. One does not have to detect the similarity between two corresponding forms in order to use both of them. As linguists, we can see the similarity in the two forms with an overview, noting that the orrery relations are the same (except for the presence or absence of a question operator) and that this economizes on the rules a language user has to employ.

Transformational theory portrays the similarity across different sentence forms as structural similarity. In transformational theory, structural similarity means similarity in the base rules that are used for the different sentences. For the syntax crystal, similarity across forms is also portrayed as structural similarity. However, for the syntax crystal, structural similarity means only topological similarity; the rules that connect topologically similar structures may or may not be the same. As we explained in Chapter 2, this is because transformational theory requires the information contained in the base rules for semantic interpretation, while our theory claims that only scope and dependency information are essential.

Negation

For negation, an optional code added to a few modules already described and two new modules can handle all the different constructions (Figure 5.19b[a]). The arrowed module for negation allows NOT to occur in the midst of the constituent it operates on. In Figure 5.19(b) the scope of NOT is IT MIGHT HAVE CREAKED; in (c) it is MIGHT HAVE CREAKED; in (d) it is TO GO. And in both (e) and (f) the scope of NOT is HAS IT CREAKED. In (e) and (f) both the N1 and X2 occur on arrowed modules. If we interpret the positional priority exception as meaning that an arrowed module

(a)

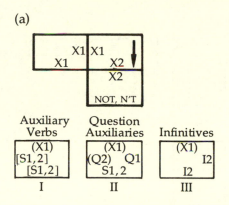

Auxiliary Verbs	Question Auxiliaries	Infinitives
(X1) [S1,2] [S1,2]	(X1) (Q2)　Q1 S1,2	(X1) I2 I2
I	II	III

(b)

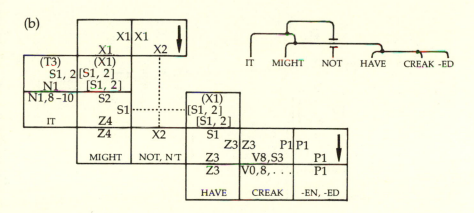

(c)

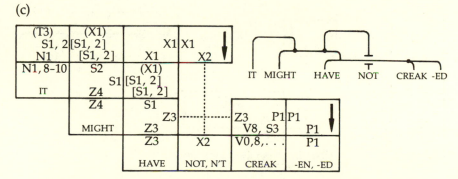

Figure 5.19. (a) Modules for negation. (b, c) Constructions using Module I. *Continued on the next page.*

(d)

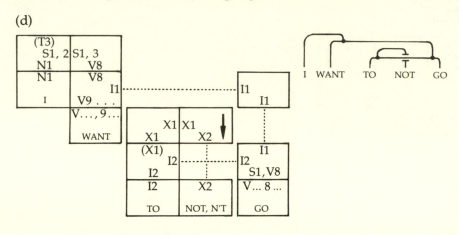

(e)

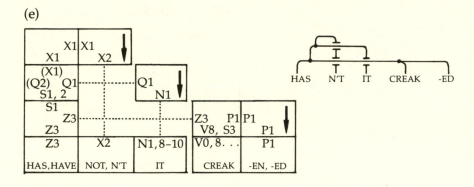

(f)

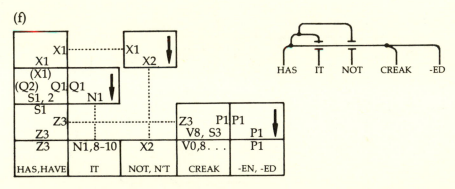

Figure 5.19 (*cont.*). (d) Constructions using Module III. (e,f) Constructions using Module II.

forces only nonarrowed modules to move out of its way, then the strings of (e) and (f) are both possible. If it turns out that this interpretation leads to unacceptable strings in other constructions, a stricter interpretation can be adopted. This would require *all* modules, including other down-arrowed modules, to move out of the way of a down-arrowed module higher up in the structure. Thus the positional priority exception would become the exact inverse of the positional priority rule itself. In such a case, additional structure modules would be required to generate the string in (f).

Relative clauses

The purpose of discussing relative clauses in this chapter is to illustrate some additional properties and some problems of syntax crystal modules. Relative clauses are very much like certain sentences, except that instead of a noun phrase in the sentence, there is a noun phrase plus relative pronoun (which is sometimes optional) preceding the relative clause. For example:

1. I JOG WITH THE GIRL
   THE GIRL (WHO(M)) I JOG WITH
2. YOU SAW THE DOG EATING
   THE DOG (THAT) YOU SAW EATING
3. I BELIEVE THAT YOU TOLD THE STORY
   THE STORY THAT I BELIEVE (THAT) YOU TOLD

And the pair discussed earlier:

4. THE HOUSE IS SMALL
   THE HOUSE THAT IS SMALL

Transformational theories treat relative clauses as embedded sentences to which transformation rules are applied. That is, they posit the same underlying structure – the same base rules – for relative clauses as for sentences. However, there are many sentences and positions of noun phrases that do not have corresponding relative clauses. Some examples are:
Questions:

DID CAROL HEAR THE DOG EATING?

★THE DOG (THAT) DID CAROL HEAR EATING

(WHAT NP1 verb) IS (VP-minus-verb) forms:

WHAT CAROL HEARD WAS THE DOG EATING

★THE DOG (THAT) WHAT CAROL HEARD WAS EATING

Coordinate structures:

> FIDO LIKES EGGS BUT TABBY LIKES CEREAL
>
> ★ THE EGGS THAT FIDO LIKES BUT TABBY LIKES CEREAL

NPs modifying the subject:

> THE WOMAN WITH THE HAT WALKED AWAY
>
> ★ THE HAT (THAT) THE WOMAN WITH WALKED AWAY[6]

NPs of some prepositional phrases modifying NP in the VP:

> I SAW THE HOUSE WITH THE GARDEN
>
> ★ THE GARDEN I SAW THE HOUSE WITH

NPs (other than of PrepPs) modifying NPs:

> I BUILT A DOG HOUSE
>
> ★ A (THE) DOG THAT I BUILT HOUSE
>
> I BORROWED THE PITCHER'S GLOVE
>
> ★ THE PITCHER THAT (WHOSE) I BORROWED GLOVE

Predicate nominatives:

> ALICE IS A LAWYER
>
> ?THE LAWYER WHO(M) ALICE IS

Few of these possibilities are eliminated by transformation rules themselves. Some are prevented by ordering the rules and making some rules last-cycle-only (or "root" transformations). Others are eliminated only by ad hoc stipulation: Do not move NPs in such and such positions (Ross, 1967).

In this section we will discuss how syntax crystal modules can handle some of the properties of relative clauses. We do not provide modules for all features of relative clauses, but we hope that this preliminary discussion will aid in the study of how local rules might handle these apparently intricate relations.

Because relative clauses and sentences are similar, for economy the syntax crystal, like transformational grammar, uses the same set of rules to construct both. Modules specific to relative clauses are added or substituted to connect the clause to the rest of the string.

The module, shown earlier, that connects nouns to the relative clauses modifying them is that in Figure 5.20(a). Where the relative pronoun is the subject of the relative clause, the module in Figure 5.20(b) connects on the right to verb phrases and through the bottom code to the relative pronoun. But a more complex structure is required when the relative pronoun is not the subject. We need modules to replace those connecting to noun

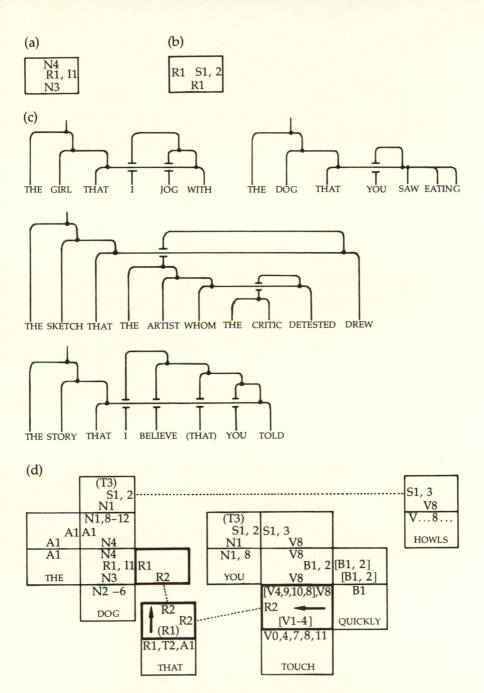

Figure 5.20. (a) Connects nouns to relative clauses. (b) Connects relative pronoun to verb phrases. (c) Orreries for relative clauses. (d) Modules for the orreries. *Continued on the next page.*

(e)

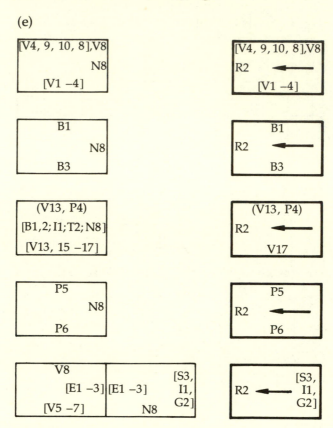

Figure 5.20 (*cont.*). (e) Modules for object noun phrases and their corresponding relative clause modules.

phrases such as direct objects, indirect objects, objects of prepositions, and those in sentoids. And we want the relative pronoun to have the same orrery relations as the noun phrase would have had in the sentence. Figure 5.20(c) shows some orreries for relative clauses.

The syntax crystal needs to make use of positional priority exceptions to handle such constructions. The relative pronoun needs to displace all other modules in the embedded clause to appear on the far left of the clause. Figure 5.20(d) shows some modules that effect constructions like those in Figure 5.20(c). The module with the leftward arrow replaces a module that would in other constructions connect to a noun phrase. This new module connects to modules that then connect to a relative pronoun in a different place. The module with the leftward arrow displaces the module to which it points until the displaced module no longer interferes with any module connected to the arrowed one. This allows THAT to precede the remainder of the relative clause. The module with the upward arrow, although its positional priority exception is not needed in this particular example, lifts the main noun phrase above the relative clause so that the main verb phrase (HOWLS) appears at the end of the string.

Corresponding to the modules with N8 codes, there must be modules with a leftward arrow and an R2 code on the left edge as shown in Figure 5.20(e). These modules cannot be assembled randomly without the risk of ungrammatical embeddings such as those discussed earlier. One way to prevent this is to use extra modules to govern the top of the embedded subject and verb columns. But this introduces a new feature, multiple scope connections. The relative pronoun connects to the verb column at both the top and some other place in the verb phrase, as well as to the noun phrase. This gives the relative pronoun several scope and dependency relations: one that corresponds to the noun phrase as it would appear in the sentence form, another indicating that it is the main term in the relative clause, and yet another connecting it to the top of the embedded subject column. It seems unlikely that these multiple scope connections are desirable; another way of ruling out unwanted constructions would be preferable Figure 5.21(a) gives the alternative relative clause modules with multiple scope connections.

In this case only two modules with upward arrows are needed to take the place of modules with N8 connections. They are shown in Figure 5.21(b). But other modules that may occur at the top of the verb phrase must be coded with an R5 or R6. These are shown in Figure 5.21(c). The extra connections that prevent such strings as ⋆ THE COAT THAT WAS I PROMISED TORE; ⋆ THE COAT THAT THE DOG WITH ATE A FLOWER; and ⋆ THE COAT THAT THE HAT THAT THE DOG WITH ATE also produce problems when used for random generation. Impossible crystals may result because the structure can grow independently from more than one place on the verb

(a)

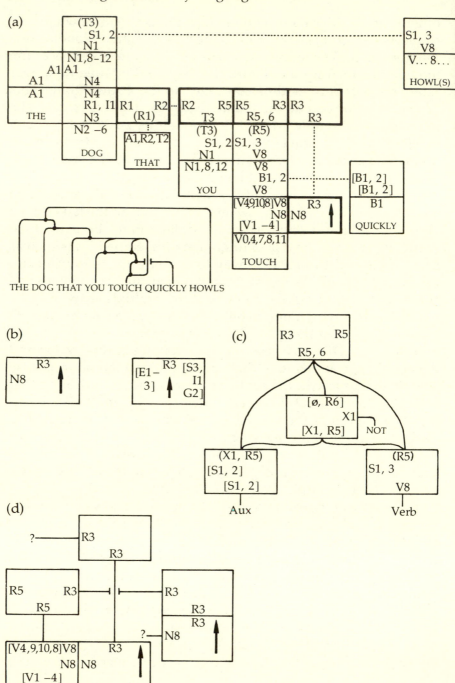

THE DOG THAT YOU TOUCH QUICKLY HOWLS

(b)

(c)

(d)

column. For example, in Figure 5.21(d) duplicate structures grow from the R3 and N8 codes without joining each other. Neither scheme for relative clauses rules out relative clauses such as:

- ★ THE HOUSE THAT CAROL WAS HEARD BY THE DOG FROM
- ★ THE CORNER I MET MY FRIEND AROUND
- ★ THE SKETCH I KNOW THE ARTIST WHO DID

If we want to eliminate these possibilities syntactically, we must construct local rules that will discriminate among different sorts of noun phrase modifiers. For example, one might begin by positing a difference in structure shown by the orreries in Figure 5.22. Then, one would need relative clause modules that would only connect to the nouns within noun phrases having the largest (or equally large) scope and/or dependency value. How such constraints might be represented in terms of syntax crystal modules is yet to be worked out. For more on relative clauses and their relation to other grammatical forms, see Appendix B.

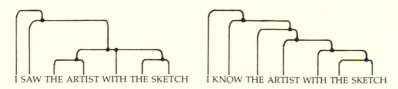

I SAW THE ARTIST WITH THE SKETCH   I KNOW THE ARTIST WITH THE SKETCH

Figure 5.22. Possible structural differences for some noun phrase modifiers.

Summary comparison of syntax crystal and transformational models

In the preceding chapter we described the basic features of transformational grammar. In this chapter we described those of the syntax crystal. Both models claim to present the essentials of a mechanism that could, with refinement, generate only and any of the well-formed strings of a natural language and also provide a correct description of their syntactic structures. Although there

Figure 5.21. (a) Alternative to modules in Figure 5.20, with orrery. (b) Relative clause modules needed for crystal in (a). (c) Other modules with R5, R6 codes needed for alternate relative clause structures. (d) An impossible crystal using relative clause modules.

are some differences, which we have pointed out earlier, both models claim the same domain of operation; they are functionally equivalent in the gross view. However, as we have indicated, there are several important differences in the operations of the two models – differences that are important in theoretical terms and also for the way in which each can serve as a model of the cognitive operations involved in language use. In this section we summarize the similarities and differences between the two models.

The two models differ as to the size of their basic local rule unit. In the base rules of transformational theory, syntactic elements are combined into rewrite rules, each of which describes a node at one level of the tree graph and its connections to at least one other node at a lower level. A module of the syntax crystal, in contrast, may provide information that lies entirely within a single node of the tree graph. The units are smaller than those of transformational theory. Modules may be combined into larger units resembling rewrite rules; however, as explained earlier, information may be lost in the combination.

A second difference is that the modules of the syntax crystal contain both scope and dependency information, while the local rules of transformational theory contain only scope information. The rewrite rule only makes use of left-to-right order in the configuration of elements. The module, on the other hand, using its geometry as a source of encoding, has both left-to-right order and dependency to contribute to syntactic structure.

The addition of dependency information to syntactic structure provides the syntax crystal with high structural resolvability without using information about the identity of individual elements and rules in the structure. In contrast, transformational theory requires that the identity of individual elements and rules be preserved for semantic analysis, for example, to distinguish subject, object, and verb. To portray similarities of paraphrases and grammatical variants that express the same relation of concepts, transformational theory has assumed it must reduce similar strings to base structures with similar rules and topology. The syntax crystal only needs to show that similar strings have similar topology.

This has an important consequence. A model of syntax must

show how the surface order of a string is related to the underlying representation that encodes the relations of concepts for semantic interpretation. In the syntax crystal this can be done in a *single* structure because of the added resolving power contributed by dependency and its ability to show the correct scope relations for discontinuous constituents. In contrast, transformational theory requires a base structure and a surface structure and a set of transformation rules that operate globally on a structure to map one onto the other.

The difference is illustrated by examining the formal operations required to change certain string forms, such as the interrogative passive, into others, such as the declarative passive form. (This does not imply that a language user would ordinarily perform such a change.) In transformational theory, rules that produce question forms are usually last-cycle-only rules to prevent them from being applied to some phrases that are given base representations as embedded sentences. Only on the last cycle – for the complete sentence – may the conversion to a question form take place. So, to convert an interrogative passive string to a declarative passive, transformational theory would start with the surface structure of the interrogative passive, apply the question transformations in reverse until a structure free from such transformations is obtained, and then change direction and apply the rules in forward order to derive the surface structure. This process might require a return all the way to the base structure to eliminate a question marker. The syntax crystal would replace the interrogative mode modules in the crystal of the first string with the mode modules for the declarative form. This would force the remaining local rule modules to rearrange themselves into the second structure *without any additional control information.*

The two models differ as to the nature, complexity, and number of global operations required for each. For transformational theory these global operations are the transformation rules and the metarules that control them. For the syntax crystal the global operations are the positional priority principle and the exception signaled by an arrow on any module that requires it.

Both types of global operations control the position of syntactic constituents or parts of constituents. Transformation rules change the position of (or insert or delete) an element from one structure to another. The positional priority rules for the syntax crystal, in contrast, only control the position of constituents during the generation of a single structure.

The variety of transformation rules was discussed in the previous chapter along with a brief description of the metarules that constrain their application. In contrast, the positional priority rule and its exception is one rule plus a corollary that can be described in a few words. This is because the positional priority rule is very general: It makes no distinctions among the different syntactic modules except for whether or not the arrow signifying an exception is present. On the other hand, the elements of transformation rules are particular syntactic constituents. These constituents, and often their syntactic context, must be recognized in order for the transformation rules to operate. For example, a simplified description for one analysis of the placement of relative pronouns is: Take the element dominated by Article and followed by Nominative in a Noun Phrase embedded in a Sentence which itself follows a Nominative that equals the other Nominative, and if the element has the feature [−wh, . . .] give it the features [+wh, +Relative, +Pronoun], erase the Nominative following the Article, and delete the Sentence boundaries of the embedded Sentence (Stockwell, Schachter, and Partee, 1969:494). To execute this rule, a series of rather detailed analyses must be performed by the syntactic mechanism in order to identify the elements to be manipulated. In the preceding chapter we argued that these additional analyses themselves require explanation and therefore transformational theory could only serve as an incomplete model of the cognitive operations involved in language use. For the syntax crystal's positional priority rule, if any (non-arrowed) module encounters an obstruction to its bottom code from any other module, it moves one space and tries again. Thus all global operations are reducible to a simple recursive procedure.

To some extent, the features of transformational grammar and the case categories of other theories are replaced by the differentiation available in the connection codes of the syntax crystal modules. The syntax crystal, however, does not claim that this information plays any but a supplemental role in semantic interpretation; its job is to eliminate the possibility of ill-formed strings.

The top codes of morpheme modules serve the same function as some lexical rules. In transformational grammar, for example, lexical rules for EAT would be: V, [———NP], [———] indicating that it is a verb, can take an object, but the object need not be present. For the syntax crystal, the top codes for the EAT module would include V4, which connects to direct objects, and V8, which connects to adverbial modifiers or the main verb phrase without connecting to a direct object. The sort of verb phrase EAT can connect to is determined by the top codes on its module. In the next chapter we will describe how this differentiation appears during language acquisition and compare its role with those of cases, features and lexical rules of other theories.

The notational variant criticism

In the preceding section we summarized some of the differences between our model and the leading syntactic theory, transformational grammar. In order to facilitate the comparison, we showed earlier how syntax crystal rules could be partly translated into rules somewhat similar to those used in the base structure of transformational grammar; how similarities across different grammatical forms explained by transformational grammar could also be explained by syntax crystal;[7] and how the syntax crystal, like transformational grammar, often requires just a few differences in the rules for different grammatical forms.[8] These comparisons were made in order to clarify the differences between the two models. However, once we have shown any similarities between the two models, defenders of transformational grammar may be tempted to claim that our model is "merely a notational variant" of the established model. This is a standard challenge directed toward any new proposal in linguistic theory.[9] Since we are presenting a new theory, we wish to anticipate this kind of criticism and show that it does not apply to the orrery–syntax crystal model. To do that, we need to analyze the notational variant criticism more closely.

There are at least three different kinds of similarities between theories that might provoke the notational variant charge. We can call them (1) term-by-term equivalence, (2) rule-system equivalence, and (3) domain equivalence. A model that is *term-by-term* equivalent to an established model is the most vulnerable to the notational variant criticism. A simple example would be a new model of arithmetic that substitutes a different set of symbols for the numerals "0" through "9." On a formal analysis, the new system would perform arithmetic operations identically with the current system. Such an innovation might be dismissed on the grounds that it was merely a notational variant. However, even this serious charge should not cause the new model to be dismissed out of hand. There may be empirical grounds on which the new model is superior. For example, the new symbols might have acoustic and visual representations that give them higher mnemonic and discriminative value, perhaps making it easier for machines or the visually handicapped to identify them. Of course, it would be up to the proponents of the new system to demonstrate these advantages.

When a new model is *rule-system* equivalent to an established model, each of its operations is translatable, without losing or gaining information, into one of the operations of the old model. For example, the *defining* and *computational* formulas of statistical parameters such as variance are equivalent. The computational formula for variance can be translated, with no loss or gain of information, into the defining formula. In the formal sense, the two systems of formulas may be considered notational variants of each other. However, there are important differences that justify the existence of both systems: The defining formulas are heuristically more useful – it is easier to see what they mean; while the computational formulas are much easier to use on numerical data. Another example of rule-system equivalence is that of the rules for natural deduction and for truth trees for logic. Proofs with truth trees are more mechanical and easier to do, but proofs with natural deduction are easier to understand.

A new model that agrees with an established model about what is to be included in the phenomenon to be explained is *domain* equivalent to the established model. Since the end products of both models are the same, the new model may be accused of being a notational variant, although the intermediate processes differ in important ways.[10] If there are significant differences in the intermediate processes, there are really no grounds for the criticism. For example, it is in this sense that binary arithmetic is a notational variant of decimal arithmetic. The results of any computation in either system will be the same: If N people take an equal portion of M pies, they each end up with M/N pies, regardless of the computational system used to effect the division. However, the basic units and the actual method of computation are different. And the differences are very important: Binary computation allows the integration of logic and arithmetic and also can easily be implemented in electronic circuitry, which can reliably transmit information in two states, on and off. Binary arithmetic's use of units of a different size is essential to Boolean algebra and practical computer design. Without the new notation, these would not exist.

In summary, a new model may be like an established model in several ways. It may be identical except for the names of individual terms. It may employ different terms but combine them in ways that are translatable into the combinations of the established model. It may differ in both terms and internal mechanics but agree as to the data or phenomena to be explained.

A notational variant may be equivalent to an established model in these three ways. A new model that differs from an established one on all three grounds – terms, mechanics, and definition of subject matter – cannot be called a notational variant. We believe that we have demonstrated in this chapter that the orrery–syntax crystal differs from transformational theory in all three ways. Nevertheless, since there are some important aspects that the two models share, it will be helpful to compare other models of syntax that no one takes to be merely notational variants of each other, although they share many important features.

Transformational grammar is not considered a notational variant of phrase structure grammar because it introduced some important features not shared by phrase structure grammar. We described these innovations earlier, among them, global transformation rules and metarules, an underlying syntactic structure that differs from the surface structure, shared underlying structure to explain paraphrase similarity. But note that transformational grammar and phrase structure grammar are similar to each other in important ways: They agree on the end product of their operation, the grammatical strings; surface structures (phrase markers) are essentially the same. Both models employ many of the same grammatical categories; both employ production rules and recursion. They differ not in their output, nor in the kinds of elements or categories they operate on, nor even in *all* the rules and properties of rules they use. What keeps transformational grammar from being considered a notational variant of phrase structure grammar is the nature of *some* of its rules.

The preceding section comparing the orrery–syntax crystal with transformational theory described analogous similarities and differences. The models agree about what strings are to be produced and show the same hierarchical, recursive, and scope properties in their final surface structures. However, on the possible kinds of equivalence discussed at the beginning of this section, the orrery–syntax crystal shows important differences. The basic units of syntactic categories are roughly equivalent. This is a consequence of an essential property of language. Although we used letter-number combinations for morpheme codes, we tried to stress their similarity to established element forms by using conventional letter abbreviations for syntactic categories. Many of the syntax crystal modules could be translated into conventional category names, plus a set of syntactic features. The use of letter-number codes instead of category names represents our position that language users need not be aware of particular syntactic features but that they just be able to recognize similarities and differences in the distributional properties of morphemes.

When considering rule-system equivalence, we can see that the models are considerably different. The orrery–syntax crystal introduces a feature, dependency, not found in transformational theory. It is carried in the geometry of the cellular automaton basis of the crystal. Dependency could be added to transformational theory, but a new system of rules would have to be introduced and many transformation rules would then become unnecessary. The rules of our model correspond more closely, not to the rules of transformational grammar, but to the elements of its rules. In Chapter 6 we shall demonstrate how these smaller units make possible an explanation of the learning of hierarchical syntactic structure. Another difference is that our model generates surface structures directly in one step as opposed to the multi-stage processing used by transformational theory. Instead of many different global transformation and metarules, our model has a single general principle, the positional priority rule. While it is possible to interchange the syntax crystal rules in a way that mimics transformational operations, it is *not* possible to manipulate the rules of transformational theory to generate strings in a single step as does the syntax crystal.

With respect to the third way in which models may be equivalent, in terms of how they define the phenomenon to be explained, there are also some differences between our model and transformational theory. For example, transformational theory holds that every relation of concepts must have a different underlying structure; that is, syntax must resolve all differences in sentential semantics. In contrast, we have allowed the possibility that some underlying structures may be ambiguous, just as some words are. Since we use classic transformational examples to show how the orrery–syntax crystal can provide distinct structural interpretations for different relations of concepts, this difference between the models needs to be remembered.

In this section we have tried to demonstrate that (1) the notational variant criticism is complex, and even where it may be applied to a limited extent, there are often good formal and empirical reasons for the introduction of a new notation system; (2) that the orrery–syntax crystal is not merely a notational variant of transformational theory, even though the two models share several properties that are essential to a theory of language.

6

Syntax acquisition

In the preceding chapter we introduced the syntax crystal model, demonstrating how it worked and how it could be used to generate and parse natural language strings. We showed how the model could handle many of the linguistic structures that have been used to illustrate the power of transformational grammars. We argued that the local rules of the syntax crystal were more accessible to explanation at the cognitive level. And especially important, the syntactic rules of the model use a minimum of essential features and thus are easy to map onto the conceptual structure underlying language strings.

In this chapter we are going to show how the syntax crystal model makes it easier to explain the acquisition of syntax. With very few assumptions, the model demonstrates how the information used to construct the complex hierarchical structures of syntax can be gradually acquired using a simple mediated learning principle. In advocating a model to account for syntax acquisition by learning theory principles, we are moving counter to the nativism allied with transformational theories. Therefore, we are going to divide this chapter into two parts. The first part opens the territory for a learning account of syntax acquisition by examining and challenging the view held by Chomsky and others that there are innate, specifically linguistic mechanisms for syntax. The second part discusses the acquisition of syntax using the syntax crystal model.

Where do language abilities come from?

Dating from Chomsky's (1957) early work, transformational psycholinguists have suggested that children acquire syntax by making use of an innate Language Acquisition Device (LAD). Examples of such approaches are those of Lenneberg (1967), McNeill (1970), Fodor, Bever, and Garrett (1974), and Fodor (1975). The nature of such a device is specified only in general terms: The LAD is presumed to be species-specific, a part of the genetic endowment of the human infant. It is thought to be specific to language rather than a more general mechanism that could handle other complex cognitive skills. It is not believed to be a store of all linguistic information, but its job is to direct or restrict the formation of syntactic rules.

Since a child acquires the syntax of the particular language it is exposed to, the LAD does not determine the particular rules of syntax that are acquired. Instead, it is thought to operate on a more general level, guiding the child to make generalizations from the language it is exposed to. But the LAD would allow these generalizations to only occur along particular dimensions and only be of certain sorts. Like other innate mechanisms posited to explain animal behavior (cf. Tinbergen, 1951), the LAD is supposed to be triggered by environmental conditions at some stage of development. The notion of critical periods in language acquisition was developed most fully by Lenneberg (1967). The child is not viewed as "knowing" syntax at birth, nor as being able to use or develop syntactic rules without being exposed to a natural language. Rather the process is thought to be epigenetic, an interaction between innate and environmental factors.

According to those who posit an innate LAD, it is thought to have evolved, like the apposable thumb, through evolutionary selection pressure and to be the exclusive property of the human gene pool. Support for this view was once mustered from the claim that language was only possible for members of the human species (Lenneberg, 1967; Chomsky, 1972). This claim was based on the fact that only humans exhibited language despite serious efforts to teach other animals, especially primates, to talk (e.g., Hayes and Hayes, 1952). The inference derived from the comparison between humans and other animals was that nonhumans must be lacking some piece of cognitive machinery essential to learning language. And this mechanism was species-specific only to humans. However, as the work of Gardner and Gardner (1969) and others has shown, there was a confusion between "language" and "speech." The mechanism primates (at least) were lacking was that which gave them adequate control of the organs for speech. As soon as another modality was selected – manual transmission – primates began to make astounding gains in the acquisition of language. The debate still continues, usually focusing on some property of adult human language not yet exhibited by the subjects in the nonhuman language studies. However, new discoveries about the linguistic abilities of other primates are being made; their linguistic limitations are not yet known. Logically, the claim that the LAD is species-specific is independent of the claim that it is innate; the LAD might be shared by all members of the primate order. However, strategically, a species-specific mechanism was much easier to claim innateness for.

There are also other arguments for an innate LAD. Since we are going to argue that syntax acquisition can be explained on the basis of a simple learning mechanism, we are going to examine the remaining arguments for an innate LAD. They can be divided into four categories based on the approach taken by each:

1. Arguments against empiricism – the view that all cognitive abilities arise through experience. We will look at the way the nativism-empiricism debate has changed with respect to language.
2. Arguments against behaviorism – the view that internal processes are irrelevant to an explanation of learning. We will discuss how arguments against linear (word-word) association models to account for syntax learning have been mistakenly thought to extend to all associative learning models for language acquisition.
3. Arguments that syntax is not learned and/or taught. Here we consider arguments to the effect that syntax is too difficult to be learned in the time a child has available; that there is not enough information available to the child in the speech of adults; that syntax is not deliberately taught, therefore it could not be learned; and that learning in general requires an innate "language of thought" (Fodor, 1975).
4. Arguments that there are universals across languages, and language users, for which the only plausible explanation is an innate LAD. We will discuss a number of the universals that have been proposed in this argument and examine whether or not they imply an innate basis.

The nativism-empiricism debate

The debate about innate ideas has been raging for centuries. In the past, nativists were those who claimed that some ideas, for example, the concepts of God, or of causation, were innate. However, even the staunchest empiricist (e.g., Hume, 1739) believed that there were some prior principles used to connect ideas – for example, to associate ideas that were similar or occurred close together in time. Leibniz (1704), while arguing against empiricism, reached the perfect compromise in the debate. He claimed that although particular concepts were not innate, there were innate propensities that directed learning and played a role in selecting the ideas one acquired.

The contemporary nativism-empiricism debate in the realm of language has changed in the direction of Leibniz's compromise. It is no longer a debate about whether or not there are innate ideas – concepts, conscious thoughts – that are innate, but whether there are principles of syntax that are innate. As in many debates, the opponents often exaggerate the positions of their antagonists. Contemporary linguistic nativists often point to empiricism as denying that there are *any* innate linguistic principles or properties. Chomsky (1975) hoped to win the argument by demonstrating that there are some cognitive properties which are indeed innate. He cites the work of Hubel and Wiesel (1962), who found specialized cells in the brains of very young cats and monkeys that responded selectively to features of visual input such as vertical and horizontal lines and contours. This was taken as evidence that animals inherit at least some cognitive structure to parse the visual world. From this Chomsky suggests that it is reasonable to assume that some of the cognitive structure for processing language may be due to innate properties as well. (It is interesting to note that the argument for the species-specificity of language would not be supported by this transspecies argument.)

However, later research challenged the conclusion of Hubel and Wiesel in a way that may have a lesson for the debate over innate linguistic properties. Blakemore and Cooper (1970), Hirsh and Spinelli (1970), Barlow and Pettigrew (1971), and Blakemore and Mitchell (1973) have shown that kittens exposed only to either horizontal or vertical lines during critical periods in their infancy develop brain cells that respond selectively to those stimuli they were exposed to. Since atrophy was ruled out, what seems to be innate, then, is the *ability* to develop specialized cognitive structure as a result of experience. Language theorists should be very cautious at least in arguing for innate linguistic structure by appealing to demonstrations of innate cognitive structure in other areas of information processing. On the other hand, it is easy to accept that some innate characteristics of the human species facilitate or are necessary for language acquisition, for example, high intelligence, an innate affinity for fellow humans, possibly even predispositions to respond to human speech sounds more readily than other sounds. The later work in visual perception suggests, then, that even if the acquisition of language were shown to depend upon some uniquely linguistic abilities, these abilities themselves may have been learned as a result of early experience guided by other properties, which themselves may be nonlinguistic.

Arguments against traditional learning approaches to language acquisition

The argument for an innate language acquisition device seems to be aimed in part against behaviorist accounts of language acquisition such as those of Skinner (1957), and more recently, Winokur (1976). Behaviorists have suggested that language and its acquisition can be explained without appealing to any cognitive structure beyond the linear organization that appears in strings of words. But the arguments that externally observed behavior and environmental correlations are not sufficient to explain language is independent of arguments for an innate LAD. We argued against the former claim in Chapter 1.

Chomsky has always made clear that internal cognitive structure is essential to the understanding of language behavior and acquisition. He asks, "What initial structure must be attributed to the mind that enables it to construct . . . a grammar from the data?" (1972:79). In other words, what abilities, properties does the child need to have to learn the syntax and phonology of a particular language? We agree with Chomsky that this question is an important one. However, Chomsky assumes that any initial structure that guides learning must be specifically linquistic and genetically determined. It is here that we disagree.

Chomsky (1959 and elsewhere) has argued that traditional learning theory is inadequate to explain language, and at the same time he posits innate cognitive structure. Although the connection is not made explicit, Chomsky and others seem to be saying that the only alternative to innate structure is traditional learning theory. Therefore, if traditional learning theory can be shown to be inadequate, what remains as the only alternative explanation is innate structure. This reasoning has been ridiculed by G. Lakoff (1973), who pointed out the weakness in the implied argument by saying that "nothing follows from a lack of imagination." As Osgood (1963) and others have pointed out, learning theory need not be limited to associations between contiguous elements but may invoke mediated hierarchical associations. In this chapter we are going to show that such mediated hierarchical connections can serve as an adequate explanation for language acquisition.

A paradigm of the criticism directed against learning theory explanations for language acquisition is the inability to explain how a language user can generate, and parse, novel strings (Chomsky, 1957). As we pointed out in Chapter 1 and elsewhere (Robinson, 1977), the surface properties of language strings do not provide a basis for generalization from familiar to novel strings. It is only by looking at their underlying hierarchical properties that a basis for generalization can be found. Chomsky (1957) used the example of a "language" with just two elements, A, and B, and one rule of symmetric combination to illustrate this problem. In this language, AA, ABBA, and BAAAAB are well-formed strings. Generalizations from the surface properties of these strings, that is, the linear order of the string taken as a whole, does not provide the information required to allow other strings such as BBBB or BABBAB to be produced.

Even if we allow that the context can act like a discriminative stimulus and place conditions on the appearance of elements in the language, this is still inadequate. For example, let us suppose that BA could be produced in the context of AB, allowing AB BA; similarly for BA AB. But now we need to have a global stopping rule to prevent strings such as BA AB BA. That is, if AB is produced in the context BA, and BA in the context AB, then strings that are *not* symmetric (and therefore not well formed), such as BAABBA, might be produced, unless there are other principles of combination. The only alternative is to use an organizing principle that goes beyond the linear properties of the string. For example, one could allow contexts that are made up of elements that are not adjacent in the string. One could produce BB in the context of A ———— A, allowing ABBA, and AA in the context B ———— B, allowing BAAB. This would prevent strings that are not symmetric from being generated. But it presupposes a principle that organizes elements into contexts hierarchically, rather than by their linear order in the string. Thus, to the extent that natural languages have the properties of this symmetric language, which permits recursive embeddings of elements and phrase types in expansions, the symmetric language example shows that more has to be learned than which elements follow which other elements. In the preceding chapter we showed how syntax crystal modules can produce Chomsky's symmetric language from a structure that has simple associative connections between modules. But the association is not the linear sort, connecting contiguous elements in the string. It is a mediated hierarchical connection as described in the preceding chapter.

Arguments against the learning of syntax

Those who hold that there is an innate, specifically linguistic LAD use other arguments in addition to those based on the inadequacy of traditional learning theory and the appeal to innate structure that might underlie nonlinguistic activities. Another argument is that syntax is not learnable because the child is not exposed to enough information that could serve as the basis for learning. Of course, this view acknowledges that the details of syntax for particular languages are learned, but claims that the child must have a big head start in terms of general principles of syntax wired into the LAD. This is the *impoverished data thesis*. A second argument is that language is not *taught* to children, therefore language is not learned. This argument is usually presented as a complement to the impoverished data thesis. Still another argument claims that all learning requires theory construction and hypothesis testing about what is to be learned, and that theory construction and hypothesis testing require an innate "language of thought." A fourth argument is that there are properties of syntax that are universal to all languages, and the best explanation for the existence of such universals is the universality of a genetically given LAD. In the following subsections we will examine each of these arguments.

The impoverished data thesis.   Katz (1966) argues that the information available in any finite sample of language strings is inadequate to enable someone to generate novel strings correctly. And this would be so, he says, even if we granted the language learner the ability to recognize which features of the language are relevant syntactic cues. The problem, according to Katz, is that any finite set of data would allow several alternative hypotheses that could account for the structural properties of the sample strings. Since children choose the "correct" hypothesis, that is, the correct set of syntactic rules, there must be some innate predisposition to direct them.

What Katz says about language learning, Hume argued in 1739 was true of all knowledge: The data experienced are never sufficient to guarantee a generalization that goes beyond our experience. According to Hume, we have no real justification for any of our theories or beliefs about future events. The contemporary response (e.g., Goodman, 1955) to general skepticism such as Hume's is to point out that we do not make generalizations based on particular data alone, but related to what we know about the world, and our other theories and conceptual organizations, and that we have the opportunity to test our generalizations by continued experience and experiment. Although this does not give us complete certainty, in the skeptic's sense, it gives us good reasons for our hypotheses and generalizations. This is relevant to Katz's claim because he has supposed that the only data available to the child in making generalizations are language strings in isolation.

Performing a language induction task in isolation is analogous to trying to decipher tape recordings or hieroglyphs of an unknown language. As we discussed in Chapter 1, the only way to solve this problem is to do a distribution analysis without access to semantic information. As demonstrated by Miller and Stein (1963) and Moeser and Bregman (1972), the induction of syntactic rules without access to meaning is extremely difficult. Table 6.1 provides a sample of strings from an artificial language. Below

Table 6.1. *Sample strings and test questions in an artificial language*

Sample strings

1. re derfin	6. rek chamial crimek resket premin
2. re termas	7. rek derfinle crimek reket termasin
3. res loum	8. rek derfinle figek resket lumtin
4. re chamin	9. rek urjle figek resket loumin
5. re chamia	

Test

1. rek ——— crimek resket daltin
   a. resketle
   b. derfial
   c. loumle
   d. premle
   e. preminle

2. rek chamial ———
   a. figek reket chamian
   b. figek
   c. figek resket
   d. figek resketin

3. rek termasle crimek ———
   a. reket loumin
   b. reket termasinin
   c. resket urjlen
   d. resket derfian

---

the sample are three multiple-choice test questions. Before looking at Figure 6.1, try to abstract the syntactic principles and correctly answer the multiple-choice questions.

Now use the semantic information in Figure 6.1 and see how
much easier it is to learn the syntactic rules that allow you to answer the questions correctly.

Fortunately, language learners *do* have more information than
the syntactic data alone, which Katz correctly claims to be inadequate. What is available is the connection of linguistic elements
with the nonlinguistic environment. Syntactic structure encodes
the relations among the concepts named by the lexemes in a
string. If the language learner can understand any of the lexemes
in the string and can derive from the nonlinguistic context some
idea of what is expressed by the string, a knowledge of syntactic

rules can be developed. Later in the chapter, we will show in detail how this can be done.

The examples Katz uses to stress the necessity of an LAD raise just the sorts of problems that meaning and nonlinguistic context can help to solve. For example, Katz claims that the language learner would not be able to figure out that strings such as HELP THE MAN mean the same as YOU HELP THE MAN, rather than THEY HELP THE MAN or some other combination. He denies that:

> the language learner can make an inductive extrapolation of a second person pronoun subject from cases of sentences interpreted as requesting (commanding, etc.) something of the person addressed in which there is an explicit occurrence of "you" to cases also interpreted in this manner but in which there is no explicit occurrence of "you" . . . because as well as strings such as YOU HELP THE MAN and HELP THE MAN, there are also strings like (a) JOHN JONES HELP THE MAN, (b) EVERYONE HELP THE MAN, (c) NO ONE HELP THE MAN, (d) EVERYONE WITH A SERVICEABLE BOAT HELP THE MAN and indeed any of indefinitely many similar sentences with different noun phrase subjects also occur . . . Without an LAD there is nothing in the language learner's inferential equipment that prevents cases like (a)–(d) from leading to incorrect inductive conclusions about normal imperatives. [Katz, 1966:256, 258]

But surely the meaning of the individual words and the context in which a string such as HELP THE MAN occurs will make clear who is supposed to do the helping. However, Katz dismisses appeals to meaning:

> In each case, it is presupposed that the language learner understands a sentence $\underline{S}$ (whose final derived phrase marker is itself too impoverished to account on associationist principles for how he understands $\underline{A}$) because he can correlate $\underline{S}$ with another sentence $\underline{S}'$ whose final derived phrase marker is not too impoverished (it being the same as the underlying phrase marker for $\underline{S}$). [Katz, 1966:260]

What Katz is worried about is that $\underline{S}$ might be a string like HELP THE MAN and $\underline{S}'$, YOU HELP THE MAN. But he has missed the point: Understanding $\underline{S}$ does not require associating it with some other *string*, but with some relation of concepts, with an idea. The last quote above reveals an important assumption underlying Katz's impoverished-data argument against the learnability of syntax. He claims that "associationist principles" – and here he means linear, word-word connections – do not have enough information to make the generalizations needed for natural language

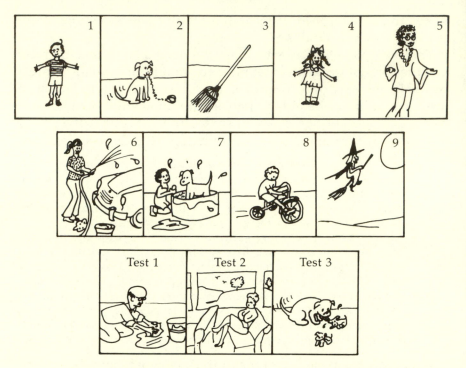

Figure 6.1. Semantic content for the strings and tests in Table 6.1.

syntax. If we accept his argument, it follows only that language learners need to use more than linear, word-word connections in order to learn language. It does *not* follow from his argument that the data available to the language learner – when nonlinguistic data are included – are too impoverished to allow the needed generalizations.

The argument that language is not taught.   Another claim used to support the innate LAD is that language is not taught and therefore is not learned in any ordinary sense. Chomsky (1975:161) says: "Language is not really taught, for the most part. Rather, it is learned, by mere exposure to the data. No one has been taught the principle of structure-dependence of rules, etc. . . . . Nor is there any reason to suppose that people are taught the meaning of words." The only alternative, according to Chomsky (1972:53) is an "innate schematism that determines the form of knowledge of language." Using this LAD he says that "we can account for certain aspects of the knowledge of English possessed by speakers who obviously have not been trained and who have not even been presented with data bearing on the phenomenon in question in any relevant way, so far as can be ascertained."

What Chomsky denies is that the ordinary child requires a controlled training or "shaping" program (cf. Premack, 1971) in order to master linguistic skills. While it is debatable exactly how much deliberate shaping the average child receives, no one would claim that deliberate feedback and control over the child's linguistic experience is necessary. The power of the argument that language is not taught and therefore not learned seems to depend on our feeling that "teach" and "learn" are reciprocal concepts, that anything which is learned must be taught, analogous to terms such as "bequeath" and "inherit." But, that someone learns something does not necessarily imply that someone else is teaching that something.

The "bootstrap problem": an internal representation must already be present in order to acquire language. Fodor (1975:58), defending the hypothesis of an innate LAD, says, "The first point to make is that we have no notion at all of how a first language might be learned that does not come down to some version of learning by hypothesis formation and confirmation." He then argues that hypothesis formation and confirmation presupposes that there already be some representational system. In other words, to learn language (or anything else for that matter) the hypotheses and their tests must be mediated by some preexisting cognitive structure. Fodor then argues that this representational system is either innate or is itself learned through some other representational system. Therefore, *some* representational system must be innate. He calls such a representational system that mediates language acquisition, the "language of thought." He says: "It follows immediately that not all the languages one knows are languages one has learned, and that at least one of the languages one knows without learning is as powerful as any languages that one can ever learn [in order to be able to formulate the hypotheses and confirmations]" (Fodor, 1975:81).

One can interpret Fodor's argument charitably to be saying

merely that: For learning to occur there must be some internal processing and for internal processing there must be something inside to do it. In this sense his claim is true, but vague and uncontroversial. However, his terminology – "language of thought"– and his other arguments indicate that his claim is a much stronger one. Therefore, it is appropriate to challenge whether learning, in particular, language learning, requires hypothesis testing that must be mediated by a preexisting languagelike representational system.

Some things we learn by formulating and testing hypotheses that can be explicitly expressed in linguistic or some other symbolic form. But this is not true for all learning. Fodor's assumption that all learning can be reduced to hypothesis testing is either incorrect or is true only in a very extended sense. It is possible to demonstrate that learning, even quite complex learning, can take place without any process that could be reasonably called hypothesis formulation and testing. One early example was D. O. Hebb's (1949) cell assembly model. Hebb's model of neural firing patterns explained how an initially random system could develop cognitive structures merely on the basis of experience. Because Hebb's formulation was expressed in general and somewhat vague terms, Rosenblatt (1962) constructed an actual working model. This electromechanical device, the *Perceptron*, could automatically classify input stimuli into perceptually similar categories or into conventional categories, such as those used in learning to discriminate the letters of the alphabet. Since it can do this even when the input patterns are distorted and noisy or even when it receives inconsistent information about the proper categories, the task is not unlike what might be required to learn the syntactic categories of a natural language and the relations among them. Another example is the simple mechanical devices of Block (1965), which, although initially random, can learn how to extract the optimal strategies of several games, in many cases faster than humans can. Unless one wanted to say that an initially random structure is a representational system, these models falsify Fodor's claim. In none of the models would one wish to say that hypotheses are being formulated and tested.[1]

From this consideration of Fodor's argument, we can conclude

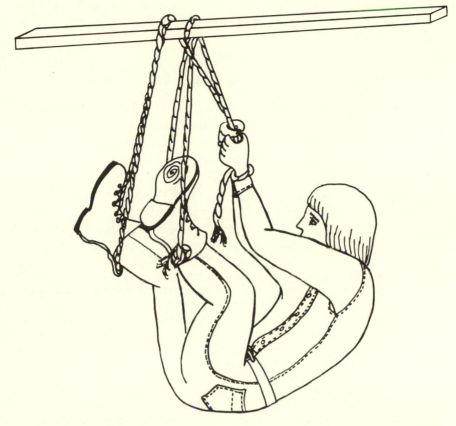

Figure 6.2. Solving the "bootstrap paradox."

that in order to show that language learning, in particular syntax learning, does not require a preexisting representational system (an LAD) one must show how syntactic structure can be developed from initially random connections.

The problem of seeming to require a language in order to learn a language is analogous to the old paradox involved in "pulling oneself up by one's bootstraps." The bootstrap paradox is resolved in a very simple way, as shown by Figure 6.2. Something outside the boots and the person is needed. For language acquisition without supposing that language structure preexists, the additional factor is the nonlinguistic environment. Later in the chapter we will demonstrate how syntax can be learned when we allow the nonlinguistic environment to provide information to the language learner.

Nativist arguments based on linguistic universals

The claim for an innate LAD is often supported by appeals to the existence of linguistic universals. The argument is that if a certain property is found in all languages, including those that are historically unrelated, then the best explanation for this universal property of language is a universal property of language users. What all human language users share is their basic genetic endowment. Therefore, there is an innate LAD.

Chomsky describes the relationship between language acquisition and putative universal properties like this:

> The native speaker has acquired a grammar on the basis of very restricted and degenerate evidence; the grammar has empirical consequences that extend far beyond the evidence. At one level, the phenomena with which the grammar deals are explained by the rules of the grammar itself and the interaction of these rules. At a deeper level, these same phenomena are explained by the principles that determine the selection of the grammar on the basis of the restricted and degenerate evidence available to the person who has acquired knowledge of the language, who has constructed for himself this particular grammar. The principles that determine the form of grammar and that select a grammar of the appropriate form on the basis of certain data constitute a subject that might, following a traditional usage, be termed "universal grammar." The study of universal grammar, so understood, is a study of the nature of human intellectual capacities. It tries to formulate the necessary and sufficient conditions that a system must meet to qualify as a potential human language, conditions that are not accidentally true of the existing human languages, but that are rather rooted in the human "language capacity," and thus constitute the innate organization that determines what counts as linguistic experience and what knowledge of language arises on the basis of this experience. Universal grammar, then, constitutes an explanatory theory of a much deeper sort than particular grammar, although the particular grammar of a language can also be regarded as an explanatory theory. [1972:27]

According to Chomsky, the search for linguistic universals is done both to strengthen the evidence for an innate LAD and also to discover the innate structure of the human mind. We are going to concentrate on the first goal, which is logically prior to the second. First, we will show that universals do not necessarily depend on innate cognitive structure. Then we will critically examine a sample of those properties that have been claimed to be linguistic universals.

Universals from sources other than innate cognitive structure

The argument for innate cognitive structure based on the existence of universal properties of human behavior is at best a heuristic one: Innate cognitive structure just seems to be a good candidate to be the explanation for universals. However, the lack of rigor in the argument is not mentioned by proponents of an innate LAD. One way to undermine the argument is to show that there are reasonable alternative explanations for universals in language. Consider an analogy:

All around the world there are games in which balls are used. Let us call them "ball-playing games." There is an enormous variety in the details of ball-playing games: bocce, pachinko, soccer, golf, and so on. However, there are some properties that all ball-playing games have in common, even those that have been developed in historically unrelated cultures. Let us call these common properties "ball-playing universals." Some of these are: the ball is always thrown or propelled in some way; the trajectory of the ball is critical to the outcome of the game; there are criteria for good performances; skill is involved that is learned gradually and, sometimes, in stages of proficiency, for example, a child can throw before it can catch.

Now we can ask whether the universals in ball playing support the existence of an innate "Ball-playing Acquisition Device" (BAD). In other words, is there something in the human genetic endowment that specifically facilitates the acquisition of ball-playing skills? There are certain innately determined capacities of ball players that influence the kinds of games they can play: perceptual-motor coordination, strength, grasping ability, competitiveness, and so on. However, these are general capacities that are not specific to ball playing.

In addition to these general capacities, there are other factors that may have affected the universal appearance of ball games. These factors include the rolling and ballistic properties of spheres (and their prolate variants), the universal effects of gravity, friction, elasticity, and the laws of dynamics.

Considering the general human capacities and the properties of balls and their physical environments, it is not convincing to claim that the universality of ball playing is evidence for the existence of an innate acquisition device specific to ball playing. Analogously for language behavior, there are certainly innately determined capacities (such as short- and long-term memory capacities, limits to perceptual and motor resolution of sounds or gestures), and some universal constancies in the physical and social environment of the child which determine or constrain the type of language that can be developed.

The analogy should make us suspicious of the nativist argument from universals. However, by itself the analogy does not prove that no linguistic universal can serve as evidence to support the existence of an innate LAD. There might be important differences between universals in language and universals in ball games. In what follows we shall consider some of the specific linguistic universals that have been proposed and see if they suggest the presence of innate, specifically linguistic, cognitive structure.

Some proposed linguistic universals

Syntactic universals.   Medieval philosophers made strong claims about the universality of syntactic relations. Roger Bacon said: "Grammar is substantially the same in all languages, even though it may vary accidentally" (Lyons, 1968:15–16). And from an anonymous scholar who was a contemporary of Bacon: "Whoever knows grammar in one language also knows it in another so far as its substance is concerned. If he cannot, however, speak another language, or understand those who speak it, this is because of the difference of words and their formations which is accidental to grammar" (Lyons, 1968:16). Lyons interprets these statements as follows: "When they are stripped of their metaphysical expression in terms of 'substance' and 'accidents,' [they mean]: all languages will manifest the same parts of speech and other general grammatical categories" (Lyons, 1968:16). Under this interpretation, the medieval claims are false; it is clear that languages differ in the grammatical categories they use. In Chapter 2, we reviewed some of the evidence against the universality of grammatical categories.

However, if we interpret "accidents" to mean surface structure and "substance" to mean deep structure, then the medieval claim is close to the modern position expressed by Chomsky (1965:118):

> It is commonly held that modern linguistic and anthropological investigations have conclusively refuted the doctrines of classical universal grammar, but this claim seems to me very much exaggerated. Modern work has, indeed, shown a great diversity in the surface structures of languages. However, since the study of deep structure has not been its concern, it has not attempted to show a corresponding diversity of underlying structures, and, in fact, the evidence that has been accumulated in modern study of language does not appear to suggest anything of this sort. The fact that languages may differ from one another quite significantly in surface structure would hardly have come as a surprise to the scholars who developed traditional universal grammar. Since the origins of this work in the *Grammaire générale et raisonnée,* it has been emphasized that the deep structures for which universality is claimed may be quite distinct from the surface structures of sentences as they actually appear.

And in summary, Chomsky says (1965:209–10): "In general it should be expected that only descriptions concerned with deep structure will have serious import for proposals concerning linguistic universals."

The constituent relations in surface structure can be very different from that of the deep structure, so it would be possible for languages to differ greatly on the surface yet have the same or similar deep structures. Since deep structures are never observed, only inferred, their form is restricted only by formal criteria – simplicity and consistency. For example, if it were less complex to assume that all languages used a verb-subject-object order in deep structure, then such an order could be considered a linguistic universal.

More frequently it is the *categories* of deep structure that are claimed to be universal. Transformational grammar aims to show similarities among the syntactic relations of different forms such as object of active verb and subject of passive verb. If this is done by positing a similar deep structure for active and passive, then the relations of subject and object in deep structure are considered linguistic universals (Chomsky, 1965). If this is done by positing agent and object relations in deep structure, then these are considered linguistic universals (Fillmore, 1968). And if this is done by positing lexical rules that relate active and passive forms, then active and passive are proposed as linguistic universals (Bresnan, 1978).

Other properties that are not directly a part of deep structure have been proposed to be universal: some because they allow a more economical set of transformation rules and others because restrictions on transformation rules are required to eliminate ungrammatical strings. Examples of the latter include Chomsky's "A-over-A" (1972:53 ff.) and "subjacency" (1975:78–118) principles, and Ross's "constraints on transformations" (1967). In a very curious argument, Chomsky (1965:209) claims that since such restrictions on transformations do not follow from transformational theory itself, they must be indications of the innate determinants of syntax, and therefore are universal. Ross's (1967:180) argument is simpler: Since no transformation rules exist that violate the restrictions, he suggests such restrictions be considered universal.

The argument that restrictions are embodied in an innate LAD because they are universal is nowhere spelled out clearly. But it is not enough to show that no existing rules violate the restrictions. Syntactic rules do not violate the laws of thermodynamics, nor the constraint that no relative clause may have only one consonant and no vowels. But neither of these are likely candidates for incorporation in an innate LAD. To some extent the whole argument is circular. The attribution of universality, and hence innate status, depends on the assumption that there *is* an innate LAD that restricts the hypotheses a language learner can formulate, which in turn restricts the rules and/or metarules possible for language. The existence of an innate LAD need not be presumed. It is easier to suppose that the need for such "universal" restrictions on transformation rules is an indication of a consistent, and therefore universal, shortcoming of the theory rather than highlighting the discovery of some components of innate cognitive structure.

In addition to constraints on the general properties of rules, the very operations performed by transformation rules are also seen as candidates for universals. According to Slobin (1971:17), "Such operations are linguistic universals, characteristic of all known human languages." In other words, transformational theory requires operations such as substitution, displacement, and permutation (ibid.) in order to achieve its goals of economical generation and the representation of similarities across different types of language strings. Independent of transformational theory, it is true that all languages can express the same relation of concepts in more than one way. Transformational theory explains this fact in terms of the operations performed by transformation rules. Other theories explain this fact without transformation rules, as we did in Chapter 5. Thus, only if we already accept transformational theory's explanation for the universal phenomenon that the same relation of concepts can be expressed in more than one way, could we accept transformational operations as linguistic universals.

On still another level of analysis, Osherson and Wasow (1976) have proposed that the use of order and inflection to express the thematic relations of subject, object, and indirect object is an innate, specifically *linguistic* universal. For a universal to be specific to language, it must not also be shared by other cognitive systems. This is what Osherson and Wasow (1976:211) argue: "For, neither the ordering of a set of elements, nor changes in their morphology [inflections] are employed to represent thematic relations in other cognitive systems (so far as we know), not even in nonlinguistic systems like Israeli Sign and Classical Chinese that share with natural language essentially identical purposes, namely, the expression and communication of thought." And there is no doubt about what Osherson and Wasow (1976:212) mean by an innate universal; it is something that is determined by "psychological and neurophysiological circumstances."

However, there are some reasons to be uncomfortable with their claim: In order for it to be true, some linguistic systems must be excluded from the class of natural languages. They admit that their claim for universality forces them "to construe the language faculty more narrowly than usual, as concerned with systems of sound–meaning correlation. Nonspoken 'languages', such as Israeli Sign and Classical Chinese (which only has a written form) are thus excluded from the class of natural languages" (Osherson and Wasow, 1976:210).

Further, the particular thematic relations they consider – subject, object, indirect object – represent a small subset of possible thematic relations. Other symbolic or representational systems, such as music and arithmetic, use order and inflection to express different thematic relations. And Osherson and Wasow's claim that the expression of thematic relations is universal depends upon a theory that portrays inferred thematic relations in the deep structure of strings that do not express such relations on the surface. For example, HELLO might be represented as, for example, I (subject) SAY (verb) HELLO (object) TO YOU (indirect object) in deep structure. In other words, the universality of the expression of thematic relations such as subject, object, and indirect object is not obvious. The universality only appears in an inferred theoretical structure that has no status independent of particular versions of transformational theory. Bresnan's (1978) version, for example, provides "functional structures" in the lexicon to handle subject-object relations, claiming instead that the active-passive relation is a linguistic universal.

Phonetic and developmental universals.   Proposed candidates for language universals have not been restricted to deep structure or even to the realm of syntax. For example, Lenneberg (1964:588) proposes as evidence for an innate LAD: "The absolutely unexceptional universality of phonemes, concatenation, and [the existence of] syntax and the absence of historical evidence for the slow cultural evolvement of these phenomena lead me to suppose that we have here the reflection of a biological matrix or Anlage which forces speech to be of one and no other basic type." The ball-playing analogy developed in the preceding section is helpful here. It may be that the properties Lenneberg mentions are indeed part of what we refer to as a natural language. In other words, such properties are universal because they are *defining* properties, just as certain properties are essential to our definition of a ball game. There are many systems of communication and symbolization that are not called "natural language" because they do not have one or enough of these properties (see Hinde, 1972). From bee dances to cave paintings, all these communication systems are related (MacKay, 1972). But only the ones with phonemes, concatenation, and syntax (of hierarchical, generative form) are called "languages" in the strict sense. It still remains for people who take such universals as evidence for an innate LAD, the "biological matrix or Anlage," to show that such properties of language do indeed arise from a language-specific genetic source.

When Lenneberg brings up the "absence of historical evidence for the slow cultural evolvement" of language properties he considers universal, he is suggesting that language appeared as the result of genetic mutations in the direction of an innate LAD. Leaving out extraterrestrial intervention, mutation would be a plausible explanation for a relatively sudden appearance of language in the history of the human species. However, it is not clear that the appearance of language was relatively sudden in human evolution. The absence of historical evidence for the slow cultural evolution of language is not surprising, given that speech and/or gesture communication undoubtedly preceded written forms for which there could be such a historical record.

The strongest argument for an innate LAD is based on claims that there is a universal regularity in the time-course of language development. Lenneberg (1967) presents the most complete argument, which is based on two main premises. First, he claims that regardless of wide differences in environment and general intellectual ability, each human child develops language skills following the same timetable. Second, he argues that there are critical periods during which the child must be exposed to language stimuli in order to develop linguistic skills. This is analogous to the critical period described by ethologists (Lorenz, 1957) wherein an animal, in order to develop normally, must be exposed to some particular stimulus conditions.

Although the timetable and the critical periods in language development are not as well defined as Lenneberg suggests (see Taylor, 1976, for a brief review), we can still acknowledge their existence without agreeing that they are the result of an innate, language-specific mechanism performing its program from genetic code. The order in which language rules and forms are mastered can be analyzed into a number of acquisition priorities such as simplicity, essentialness, saliency, concreteness, generality (Taylor, 1976:235). When looked at this way, it becomes easy to agree with Taylor when she suggests that these priorities "may occur in acquisition of other cognitive tasks than language" (1976:235). Clearly, Piaget's work has suggested that some simple principles describing the increase in information-handling ability of the child can explain the orderly development of general cognitive skills. We believe that it is most sensible to consider the developmental sequence of language as just one aspect of general cognitive development rather than presuming a specific innate mechanism guiding just this one skill.

The ball-playing analogy is again helpful. Consider the acquisition of skill at pocket billiards. Direct shots to sink one ball are acquired before shots made at greater angles; single cushion shots before multicushion shots; straight rolls before english spins; and so on. For billiard players all over the world, this acquisition sequence is universal. But we would not want to say that this was evidence for an innately programmed billiard acquisition device. Rather, the growth of general abilities, strength, coordination, reach, and the order of difficulty intrinsic to the various shots make the explanation of these developmental universals much simpler. So also for language development.

Innate versus learned structure: general considerations

Many language theorists have readily assumed that language acquisition depends upon a genetically programmed neural mechanism. We discussed how the inability of simple stimulus-response learning theory to explain hierarchical language structure helped to support the beliefs in innate structure. Then we looked at other arguments for the nativist position: the impoverished data thesis, the argument that language is not taught and therefore not learned, the "language of thought" bootstrap argument, and the arguments from universals. Each argument was criticized as we discussed it. Now we are going to raise some general issues to put the nativist position in critical perspective. Some of these criticisms were mentioned in connection with the individual arguments presented earlier.

First we will treat the problem of the *reduction* of linguistic properties. Here we will suggest that what have been considered to be specifically linguistic properties can often be explained in terms of more general properties. Next we will deal with the relationship among generality, universality, essentiality, and innate structure. Then we will discuss the distinction between theoretical priority and temporal priority showing how these have been confounded in nativist arguments. Finally, we will describe what we believe to be the necessary properties of language acquisition. This will lead us into our own formulation of language acquisition, which uses the syntax crystal model to show how syntax can be acquired without the need to postulate innate specifically linguistic structure.

Reduction of linguistic properties

As we discussed earlier in the chapter, several properties of language have been proposed as linguistic universals. Nativists have argued that any universal property that is specific to language is evidence for an innate cognitive mechanism specialized for language acquisition. Most of the universal properties discussed by nativists are syntactic, defined in terms of the hierarchical structure underlying language strings.

As we and many others have discussed, hierarchical structure is not the exclusive property of language: All complex motor and cognitive operations involve hierarchical organization. What is specific to language are the particular theoretical entities that are used to describe language structure. If, however, these theoretical entities could be shown to be reducible to, or to arise from, other, more general properties, it would be much harder to take the theoretical entities as evidence for an innate language acquisition device.

Reducing theoretical entities is an accepted goal in syntactic theory. Transformational theory does not define its theoretical entities in terms of other, more basic properties but it does not rule out the possibility of their being explained or reduced in this way. As Chomsky (1965:35) puts it: "Real progress in linguistics consists in the discovery that certain features of given languages can be reduced to universal properties of language, and explained in terms of these deeper aspects of linguistic form." Now, if we have reason to believe that universal syntactic properties can be reduced to, explained in terms of, *general* hierarchical properties, there is little reason to assume they arise from innate cognitive structure specific to language.

Universality, generality, essential properties, internal and innate structure

As we have shown, the arguments for innate linguistic structure are intertwined with arguments about universals and arguments for the necessity of considering the internal cognitive structure of the language user. By unraveling these arguments and by distinguishing between universal and essential properties, we can clarify the issues and show in what way our theory of language acquisition is related to the nativist view.

According to Chomsky, the several universal properties of language that have been discovered should not be treated in isolation. Rather, they should be considered part of a single system that could explain the common properties of all languages and how variation across languages could arise from those common properties. This is called a universal grammar. Chomsky defines it this way:

> Let us define "universal grammar" (UG) as the system of principles, conditions, and rules that are elements or properties of all human languages not merely by accident but by necessity – of course, I mean biological, not logical, necessity. Thus UG can be taken as expressing "the essence of human language." UG will be invariant among humans. UG will specify what language learning must achieve, if it takes place successfully. [Chomsky, 1975:29]

This definition fits our approach to language acquisition with the important exception that the necessity is not biological in the sense of an innate LAD, but a necessity because the properties in question are essential to syntactic processing. As we argued in Chapter 4, a theory of syntax should be based on the minimally essential properties necessary to explain the operations of syntax.

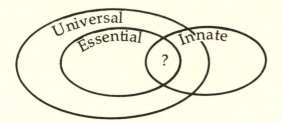

Figure 6.3. Relationship among essential, universal, and innate properties.

Additional properties should be added to a psychological theory of syntax only when they can be supported by independent empirical evidence. Thus our model is a universal grammar rather than a theory specific to a particular language. The value of a universal grammar is its generality, that a single theory can cover more territory. Sometimes the search for a general theory needs justification: Not all phenomena can be explained by a single theory. But a universal grammar does not require a biological justification, an innate LAD; there are essential similarities in all the phenomena we call languages. The quest for a universal grammar is like the search for general principles in any field. A universal grammar is analogous to Newton's laws of motion, which comprise a characterization of the essential (and hence universal) properties of the phenomena they apply to.

A universal theory of syntax will make claims about essential properties. Properties that are shown to be essential will necessarily be universal. For example, in transformational theory, transformation rules are taken to be essential. For the syntax crystal model, scope and dependency are taken to be essential. It is important to realize that not all universal properties are essential. And since both universal and essential properties might be the result of similarity across the phenomena, rather than biological necessity, neither universal nor essential properties have to be innate. Figure 6.3 shows the relationship among these three kinds of properties.

If a property is merely universal, it may not be crucial to a theory of syntax. It is only if the property is universal *because* it is essential that it must be included in syntactic theory. Note that Chomsky would agree with this except that he would also claim that essential properties derive their necessity from an innate biological mechanism that is an essential property of language users.

The analogy with a general theory of motion can help to clarify the relationship between universal and essential properties. Empirically, friction is a universal property associated with moving bodies in the range appropriate to Newton's laws.[2] But friction is not itself an essential property of motion. It is important to the power of Newton's laws of motion that they disregard friction. In fact, earlier theories of motion, such as Aristotle's, were inadequate because they tried to explain what turned out to be the effects of friction. The idealization required for an adequate theory of syntax is exemplified in the competence/performance distinction (Chomsky, 1957; see the discussion in Chapter 4 on the ideal language user).

Theoretical versus temporal priority of language properties

There is a further difference between properties that are essential to language acquisition and those that are assumed to derive from innate cognitive structure. Essential properties are theoretically prior. That is, other properties of language are explained in terms of the essential properties. But such explanations do not assume that the essential properties exist earlier in time than the other properties. This contrasts with innate properties, which are assumed to be temporally prior. That is, other language properties are supposed to arise from the innate properties in the course of development. In the arguments for an innate LAD that confound universal, essential, and innate properties, there is an assumption that essential properties, which are *theoretically* prior, will be temporally prior as well, that is, exist in the organism as innate properties before language is acquired. The converse is also assumed: Properties of language that are innate, and so *temporally* prior to language acquisition, would be theoretically prior as well, and therefore essential to language. We hope we have shown that a theory of language that makes claims about essential properties need not be making claims about innate cognitive mechanisms.

Essential properties for language acquisition

Although nativists have not succeeded in proving the existence of an innate LAD, a number of important conclusions for language acquisition can be drawn from the arguments they have used.

First, an account of language acquisition must consider the underlying structure of language, in other words, the internal hierarchical connections made by the language user. In earlier chapters we argued this point strongly, and many linguists and psychologists have argued for the same conclusion. Chapter 5 and this chapter raised this point again, using Chomsky's focal argument that recursive embedding cannot be explained without hierarchical structure. This is the valuable part of the argument for innate structure based on the inadequacies of traditional learning theories: Linear associations are inadequate. A theory of language acquisition that does not presume innate linguistic mechanisms must show how hierarchical structure can develop by learning.

Second, the internal connections need to be developed from initially unstructured, random connections operated on by simple principles whose nature must be made explicit. Otherwise, if an initial organization is required for language organization, that organization must itself be explained. This is the point that is valid in Fodor's language-of-thought argument.

Third, we cannot suppose that first-language learning requires specific feedback about correct and incorrect syntactic construction. Some feedback can be required, but it must be general enough to encompass the wide range of learning environments of first-language learners. This is the empirically reasonable claim that, except for very special cases (e.g., Premack, 1971) first languages are not acquired under carefully controlled conditions of laboratory learning experiments.

Fourth, language learning is done in conjunction with episodes in the environment. That is, the language learner has access to nonlinguistic information. If we can demonstrate how this nonlinguistic information enables the first-language learner to make syntactic connections, we will have overcome the objections raised by Katz's impoverished data argument.

Syntax crystal model for syntax acquisition

In this section we take up the challenge to provide an alternative to the nativist position on syntax acquisition. First we will reintroduce the syntax crystal model described in Chapter 5. We will show how it is a universal syntax because it is based on essential properties that can explain how the syntactic structure of any natural language can be acquired. Then we will describe how the model portrays the connections that are formed during syntax acquisition and how hierarchical structure arises from considerations of generality mediated by the principle of use versus disuse. Next we will give a general sketch of how some basic syntactic structure is acquired by principles of association. Then we will formalize the operations required to learn syntax, presenting them in the form of an algorithm.

The syntax crystal as a model for universal syntax

A universal syntax must be described in terms of properties that can portray the syntactic structure of any and all natural languages. In Chapter 5 we demonstrated how the syntax crystal could generate and parse both languages that use order to encode conceptual relations (e.g., English) and languages that use inflection (e.g., Latin). Morpheme order and morpheme inflection are the main coding schemes used in natural language. But even if some new method were discovered, Chapter 5 described how conceptual relations could be mapped by syntax crystal modules operating in a "space" of any dimension and any variables.

The syntax crystal model does not presuppose particular grammatical categories as basic properties of the theory. Traditional categories such as noun phrase and relations such as subject-verb-object can be *derived* from properties of a crystal. For example, a sentence could be defined as any completed crystal. For convenience, the modules presented in Chapter 5 translate easily into the syntactic categories of English. But the model could apply to languages that use different sorts of syntactic categories.[3]

The acquisition of a coded set of syntax crystal modules represents the acquisition of syntactic competence. We are going to show how a set of coded modules can be developed by exposure to well-formed language strings when the nonlinguistic context provides the language learner with some information about the idea expressed by the string. In other words, the nonlinguistic context provides some data about the scope and dependency of the conceptual relations expressed by the string, while the well-formed utterances of competent language users provide information about morpheme sequence and inflection. Thus our model reduces linguistic properties to scope and dependency. As we argued earlier, scope and dependency are not essentially linguistic properties because they are also properties of other cognitive and motor abilities that are hierarchically organized. This may enable us to show how the acquisition of linguistic competence is similar to the acquisition of other skills. From a reduction of linguistic properties to the more general properties of scope and dependency, a more general theory of cognitive structure may be developed. This would lessen the plausibility that language acquisition is explained by an innate mechanism that is specialized to handle only linguistic information.

Prerequisites for learning syntax

We will start with only the most general of requirements for syntax learning:

1. An environment to provide something to converse about. The language learner must be able to perceive and understand at least some of the entities and events in the environment.
2. A competent language user to provide well-formed strings that correspond to events and ideas the language learner can conceptualize. The competent language user also provides feedback as to the general acceptability of the strings produced by the learner.
3. The language learner must be able to produce and perceive the signals that carry linguistic information.

These requirements are simplifications of the language acquisition process. For example, learning to produce and perceive the signals that carry linguistic information does not entirely precede syntax acquisition. Nevertheless, such simplification does not invalidate an explanation of syntax acquisition. That is, the simplification does not involve any essential properties of the syntax acquisition process.

In Chapter 1 we distinguished three types of information processing that are essential to language competence: lexical, syntactic, and pragmatic. During cognitive development the ability to process each type of information undoubtedly aids the acquisition of the others. For example, the syntactic form class of an unknown word helps us to discover its meaning; the lexical and syntactic information in a language string often teach us things about the world that we have not directly learned from experience. For clarity, we are going to ignore lexical information processing and its role in syntax acquisition. The development of lexical semantics is a fascinating and important problem that we have touched on elsewhere (Block, Moulton, and Robinson, 1975) and others have dealt with at greater length (see, e.g., Miller and Johnson-Laird, 1976; or Clark and Clark, 1977). However, it is not essential for syntax acquisition to consider how the child acquires the meaning of individual lexemes. Syntax is the use of relations among lexemes to express relations among the concepts they stand for. Therefore, we are only going to treat the interaction between syntactic information acquisition and pragmatic information.

Initially, language learners appear to use language in single chunks that they treat as a whole unit: single words and later small groups of words used as frozen forms. At this point syntactic information processing has not yet appeared. It is only when the language learner discovers that words can be combined in such a way that the combination expresses more than the meaning of the individual words, that syntax appears. The nonlinguistic environment is the source of this insight. Just as the child discovers that a particular word reliably co-occurs with some salient object, person, or event in its environment, so also does it discover that the appearance of two or more words in a string co-occurs with things named by the words being related in some way. For example, if the child knows what RED and BALL refer to and the string RED BALL is used in the presence of a red ball, the child has the opportunity to detect the co-occurrence between the relationship of the words in the string and the relationship of coinstantiation of the concepts in the red ball. According to Bloom and Lahey:

> Utterances in the speech of mothers addressed to their children are frequently redundant in relation to context and behavior, and language learning no doubt depends on the relationship between the speech children hear and what they see and do. For example, the statement, "Will is going down the slide," spoken to a child who has been playing with Will on the playground would be likely to cause the child to look for Will or look toward the slide. If children do not understand sentences that refer to relations among objects and events that are not immediately available, then the extent to which they analyze the semantic-syntactic structure for understanding is certainly questionable. Thus, the same statement "Will is going down the slide" or the question "Is Will going down the slide?" would most probably draw a blank if the child hears it at the dinner table or while taking a bath. [Bloom and Lahey, 1978:241–242]

While it is undisputed that the learner must be exposed to a source of well-formed language strings in the speech of competent language users, it is less clear that the competent language users must provide the learner with a source of feedback as to the acceptability of its own productions. As we discussed in the first part of the chapter, transformational theorists wish to undermine the importance of feedback in order to strengthen the claim for an innate LAD. In addition, both informal and some formal studies of language development tended to emphasize that language comprehension generally precedes language production. This is the position expressed by McNeill (1970).

Bloom and Lahey challenge the notion that comprehension is prior to production and emphasize instead that the two processes are "mutually dependent" (1978:238). We are going to take a cautious intermediate position on the role of feedback in syntax acquisition. In the initial stages of syntax acquisition, adults tend to be very tolerant of the deviant productions of children for the same reason that parents eagerly take the early sounds of children to be real words when in fact they may deviate enormously. A wide variety of studies have looked at the nature of feedback that parents provide when children have begun to produce more complex syntactic combinations. For example, Feldman and Rodgon (1970) discovered that syntactic development was helped more when parents responded only to the clear productions of their children than when they responded to all productions regardless of how acceptable they were. We are not going to assume that feedback explicitly provides syntactic information but only that the learner receives information about the general acceptability of its productions. The feedback could consist of something as general as the failure of the adult to respond to the utterance in the way the child expects. General feedback is likely to confound syntactic, semantic, and possibly stylistic acceptability. In other words, a positive response is withheld whenever the learner's utterances are ungrammatical, nonsensical, impolite, or any combination of these faults. Criteria of acceptability will vary widely across conversants, situations, and the sophistication of the language learner.

The role of pragmatic information in syntax acquisition

Earlier, we reviewed Katz's (1966) argument that even if the language learner knew all the syntactic features of its native language, there would not be enough information to learn syntax in any finite set of well-formed strings. We pointed out that Katz had ignored the role of the nonlinguistic environment. We are claiming, with Bloom and Lahey (1978), that pragmatic information from the environment frequently is redundant to the language strings the child hears. That is, pragmatic information provides clues to the relations of concepts encoded by the language string.

In Chapter 1 we demonstrated how syntactic information may not always be necessary to understand the meaning of a string. Primitive syntax – the clue that concepts are related because their lexemes are temporally or spatially related – along with pragmatic information – knowledge of how the concepts can be or are likely to be related – can often support complete understanding. For example, in RED BALL BOUNCE(S), syntactic information is unnecessary to understanding the relation of concepts expressed by the string. It is this redundancy, the fact that pragmatic information supplies clues to the relation of concepts expressed, that makes syntax learning possible. Learning syntax is learning the code that enables relations among lexemes – sequence, inflection, and function words – to stand for relations of concepts. In our view, relations of concepts can be represented by the information contained in the orrery diagram, the picture of underlying conceptual structure. The language string uttered by an adult provides the information about sequence, inflection, and function words. Where redundancy exists, the nonlinguistic context provides at least partial information about the underlying conceptual structure. The job of the syntax learner is to figure out what syntactic features present in the string correspond to scope and dependency relations among the concepts. The connections between modules of the syntax crystal is our way of representing this correspondence. Acquiring syntax then is acquiring these connections. Now we are going to describe how the connections are acquired as a result of experience. First we shall go through the process in an informal way and then we will present an algorithm, a clearly specified learning procedure which is our model for syntax acquisition. As a model, it suggests the cognitive operations that could mediate the learning of syntax. No innate, language-specific structure is presumed. Only simple mediated associations are used in the explanation, keeping global procedures to a minimum.

Generality and efficiency in the acquisition of syntactic structure

In this section we are going to use syntax crystal modules to show that a hierarchical structure is superior to a linear (Markov) structure. Consider a simple string: GIRL GOES BEHIND BOY. If the individual words are recognized, the easiest and most obvious way to connect them to preserve their sequence would be to hook them together in a Markov chain. Let each of the words be written on a syntax crystal module. We can represent the Markov chain connections by three pairs of matching codes as shown in Figure 6.4(a). Using only six codes, this would be the most efficient system possible if this were the only string the syntax needed to handle. But, as we discussed in Chapter 1, if there were many strings in the language, each string would require a unique set of connections so that parts of one string could not get mixed up with the parts of another, creating an impossible cognitive burden.

(a)

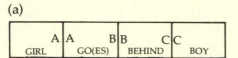

(b)

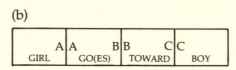

(c)

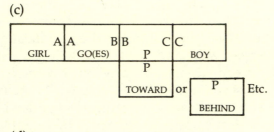

(d)

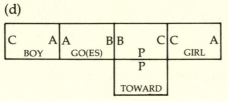

(e)

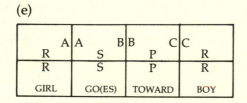

(f)

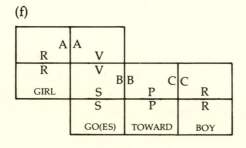

(g)

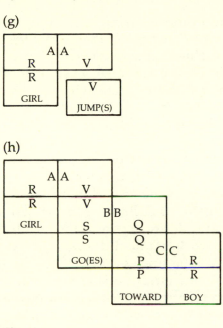

(h)

(i)

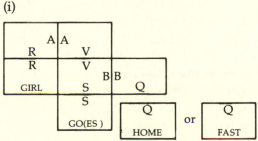

Figure 6.4. (a) Markov chain of modules. (b) Reusing codes for other strings. (c) More general scheme for generality of codes. (d) Interchanging modules. (e, f) New use of modules avoids problems and increases generality. (g) Intransitive verbs. (h) Four levels of connections. (i) Reuses B/Q modules of (h).

We might improve the efficiency of the Markov chain system by recognizing that some morphemes can be substituted for each other to produce a different string. Morphemes that are intersubstitutable can use the same connection codes. Figure 6.4(b) shows how the word TOWARD can be substituted for BEHIND using the same connection codes. Each new morpheme that can appear in the third position in the string needs only two additional codes entered on its side edges. If there are a great many such morphemes, we can achieve greater efficiency by using only a single connection code on the top edge of each morpheme. Then we can attach them to a module that itself contains no overt part of the string. This is shown in Figure 6.4(c). However, as soon as we take this step we have gone from a Markov to a hierarchical system.

Another, and more important, reason for using hierarchical rather than Markov connections is seen when we try to use the same word in a new position in the string. In our example GIRL and BOY might be substituted for each other in the first and last positions. If we give them codes that permit them to link up in either position (see Figure 6.4[d]), then the Markov system exhibits a serious drawback. The unconnected codes on BOY and GIRL in Figure 6.4(d) allow the string to keep on growing in an unmanageable and ungrammatical way: . . . TOWARD BOY GOES TOWARD GIRL GOES TOWARD. . . . We could control this problem by adding "stopping" rules that would be global with respect to morpheme-morpheme connections. Alternatively, we can abandon the Markov system and separate the string-organizing role from the string of morphemes itself. This is hierarchical organization: Each morpheme is not directly connected to the others but is connected indirectly through an intervening structure module (see Figure 6.4 [e]).

This scheme has three advantages: We have minimized the number of connection codes that need to be added for each new morpheme; we have represented the similarity in the privilege of occurrence, the syntactic category, of the morphemes that can occupy the same position in a string; and we have used only local rules to build the syntactic structure.

Hierarchical organization can be extended to additional levels in order to achieve even greater efficiency and generality. For example, Figure 6.4(f) shows the original string organized with three levels in the hierarchy. This allows the A$/$V module to be used with simple intransitive verbs as shown in Figure 6.4(g). The module A$/$V is more general than the module A$/$S$\backslash$B used in Figure 6.4(e), which requires a verb complement. Adding a fourth level as in Figure 6.4(h) allows the B/Q module to be used also in strings like the one shown in Figure 6.4(i) where the B/P\C module in Figure 6.4(e) could not be used.

Generality means more frequent opportunities for use. If we suppose that frequency of use strengthens the cognitive associations represented by the codes, hierarchical structures will be favored over linear ones because they employ structure modules that can be used in a greater variety of string forms. In the next section we examine this argument in the context of child language acquisition.

How modules become connected to represent the acquisition of syntactic structure

Let us begin by asking why a child would learn to make indirect hierarchical connections between morphemes, rather than Markov-chain connections. We believe that this is the big stumbling block to a theory of language learning. Although many psychologists recognize the existence of indirect or hierarchical relations in many kinds of behavior, to our knowledge no one has offered a detailed explanation of how hierarchical rather than Markov-chain relations are learned.

We know that language learners have available for syntax acquisition more information than the particular language strings they receive, and that chains of association linking particular sequences of symbols (echolalia) do not play a significant role in language acquisition. Let us suppose that a child understands, in some elementary sense, the morphemes WENDY and WALK, and that it receives the string NOW WENDY IS WALKING while observing the event described. The child may just attend to the morphemes it understands. To an adult the string provides syntactic information in the form of a sequence of five morphemes, NOW, WENDY, IS, WALK, ING. But to a language learner in the initial stages of syntax acquisition, most of this information is unusable. The nonlinguistic information in the environment accompanying the string provides the information that WENDY and WALK are related. The child does not have to encode the relationship as, for example, actor-action. If it recognizes that *some* relationship exists between the two concepts expressed by WENDY and WALK, it can form a connection between the two morphemes.

But we have to explain why indirect, hierarchical rather than linear, Markov-chain connections are learned. If we suppose that a *variety* of connections are formed between the two morphemes, an explanation is possible. Some of the connections will be direct morpheme-morpheme connections and some may be indirect, mediated by other associations, or by as yet uncommitted pathways. This hypothesis is consistent with neurological models of learning in which a stimulus initially excites a number of different (and perhaps random) pathways or patterns. According to these models (e.g., Hebb, 1949, 1972; Rosenblatt, 1962) once excited, the probability that a pathway will be excited again by similar stimuli increases. Some of the pathways will be excited by a range of other stimuli. Pathways that are active in the presence of more than one stimulus will become stronger than pathways that are unique. If they are stronger they will be more likely to be used than weaker connections. Frequent use will establish the stronger connections at the expense of the weaker ones.

Let us represent the connections by lines between modules as in Figure 6.5(a). The modules themselves may represent an assortment of connections or patterns. The line between two of the rectangles represents the conceptual connection the child makes between WENDY and WALK. Some of the connections may be direct, represented in Figure 6.5(a) as pathway A; some of the connections may be indirect mediated ones, like pathways B, C, and C'.

Now suppose that the child receives some new strings expressing things about Wendy, for example: WENDY EATS, WENDY WAITS, WENDY IS GOOD. If the child understands the lexemes EAT, WAIT, GOOD and guesses that the idea expressed by each of the strings represents a relation it understands from nonlinguistic context, these additional morphemes can also be connected to WENDY. The new connections for WAIT are shown in Figure 6.5(b). Imagine that the same thing happens on a larger scale for many different strings. Some of the connections formed will be unique to particular combinations of morphemes. By definition,

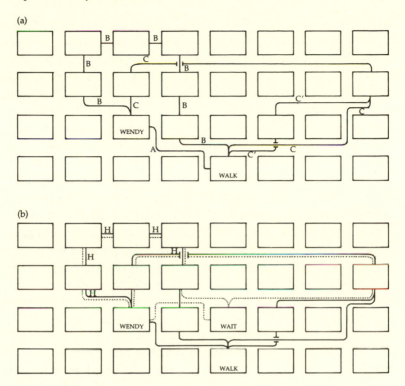

Figure 6.5. (a) Random connection among the identifiable morphemes in a string. (b) Random connections for an additional morpheme showing the reuse of a connecting pathway.

every direct morpheme-to-morpheme connection will be one of the unique ones. However, some of the hierarchical connections, that is the indirect pathways mediated by additional structure modules, will be shared by more than one pair of connected morphemes.

Because the hierarchical pathways are more general, they will be used more frequently than the direct pathways. Every connection represents an association. If we make the reasonable assumption that frequently used associations are stronger, the strength of direct morpheme-morpheme connections will diminish as the variety of strings presented is increased. Mediated hierarchical connections survive in a process analogous to natural selection.

This explanation also accords with what is known about child language acquisition. First there is a one-word stage, then a two-word stage. In the two-word stage a few words are frequently coupled repeatedly with a variety of different words. In our example the connections to WENDY might become established in this way. At the two-word stage hierarchical relations between pairs of words are learned.

Then instead of a three-word and then a four-word stage, there is a multi-word stage. At this stage the established hierarchical connections between pairs of words can be treated as units to become part of a larger hierarchical connection with several levels. Utterances are not limited to just one additional morpheme, because hierarchical connections can be made between single morphemes, between an established hierarchical connection of two morphemes and a third, between two hierarchical connections of two morphemes each, and so on. The child's big insight here is that a set of two or more words can function as a unit to join with other units.

Finally, inflections and function morphemes are added to child language. These cues that adults use to determine the hierarchical structure of language are not learned by children until considerable understanding about how lexical morphemes go together has been achieved.

Child language acquisition and the syntax crystal

Children's first utterances are, expectedly, composed of single lexemes.[4] They enlarge their lexicon, uttering one word at a time, but do not immediately begin putting lexemes together in strings. Because young children obviously can understand more than they can express, early researchers took these single-lexeme utterances to represent full sentences expressed in an abbreviated form (e.g, de Laguna, 1927). Some transformational psycholinguists claimed that the child was developing syntactic categories and relations at this stage: "There is a constant emergence of new grammatical relations, even though no utterance is ever longer than one word. Very young children develop a concept of a sentence as a set of grammatical relations before they develop a concept of how these relations are expressed" (McNeill, 1970:23). Recently, Bloom (1973) and Scollon (1974) have argued from the nature of single word utterances that children have not yet developed syntax at this stage. Bloom (1975: 267) says of one child (Alison) who was just about to enter the two-word stage: "There was convincing evidence that she did not know anything about syntax. She produced series of single words in succession which were obviously related by virtue of the state of affairs being referred to, but which appeared in variable order relative to one another and were not produced in combinations as a phrase." And in her recent language development review, Moskowitz (1978:96) says about Scollon's example: "Brenda was not yet able to combine two words syntactically. . . . She could express [complex ideas], however, by combining words sequentially. Thus the one-word stage is not just a time for learning the meaning of words. In that period a child is developing hypotheses about putting words together in [clusters], and she is already putting [word clusters] together in meaningful groups. The next step will be to put two words together to form a single sentence."

In our view, when a child puts together single lexemes in clusters it is using primitive syntax to signal that the concepts named by the lexemes go together in some way. This is distinct from true syntax, where sequential information is used to convey particular information about the relation of concepts. Bloom, Scollon, and Moskowitz argue that this begins only with the two-word stage. This contrasts with the view, once held by McNeill (1970) and others, that single-word utterances and their contexts indicate that the child has the concept of a sentence and its grammatical relations.

Children discover that they can string two words together to signal a relation of concepts. The two-word stage endures long enough to have been the focus of considerable interest. Attempts were made to abstract regularities from children's two-word utterances and present them as syntactic categories and production rules. For example, Braine (1963) described two categories, *pivot*, consisting of a small group of words that tended to be modifiers, and *open*, consisting of a much larger and rapidly growing set of words that were typically nouns and salient modifiers. McNeill (1966) presented a list of possible two-word strings that we summarize in the following production rule:

$$S \rightarrow [P, O] [O, \{P, O, \emptyset\}]$$

However, more recently, this "grammar" has been challenged. Bloom (1971) found so many exceptions that the pivot-open grammar seems incorrect. For example, she found that MOMMY, a typical open word, could function as a pivot as in MOMMY PIGTAIL, MOMMY KISS, and MOMMY DIAPER. In this child's utterances, MOMMY could also occur with other pivot words such as MOMMY BYEBYE and alone, which are exceptions to the grammar.

What is especially important for our point of view is that, even to the extent it is correct, the pivot-open grammar defies classification into any scheme of adult syntactic categories and relations. Both pivot and open classes contain members of several form classes. The combinations uttered by children also involved unsystematically nearly every case relation, including agent-action, agent-object, possessor-possessed. Thus there seems to be no way for the pivot-open categories to serve as a useful precursor to adult syntax (Moskowitz, 1978). This is consonant with our hypothesis that the child only needs the information that two concepts are related in order to establish a relationship between their lexemes. The nature of the relation between concepts is given by pragmatic information and does not need to be encoded by syntax.

Although recent work shows no systematic syntactic categorization at the two-word stage, a child will exhibit striking regularities in its particular two-word combinations. For example, one child (Braine, 1963) used ALLGONE MILK and ALLGONE VITAMINS, but not MILK ALLGONE nor VITAMINS ALLGONE. In the next section we will use the syntax crystal model to explain why there would be a tendency for children to employ relatively fixed word order for frequently used two-word combinations. This does not mean that a word is fixed as either a first- or a second-position term. A given word may appear in the first position in some combinations and the second position in others. The development of the two-word stage indicates the child's ability to form hierarchical connections between two lexemes.

In language development there is a one-word stage, a two-word stage, and a many-word stage. It is surprising that there is no three-word stage. As Moskowitz (1978:97–98) says: "For a few years after the end of the two-word stage children tend to produce rather short sentences, but the almost inviolable length constraints that characterized the first two stages have disappeared. The absence of a three-word stage has not been satisfactorily explained as yet; the answer may have to do with the fact that many basic semantic relations are binary and few are ternary."

In the next section we use the syntax crystal model to describe the cognitive operations that characterize the two-word stage and the development of hierarchical connections. In an earlier section we showed that connecting words hierarchically lead to greater generality and economy. When two words are connected as a unit, the child is then able to connect them to other units. Since one pair may be connected to another pair just as easily as to a single word, there is no stage where three-word strings appear exclusively. Thus we suggest that the answer to the riddle of the abrupt switch from two- to multi-word stages depends on the syntactic mechanism rather than on any change in the child's ability to combine concepts in a coherent way. This is supported by Scollon (1974), whose subject, Brenda, was able to express quite complex ideas by concatenating a series of two-word strings. There is also the possibility that the need to differentiate the *dependency* of two-word strings helps to promote the transition to the multi-word stage. Since the dependency relationship between two terms depends on their (potential) relationship to other terms, this would encourage the construction of strings of more than two elements.

Even though they are putting several words together, the patterned speech of young children does not sound like that of an adult. The most salient characteristic is that things are missing. Brown and Fraser (1963) called the speech of children in this stage "telegraphic." As Moskowitz (1978:97) puts it: "Early telegraphic speech is characterized by short simple sentences made up primarily of content words: words that are rich in semantic content, usually nouns and verbs. The speech is called telegraphic because the sentences lack function words: tense endings on verbs and plural endings on nouns, prepositions, conjunctions, articles and so on. As the telegraphic speech stage progresses, function words are gradually added to sentences." In what follows, we shall describe how scope and dependency relations are acquired using the syntax crystal model. Then we shall turn to the acquisition of functors and inflections to show how they also can be incorporated in syntactic knowledge.

Learning syntax: hierarchical connections and dependency relations

We are not directly concerned with how a child learns to associate lexemes with concepts in the one-word stage. In describing the acquisition of a syntax crystal, we shall be concerned with the onset of the two-lexeme stage and beyond. In Chapter 2 we used the orrery model to show that underlying conceptual structure could be adequately portrayed by a hierarchical structure characterized by scope and dependency. Now we want to show that when a language learner can derive conceptual relations from the nonlinguistic context and morpheme order from the strings of a competent language user, these two kinds of information can be combined and incorporated into a syntactic mechanism that then can be used to parse and generate language strings.

To return to an earlier example, suppose the child is watching Wendy walk. It knows the lexemes for the concepts "Wendy" and "walk," and it knows that the concepts are related in the event it is witnessing. This relation of concepts, as we explained in Chapter 2, can be modeled by the orrery in Figure 6.6(a). The morpheme sequence is given by the language string WENDY WALK(S). Let us suppose that an adult utters this string in context, and the child recognizes that the relations of the two morphemes signifies the relations of concepts it sees instantiated in its environment.[5] The child can record this correlation syntactically. The syntax crystal represents this as in Figure 6.6(b).

Remember that the codes on the modules are arbitrary – pairs of matching codes represent a simple association. However, whenever a new morpheme can be substituted for another to produce a well-formed expression of a coherent relation of concepts, the new unit is given the same top code as the original unit. This is the beginning of the formation of syntactic categories on formal grounds as discussed in Chapter 1. The substitutions may *sometimes* be characterizable on a semantic basis because semantic similarity often accompanies syntactic similarity. However, similar codes will not be limited to morphemes

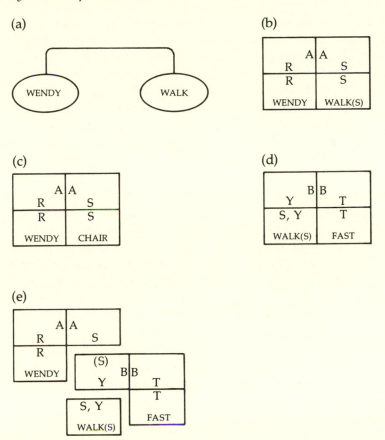

Figure 6.6. (a) Orrery for WENDY WALK(S). (b) Crystal for WENDY WALK(S). (c) Crystal for WENDY CHAIR using same structure modules as (b). (d) New modules for WALK(S) FAST. (e) Combining previously established structure modules.

with semantic similarity. Thus, while WALKS and RUNS can both follow WENDY in a string, so also can WAITS (which is not an action) and CHAIR (as in WENDY'S CHAIR). Thus the same structure modules might be used for the connection between WENDY and CHAIR as between WENDY and WALK(S). These connections would only be distinguished later (see Figure 6.6[c]).

For a new string, for example, WALK FAST, the child forms a connection if it recognizes that there is some relation between the concepts expressed by WALK and FAST. Because WALK is in a different relative position in the new string, the old structure modules cannot be used over again. Therefore, the connection must be made with a new set of modules. In Figure 6.6(d) the WALK(S) module is given an additional top code for this connection. As discussed in Chapter 5, multiple codes on a module are a shorthand for separate modules with single codes. In some cases, the child may not recognize that the same morpheme used in different ways is really the same. Morpheme identity is a complex question. While the use of multiple codes represents that a single morpheme is *able* to play multiple syntactic roles, the presence of multiple codes should not be taken as a claim that language users must treat the different uses as a single morpheme.

Now that we have simple hierarchical connections, how do we combine them? For a longer string, such as WENDY WALK(S) FAST, the phrase WALK(S) FAST forms a unit that is joined to WENDY in the same way as WALK(S) is in the string WENDY WALK(S). In other words, WALK(S) FAST is substitutable for WALK(S). So we could place an optional S code on the top of the WALK(S) FAST array of modules. (It would be optional to allow WALK(S) FAST still to be a complete phrase.) However, we need to know whether the S code belongs on top of the WALK column or the FAST column, that is, which of these two lexemes is the main one with respect to other connections. In other words, the language learner must be able to recognize and encode dependency information for this longer expression.

In many cases the language learner can use pragmatic information to distinguish the main and subordinate terms in a phrase. The nonlinguistic context is likely to provide information that is redundant to the language string to identify the main term for phrases such as FIRE ENGINE and ENGINE FIRE, or CANDY STORE and STORE CANDY. But for other phrases, discovering the dependency relations may depend on what else is said about it (the linguistic context) because the nonlinguistic context may not be enough to make clear that one is talking about, for example, WENDY'S WAIT or WAITING WENDY.

Let us return to our example, WENDY WALK(S) FAST. If it is recognized that WALK(S) is the main lexeme with respect to further connections of the WALK(S) FAST pair, then the connection will be as in Figure 6.6(e). What is required for the correct structure is that WALK(S) and FAST be connected as a unit and that the connection to WENDY be made to the column of the main term of the pair, that is, to WALK(S). If WALK(S) FAST is connected first, then the modules for connecting to WENDY will fit on top. If WENDY WALK(S) is connected first, then the modules for connecting FAST will be *inserted* into the WALK column.

For phrases that express a relation of concepts with no dependency relations of semantic consequence, the connection to other units could be made through any morpheme in the phrase. However, where such a phrase contains morphemes that appear in another phrase in which dependency does make a difference, the first phrase may come to have the same dependency relations as the second. For example, consider: THE CAT WITH THE DOG. Serial priority may make CAT seem to be more important than DOG, but it is not clear that the phrase is substantially different in meaning from THE DOG WITH THE CAT. However, in similar phrases such as THE CAT WITH THE STRIPE and THE CAT WITH LUMBAGO, pragmatic information would strongly suggest that CAT was the main lexeme. Therefore, because of the dependency relations in these latter phrases, THE CAT WITH THE DOG is likely to have the same dependency relations as the similar phrases where dependency is important. We will continue to show scope and dependency relations even when they may make no difference in meaning for the particular relation of concepts in question, as long as they do make a difference for some relations of concepts whose syntactic representations are similar.

This principle of extending scope and dependency assignments from clear examples to those which are not so clear in themselves, can be applied to the problem of explaining how subject-verb-object relations are learned. Consider, for example, WENDY PUSH(ES) DOG. Transformational psycholinguists handle the explanation by claiming that the relations are prewired into an innate LAD and all the child must do is to learn the particular sequence used by its native language to encode this relationship, for example, McNeill, (1970). Case theorists who are nativists, for example, Fillmore (1968), would claim that an agent-action-recipient relationship is innate and becomes associated with the particular sequence the language uses to encode it. Case theorists who are not nativists, for example, Brown (1973),[6] believe that the child learns to understand the world in terms of case relationships and this understanding is then matched to the language sequence. For reasons given earlier in the book, we are reluctant to assume that the child has innate cognitive structure peculiar to language, and we argued that case categories are not coherent and consistent enough to be learned with enough reliability to support syntax acquisition. This is not to deny that they may play a supplementary or facilitative role in syntax learning or that children may show evidence that they are able to use such categories (cf. Brown, 1973; Braine and Wells, 1978). But we believe that scope and dependency are adequate to explain this part of syntax acquisition.

As we have argued, there is no single semantic relation that captures all the relations expressed between subject and verb, or between verb and object. The important thing is that the relations expressed between the subject and verb are (usually) different from the relations expressed between the object and verb. What the difference is depends on the meaning of the particular verb and/or the nouns that take the subject and object positions. The orrery and syntax crystal portray this difference as a difference in scope and dependency relations, which together with the meaning of the lexemes involved, and shared pragmatic knowledge, allow the relations expressed by subject and verb and by object and verb to be communicated. However, for some verbs, the difference in meaning does not seem to be a clear difference in scope and dependency. Some relations seem to be symmetric: If A *verbs* B, then B *verbs* A (for verbs such as EQUAL, MET, WED); others, although not symmetric, seem to relate the verb concept to the subject and object equally (Levelt, 1974). In these cases, the principle of extending scope and dependency can be applied, or one could argue that a different structure is used in such cases.

Consider the following series of strings: WENDY JUMPS, WENDY WAITS, WENDY WALKS, WENDY SWINGS, WENDY PUSHES DOGS. Given experience with the first four strings, the child can use the substitution principle to assign the same scope relations to PUSHES DOGS as had JUMPS, WAITS, WALKS, and SWINGS. The syntactic structure would be represented by the crystal in Figure

6.7(a). If we consider another set of strings of similar form, the scope and dependency relations become even clearer: WENDY PUSHES DOGS HARD, WENDY EATS VITAMINS RELUCTANTLY, WENDY MET TINA INADVERTENTLY. The first string does not say that Wendy pushes hard, in general. She may push dogs hard, but push other things lightly. The second sentence does not say that Wendy eats reluctantly, but that she eats vitamins reluctantly. The phrases EATS VITAMINS and PUSHES DOGS connect as units to RELUCTANTLY and HARD respectively, and the whole phrase connects as a unit to WENDY. In the third string, while we could say that WENDY MET TINA is to say that TINA MET WENDY, as soon as the adverb is introduced, it is clear that MET TINA has the smaller scope. That is, it was Wendy's meeting of Tina that was inadvertent, although it might well have been deliberate on Tina's part. Since the same structure modules can be used for all these variants, the principle that the more generally used structures are more likely to be used in the future supplies the strings with conventional scope and dependency relations. Thus strings whose structure is unclear from pragmatic information inherit their structure from strings where the relations are obvious.

Now we return to the development of syntax crystal modules. In the string WENDY WALKS TOWARD DOG, the phrase TOWARD DOG can be substituted for FAST in the earlier string WENDY WALKS FAST. Therefore, it can be connected as a unit to the rest of the string through the same top code as in Figure 6.7(b). The codes determine the syntactic categories of the units that attach to them. Remember that the codes are assigned on the basis of acceptable substitutivity and not on any a priori or notional basis. Thus, for example, at this point in syntax acquisition, FAST and TOWARD DOG belong to the same syntactic category. Only later, when the child discovers that adverbs and prepositional phrases do not have identical substitution privileges, will their syntactic categories become differentiated. This is a general phenomenon. Consider another example: Initially, it would be possible for FAST and WENDY to receive the same codes because they are substitutable in, say, PUSH FAST and PUSH WENDY. Suppose that the language learner has not yet acquired any intransitive verbs to which FAST but not WENDY can be connected in the second

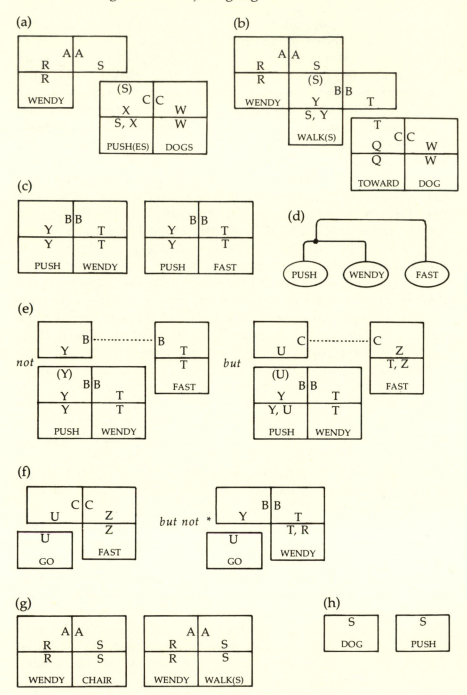

(i)

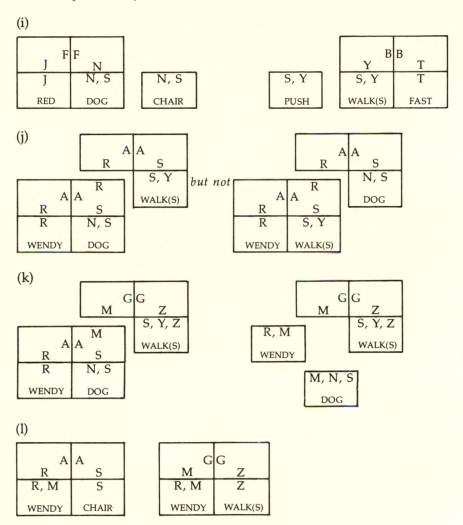

Figure 6.7. (a) New crystal formed by substitution principle. (b)
TOWARD DOG connected using same code (T) that connected FAST in
Figure 6.6 (e). (c) WENDY and FAST connected with same codes in early
crystal. (d). Orrery needed to create modules for PUSH WENDY FAST. (e)
Differentiation of codes for WENDY and FAST because they are not intersubstitutable. (f) More general U∕C and C∖Z modules can be used to
connect FAST to intransitive verbs. (g, h) Illustrating same codes for different form classes at early stage. (i) New connections result in codes
that distinguish form classes. (j) Undifferentiated codes result in unacceptable structures. (k) New modules eliminate improper structures. (l)
Different modules now distinguish form classes.

position. The learner's syntactic knowledge would be represented by the pair of crystals in Figure 6.7(c).

Now, what would happen if the child is given the string PUSH WENDY FAST? The interchangeability of WENDY and FAST breaks down because the same idea, that is, the same scope and dependency relations as represented by the orrery cannot also be expressed using the order PUSH FAST WENDY. It is not fast Wendy who is supposed to be pushed. The concept expressed by FAST operates on the unit expressed by (PUSH WENDY). The orrery for this idea is given in Figure 6.7(d). The child must learn to combine this underlying structure with the sequence PUSH WENDY FAST. We cannot connect PUSH WENDY to FAST using the same codes that connect PUSH to FAST because PUSH WENDY cannot be substituted for PUSH in other contexts, for example, in PUSH WENDY. Therefore the crystal array for PUSH WENDY does *not* receive the same top codes as PUSH and so must be connected to FAST through different modules, as in Figure 6.7(e).

At this point, FAST connects to PUSH in two different ways using different sets of modules. Since the PUSH module received a U top code, the U $\setminus$ C and C $/$ Z modules can be used for strings of the form PUSH WENDY FAST and of the form PUSH FAST. On the other hand, the "competing" Y $\setminus$ B and B $/$ T modules can be used both for strings of the form PUSH WENDY and PUSH FAST. At this stage in syntax acquisition, one set of modules is not more general than the other. However, when new strings appear, the first pair of modules turns out to be more general for connecting arrays to FAST. For example, when connecting GO to other morphemes we cannot use the modules with codes Y $\setminus$ B and B $/$ T because that would allow the ungrammatical $\star$ GO WENDY. That is, GO is not substitutable for PUSH in the structure representing PUSH WENDY. However, the pair of modules bearing codes U $\setminus$ C and C $/$ Z can be used to construct the string GO FAST without allowing $\star$ GO WENDY. Thus the pair of modules with codes U $\setminus$ C and C $/$ Z is more general and will displace the competing pair in the system of syntactic rules. We have then the modules on the left of Figure 6.7(f), but not those on the right.

In a similar way, the language learner differentiates connections that were originally the same in the two-lexeme stage. Consider, for example, WENDY'S CHAIR and WENDY WALKS. Suppose that the structure modules originally are those given in Figure 6.7(g), and that other lexemes receive the same S code as in (h). New connections will distinguish between DOG or CHAIR, and WALK or PUSH.[7] For example, RED DOG might be connected with different structure modules because substituting PUSH would make the unacceptable ★RED PUSH. It is also possible that WALK FAST would be connected with different structure modules, as in Figure 6.7(i). However, DOG and WALK still have that S code in common. An attempt to combine the structures to allow, say, WENDY'S DOG WALKS would provide the information needed to differentiate DOG and WALK, because if the codes were left undifferentiated, as shown in Figure 6.7(j), then WENDY'S WALK DOG would also be permitted (this is not the same as WENDY WALKS DOG, which has different scope and dependency relations). In order to connect WENDY'S DOG to WALKS without permitting ungrammatical forms, we need a different set of structure modules. The set in Figure 6.7(k) can also be used for other connections. The $M \backslash G$ and G/Z modules of (k) compete for the same connections as the $R \backslash A$ and A/S connections of (j). Since the $M \backslash G$ and G/Z modules are more general, they will replace the $R \backslash A$ and A/S modules participating in those connections. The $R \backslash A$ and A/S connections that do not compete will remain. So eventually there will be the modules in (l).

Learning inflections: overgeneralization explained in terms of the syntax crystal

Inflections that carry meaning, such as the past -ED or the plural -S, are usually learned after the two-word stage is past. Children learn English inflections in a predictable sequence: -ING first, then the plural -S, the possessive 'S, the third person singular -S, and the past -ED. This sequence of learning has been explained as a combination of the regularity of the morphemes, the frequency of their use, the difficulty of the concepts they represent, and/or the syntactic relations they require (see Moskowitz, 1978).

When children first learn inflections such as the plural -S they incorrectly apply it to words that take irregular plurals, such as MANS and MOUSES; for the past -ED they overgeneralize by saying GOED and SEED even if they previously had been using the correct irregular forms, MEN and MICE, WENT and SAW. This suggests, in syntax crystal terms, that the plural and the past tense are understood to apply to the whole phrase, and therefore the morphemes for these concepts are connected high up on the column of the main lexeme. Since they attach directly to the main lexeme, they are positional priority exceptions. For example, modules for the past tense, in terms of the modules constructed in learning so far, would be those in Figure 6.8(a). The structure modules for the past tense connect on the top of the verb column via the D code. The D code appears on the top of other structure modules in that column, but not on the verb modules themselves. This is fine for the majority of verbs, such as PUSH, that are regular, but for irregular verbs, such as SEE and GO, which connect to many of the same modules, this will produce mistakes. Similarly, for plurals, additional plural modules might be added to the top of the noun column with a positional priority exception module for the inflection,[8] as in Figure 6.8(b). Again, the code to connect the plural module appears on the structure modules of the noun column but is not needed on the lexeme modules themselves. Therefore, irregular nouns such as MOUSE, which had previously been substitutable for regular nouns in other syntactic contexts, will erroneously receive a regular plural ending.

Eventually, children learn to use the correct forms for irregular nouns and verbs. It is likely that much of the information used in selecting the correct plural and past forms is not incorporated into the structure but is part of the morphophonemic rules that determine the phonemic realizations of morpheme sequences. Chomsky (1975) and others are now attributing more and more things like agreement to organization at the level of the surface string. One piece of developmental evidence that this is true, is that when children first add the past -ED to regular verbs, they often omit the -ED for regular verbs that already end in that sound, such as WEED or NEED. Later they will say WEEDED and NEEDED, and sometimes this too overgeneralizes so they occasionally produce forms like HAVEDED (Moskowitz, 1978).

One interesting and unexplained phenomenon is the apparent lack of overgeneralization for the progressive -ING suffix (Brown, 1973:320–328). It is acquired before other inflections, for "pro-

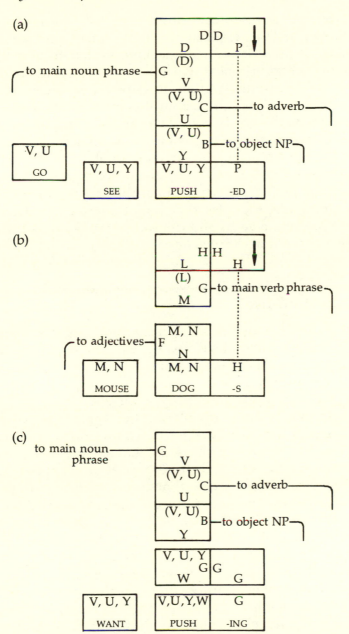

Figure 6.8. Inflections. (a) Past-tense modules. (b) Plural modules. (c) Modules for -ING.

cess" verbs such as PUSHING, GOING, WALKING, and not, according to Brown, overgeneralized to "state" verbs such as WANT, LIKE, NEED, KNOW, SEE, and HEAR. One explanation of this in terms of the syntax crystal is that the -ING suffix is not added to the *top* of the verb column: either its scope is not perceived as applying to the whole verb phrase, or it is learned before the child figures out how to encode positional priority exceptions, so its position, closest to the verb, assigns it the smallest scope, as in Figure 6.8(c). In contrast to the -ED and plural -S inflections, connection codes for the progressive -ING suffix are only entered on the tops of the particular verb modules they are used with. There are no intervening modules that might allow connections between inappropriate verbs and the -ING morpheme, as there are for the -ED and plural -S inflections.

The development of questions, negation, and verb auxiliaries

The forms children use to ask questions or express negation change as their language develops. If we look at how these developmental changes take place in terms of the syntax crystal, they make a coherent picture.

Initially, children place morphemes for questions or negation at the beginning or end of the phrase they apply to (Moskowitz, 1978). This indicates that the scope of the question or negation is understood to be the whole phrase. In terms of the syntax crystal, the structure modules for questions and negation appear at the top of the crystal. The modules shown in Figure 6.9 can be used for questions at the two-word stage, WHO 'AT? WHERE GO? and HAVE IT? (Brown, 1973:203, 207), and also at later stages, where the question adverb precedes the rest of the sentence, which remains in declarative form (WHAT WENDY CAN HAVE?) rather than the adult form (WHAT CAN WENDY HAVE?). Since question modules can have whole propositions in their scope, the morpheme and intonation modules attached to them, by the positional priority principle, will naturally fall at either end of the sentence. (From now on, letter-plus-number connection codes will be used, so that mnemonically helpful letters can be used; see Figure 6.9[a]). The Q2 code can connect to question adverbs

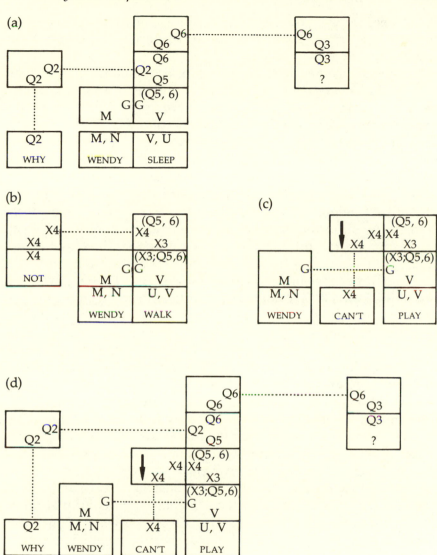

Figure 6.9. (a) Question modules for the learner. (b) Initial negation modules, without arrows but with correct scope. (c) Later negation modules with arrows. (d) Negation and question modules combined, not in adult form yet.

at the beginning of the sentence or phrase and the Q3 code can connect to a "rising tone" module at the end of the string, here symbolized by the "?".

For negation, the modules in Figure 6.9(b) allow morphemes that symbolize negation to be added to the beginning of the sentence. A similar module with a code on the right would allow the negation morphemes at the end of the string. Although the child does not hear questions and negatives in these forms, they will be produced this way because they represent the meaning as the child understands them: The scope of questions and negatives is understood to be the whole string, and the simplest way to represent this, before positional priority exceptions have been learned, is to put the morphemes for questions and negatives at the beginning or end of the string. Children studied by Bellugi (1967) initially negate by adding a NO or NOT to the beginning, and sometimes the end, of a string. Moskowitz (1978) reports that Catherine Lord (1974) even found a child who changed the *tone* of the sentence at the end, rather than adding a morpheme to negate it, treating negation the way questions are handled. This variety in children's expressions of negation is some indication that the child employs nothing more specific than scope (and perhaps dependency) information.

As a child continues to hear English, it observes the negation morphemes occurring in between the subject and verb, ignoring those morphemes, such as verb auxiliaries, that it doesn't yet understand. Bellugi (1967) found that children then acquire the ability to negate a sentence by inserting NO, NOT, CAN'T, or DON'T between the subject and the verb. At this stage, CAN'T and DON'T are treated as unanalyzed negatives, rather than a combination of auxiliary and negative. For the syntax crystal, any insertion of the negative morpheme into the middle of a string means that a positional priority exception has been employed. The same modules, except for the change in position because of the arrowed exception, can be used for the new structures (see Figure 6.9[c]). As this positional priority exception is used more frequently, strings such as WENDY CAN'T WALK, WHY WENDY NOT WALK? replace the earlier forms of NO WENDY WALK, or WHY NOT WENDY WALK? or WHY NO WALK?

Negative questions use the Q modules as in Figure 6.9(d).

Bellugi (1967) reports that this insertion takes place (1) before children learn the correct pronouns for negation (I HAVE SOME, negated, yields I HAVEN'T ANY); (2) before they learn to use the auxiliaries such as DO and IS, saying I NOT HURT HIM and THIS NO GOOD (this should be plausible for any theory of language, as it is easier to learn the more regularly used words for negation, NO, NOT, first and to learn the auxiliaries with less, or subtler meaning, such as DO and IS, later); and (3) before they learn that the second verb morpheme does not carry the past tense, saying IT MIGHT FELL DOWN or I DIDN'T DID IT.

In our view, coordinating the correct pronouns often requires a combination of structural and surface sequence information. The syntax crystal represents the rules for structural information. Rules or procedures for combining these structural rules with globally used surface sequence information are beyond the present discussion. But it is consistent with what is presented here that learning correct pronouns for negation takes place later than learning the correct structure and order.

And the learning of negation morphemes (NO, NOT) and some auxiliaries may well precede the learning of past morphemes (-ED), so that a past form of a verb will be treated as a unit and used with an auxiliary. In fact, the learning of negation as a positional priority exception may well facilitate the later learning of the past morpheme.

Children begin to learn that verb auxiliaries precede the subject phrase in questions and that verb auxiliaries are required before (or in conjunction with) the negative morpheme (Bellugi, 1967). In order to show how this is done, we must first discuss verb auxiliaries.

Let us suppose that verb auxiliaries are syntactically distinguishable from other verbs when they are learned. Although substitutable for the verb in WENDY EATS to produce WENDY CAN, verb and auxiliary are not substitutable for each other in WENDY CAN EAT – there is no ★WENDY EAT CAN. So auxiliaries must be connected to subject phrases and to verbs by new structure modules, as in Figure 6.10(a). Other modules that connect to the subject and to verbs will receive new top codes as the children test and expand their sentences. For WENDY CAN EAT, we add an S code to get the structure in Figure 6.10(b). For questions in which

(a)

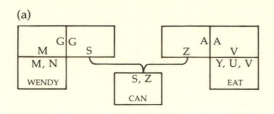

(b)

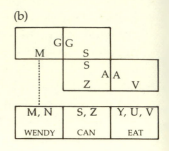

(c)

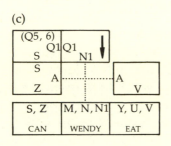

(d)

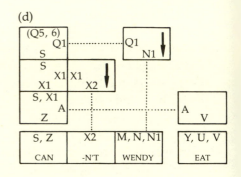

(e)

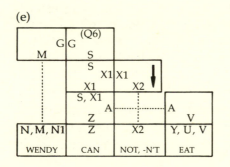

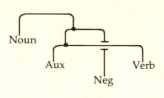

(f)

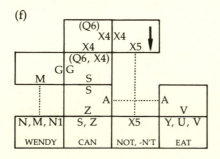

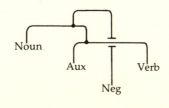

verb auxiliaries precede the subject, such as CAN WENDY EAT? two new modules (the ones with Q1 side codes) with a positional priority exception are used, leaving the other structure modules as they were for declarative connections (see Figure 6.10[c]). The Q5 and Q6 codes on the top of the S\Q1 module connect to question adverbs and interrogative tone marker for WHY CAN WENDY EAT? In order to continue to allow question modules larger scope than negation modules, new negation modules must be inserted under the S\Q1 module, as in Figure 6.10(d). In declarative form the same negation modules could be used (see [e]). This arrangement of negation and question modules requires a minimum of new modules and preserves the scope relations of these forms with respect to each other. However, it does assign a different scope to the negation in WENDY CANNOT EAT than in IT IS NOT THE CASE THAT WENDY CAN EAT. In the former, the scope of the NOT is the predicate phrase; in the latter, it is the whole sentence, WENDY CAN EAT. The apparent synonymy of these two forms may indicate that the scope of negation in declarative sentences should be as in Figure 6.10(f). Tag questions (such as WENDY CAN EAT, CAN'T SHE?) require the coordinating of the auxiliary, negation, and the pronoun for the subject. Like coordinated pronouns for negation, it is to be expected that both the structural rules of the syntax crystal and the surface morpheme sequence are employed in generating tag questions. Other question forms that use only structural information are, predictably, learned first (Bellugi, 1967; Moskowitz, 1978).

An algorithm for coding syntax crystal modules

The preceding sections described the acquisition of some syntactic structures. There are many structures that have not been discussed. Nevertheless, the same principles used to code modules can be applied to other structures. We will present these princi-

Figure 6.10. (a) Auxiliary connects to subject NP and/or main verb. (b) Auxiliary modules with greater differentiation. (c) Auxiliary precedes verb for questions. (d) Negation scope smaller than question scope with new modules. (e) New negation modules for declarative sentences. (f) Alternative crystal in which negation modules have larger scope.

ples in the form of an algorithm, specifying each step in the process of creating coded modules for a syntax crystal. This algorithm will not distinguish the developmental stages discussed earlier, nor will it include the heuristic strategies of learning that children use for language and other skills. The purpose of presenting this algorithm is to show that creating coded modules can be an automatic mechanical operation requiring no hidden cognitive apparatus.

The algorithm supposes that the scope and dependency relations of an orrery and the order and inflections of a language string are both available. The orrery relations may be evident from the nonlinguistic context when the string is presented, or the orrery relations may be a creation of the language learner and the string an attempt to express these relations using some previously learned modules and some new ones. Basically, then, three kinds of information are needed to create modules: scope information, dependency information, and some information about the position of a morpheme in a string.

The algorithm for coding modules follows the same steps for all connections: Use existing structure modules to make the connections if possible. If not, try to make the connections by adding top codes alone. Test these connections by substitution in different contexts. If they do not work, try to make the connections by using one existing structure module, and one newly coded structure module connected by a new side code. If substitutions are not acceptable, then create all new structure modules for the connections.

Here is the algorithm. To connect morphemes whose concepts are related perform the following steps in order, unless noted otherwise:

1. Are the morphemes to be connected those with the smallest scope that have not yet been connected by structure modules? If *yes*, go to 3.
2. Find unattached morphemes with smaller scope and go to 1.
3. Are the morphemes to be connected already represented on existing modules? If *no*, go to 14.
4. Can the morpheme modules, or arrays of already connected modules, be connected in the proper order by existing structure modules that have not been tried before for this connection and rejected? If *yes*, tentatively make the connection. If *no*, go to 9.
5. Do the structure modules attach either above the column of the main

morphemes or arrays to be connected, or to morpheme modules directly? If *no*, reject these tentative structure modules and go to 4.

6. Does the structure module that attaches to the subordinate morpheme column of the whole connection have a top code? If *yes*, reject these structure modules and go to 4.

7. If a morpheme, or array, occurs in between (rather than entirely on one side of) an array it is scoped with, is the structure module above it one with a downward arrow? If *no*, reject these tentative structure modules and go to 4.

8. Can the connection made with these structure modules be substituted in other constructions? If the substitutions are acceptable, go to 16. If the substitutions are unacceptable, reject these tentative structure modules and go to 4.[9]

9. Can a connection not already tried and rejected be made to existing structure modules by entering either top codes on the morpheme modules, or optional top codes on the top modules in the main morpheme's column of arrays to be connected, such that:
   a. The structure modules have top codes only above the main morpheme of the whole connection, and
   b. The structure modules connect either to the column of the main morpheme of arrays to be connected, or directly to morpheme modules, and
   c. The structure module above a morpheme or array that occurs in between an array it is scoped with has a downward arrow?[10]
   If *no*, go to 11.

10. Can the connection made with these structure modules be substituted in other constructions? If the substitutions are acceptable, go to 16. If the substitutions are unacceptable, reject these tentative structure modules and go to 9.

11. Is there an existing structure module that has a side code in the direction of the other modules to be connected such that:
   a. It connects either to a morpheme module, or to an array on the top of the column of the main morpheme of that array; and
   b. It has a top code only if it is above the main morpheme of the whole connection; and
   c. If it is above a morpheme or array that occurs in between an array it is scoped with, it has a downward arrow?
   If *no*, go to 15.

12. Tentatively assign a new side code to that structure module in the direction of the other morpheme modules or array. Place blank modules above the morpheme module or main column of an array of modules that are to be connected to the existing structure module with short edge apposing the existing module. Put the same new side code on the edge of the blank module directly facing the other structure module. Assign a new code to the bottom of the previously blank module and the same code to the top of the module under it.

13. Can the connection made with these structure modules be substituted in other constructions? If the substitutions are acceptable, go to 16. If the substitutions are unacceptable, reject these tentative structure modules and go to 15.
14. Place blank rectangular modules with short edges facing each other. The first morpheme is entered on the bottom of the left module; the second, on the bottom of the next module to the right, and so on. Go to 9.
15. Codes that have not been used before are assigned to the top of each top structure module in the main morpheme column, or to the top of each morpheme module to be connected individually. Blank modules with short edges facing each other are placed either above the morpheme modules, or above the top structure module in the main morpheme column of an array to be connected. These blank structure modules are given codes on their bottom edges to match the codes on the top edges of the lower modules. The apposing edges of the upper modules are given matching codes. If one of the morphemes or arrays just connected occurs in the surface string *within* the constituent it is connected to, add a downward arrow to the top structure module of the intervening morpheme or array.
16. Retain these modules. If there are any morphemes left to be connected, go to 1. Otherwise, *stop*.

The algorithm is a first approximation to a mechanical procedure for coding modules. It does not produce modules for the double scope connections proposed for some relative clauses (in Chapter 5). It undoubtedly could be supplemented by some additional instructions and heuristic strategies about the variety of substitution tests to perform. It may need additional instructions to interpret phrases such as "previously rejected." It may need additional instructions to handle grammatical morphemes such as -ING and OF. Although every morpheme provides some semantic hints about its scope and dependency, this information may be too sparse for some inflections and function words. Therefore, scope and dependency relations must be determined, at least in part, by the way in which such grammatical morphemes relate to other units in the string.

But we believe that this algorithm shows the main principles of how modules may be coded, and that the coding can be done without using cognitive operations that are hidden or so specific that they could only be applied to language and not to other, nonlinguistic abilities.

Concluding remarks

In the second half of this chapter, we demonstrated how the syntax crystal model could be used to explain the basics of syntax acquisition. We did not assume that any of the cognitive structure for syntax was innately given. We did assume with Bloom and Lahey (1978) and Moskowitz (1978) that the nonlinguistic environment provides the language learner with clues to the relations of concepts encoded by syntax. This means that the child can at least partly construct the scope and dependency relations of the concepts named by the lexemes in the string it hears. From the string itself comes information about the sequence of morphemes comprising a well-formed utterance. What the child must do is to put together these two kinds of information. A cognitive structure that combines concept-relation information with morpheme-sequence information is a syntactic mechanism. Using our syntactic model, the syntax crystal, we described how this information is combined. First, we went through the acquisition process in an informal way, using examples from the language-development literature and describing how associative connections, working in concert with the sequence, could be formed to represent this information. Then we formalized the module-coding procedures and presented an algorithm for producing coded modules that constitute the syntactic rules.

SCRYP, the syntax crystal parser: a computer implementation

PAUL J. GRUENEWALD

The Syntax CRYstal Parser (SCRYP) is a computer program that uses syntax crystal rules to parse sentences of a natural language. The procedures developed for the parser constitute a set of heuristics for the bottom-up, as opposed to top-down, analysis of sentence structure. We believe such procedures reflect some processes that take place in human language comprehension. This appendix will outline some advantages the parser has over other procedures as well as presenting a description of the program itself. An important consideration is the applicability of SCRYP to descriptions of human language performance. For this reason, we emphasize parsimony of description and the applicability of structural and procedural assumptions to human language performance.

Local rules and global procedures

Parsers for descriptive and interpretive grammars

The problem of constructing a parser to derive syntactic descriptions of sentences on the basis of word order and inflections is largely the problem of selecting and implementing appropriate *global procedures* to coordinate the operations of *local rules* (see Chapters 1 and 4). Various types of local rules may be used in global procedures. The rules specify the elements of syntactic form, the procedures and their application. Whether one wishes to describe a sentence using the case relations of Fillmore's (1968) grammar or with the structural relations of classic phrase structure grammars, for example, the procedures selected to perform the analysis will not be necessarily determined by the formal rules themselves. For example, the left-to-right processing assumption of augmented transition networks (ATNs) is applied to simple phrase structure grammars (Linn and Reitman, 1975) and to Fillmore's (1968) case grammar (Norman, Rumelhart, and the LNR Research Group, 1975).

The types of grammars used in parsing systems may be conveniently characterized in a way suggested by von Glasersfeld (1975). The field of grammars may be divided into two parts: descriptive grammars, which attempt to formally characterize the "grammatical" sentences of a language, and interpretive grammars, which "should be a complete mapping of the semantic connections of the

300

elements and structures of a language . . . and the elements and structures of conceptual representation" (von Glasersfeld, 1975:22). A similar distinction divides the field of parsing systems into those that primarily aim at an appropriate syntactic characterization of a sentence (descriptive parsers) and those that attempt a direct semantic interpretation (interpretive parsers).

The implementation of descriptive grammars has been primarily along two lines, the top-down parser and the ATN system. Top-down parsing systems rely on grammatical rules to generate a syntactic structure beginning at the topmost node (the root or base of the tree) and ending with the morphemes of the string (the terminal nodes of the tree). One may imagine this process as the successive application of rewrite rules beginning with a rule describing the most abstract aspect of the sentence: S → NP VP. The surface structure of the sentence is generated from this point by successive applications of the underlying phrase structure rules. In a complementary way, sentences are parsed by searching for the successive rule applications that will yield the appropriate surface structure. Such rule searches may be executed serially or in parallel. Some typical examples of top-down parsing techniques may be found in Harris (1972), Anderson and Bower (1973), Kimball (1973), and Palme (1971), who includes a description of one of the few bottom-up parsers applied to descriptive grammars. See also Kaplan (1973).

By far the most popular parsing technique to date, however, has been that developed through the application of ATNs (Woods, 1970). An ATN parser describes the successive stages of sentence processing as transitions from one state to the next. Each state transition may be viewed as a program that evaluates some portion of the sentence structure (see Winograd, 1972, 1974). Thus, in parsing a string of morphemes, the ATN grammar will seek to identify the form class of the first morpheme, then the second morpheme and so on. The network guides the process to the next form class in the string based on the occurrence of previous words or word groups. Such simple (usually left-to-right) parsing systems have the advantage that, given an appropriately simple grammar, input strings may be parsed extremely efficiently. But, given more complex grammars, these networks tend to get caught in back-tracking problems where incorrect state changes may lead to seriously incomplete structural descriptions. To derive the correct structure, the program may have to back up many times through the network. Typical applications of ATNs can be found in Woods (1970), Linn and Reitman (1975), and Norman, Rumelhart, and the LNR Research Group (1975).

Before moving on, a closer look should be taken at ATN parsers. Figure A.1 presents a network implementing a simple, recursive, context-free grammar. The network consists of states, indicated by circles, and labeled transitions, shown by arrows. In order to pass from one state to the next, the requirements of the transition must be fulfilled. Successive words in the string are tested for membership in the succeeding syntactic form classes defined by the labeled transitions of the ATN. Thus the transitions can be interpreted as instructions to be implemented by the parser (Winograd, 1972, 1974).

Let us analyze the string ROBOTS CAN BE FUN using the network of Figure A.1.

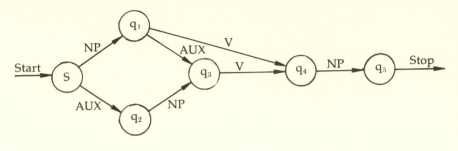

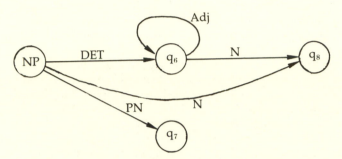

Figure A.1. A simplified augmented transition network (ATN) adapted from Woods (1970).

Beginning at state S and examining the words of the sentence from left to right, the network first requires a test for the presence of a noun phrase, NP, in the string. This transition requires the application of the second network in the figure. Here, the first constituent of many NPs, a determiner, DET, is the first form class expected. Since ROBOTS is not a member of the DET form class, the optional second transition is taken in which ROBOTS is tested as a plural noun, PN. As ROBOTS is found to be a member of this form class, the NP network reaches its terminal state and control is returned to the original transition network. The NP transition having been completed, the second word of the string, CAN, is tested for its membership in the verb, V, form class, which fails, and then in the auxiliary, AUX, form class, which succeeds. The next word, BE, is tested as a verb, which succeeds, and the NP network is again called in and identifies FUN as a member of the noun, N, form class. The sentence is successfully parsed when an exit from the transition network occurs simultaneously with the classification of the last element of the string.

An important aspect of ATN parsers, not often noted, is that they frequently exhibit properties normally attributed to top-down parsers. Strings are parsed in terms of successively more specific parts of the constituent structure. Thus the initial ATN of Figure A.1, identified with beginning node S, may call the NP ATN to perform an analysis of a noun phrase. Similarly, other ATNs for verb phrases, prepositional phrases, and relative clauses may be constructed. These ATNs, called in from the main network, S, effectively act as separate subsets of rules for parsing different phrases of a string, much like the separate sets of rules defining phrases accessed in top-down parsers.

As already noted, the most common criticism of ATN parsing systems is their need for extensive backtracking. The backing up of the parser to a previous state is caused by a failure in the currently evaluated transition. In the simple grammar used in the example above, this occurred when CAN was tested for its membership in the V form class. Since CAN was not a member of this class, backup to state q_1 was required and a test for its membership in the alternative AUX form class was made. This rather trivial example can be extended to cases where backup is required through most of the entire network.

While the implementation of descriptive parsers has tended toward top-down, left-to-right procedures, interpretive parsers have not. Interpretive grammars, as suggested by von Glasersfeld (1969), attempt direct mappings from strings to conceptual representations. Because of this emphasis, parsers for these grammars tend to be of the bottom-up variety. That is, they begin with the morphemes of a string and attempt to form a description from their elementary structural relationships. As a simple example, take the string THE BLUE ROBOT. Initially, the bottom-up parser has available to it only the binary relationships, restricted by order, of THE BLUE, THE ROBOT, and BLUE ROBOT. Each of these is an acceptable fragment of a potentially complete parse (relating the form classes DET ADJ, DET N, and ADJ N respectively). However, a complete parse can be achieved only by the parser recognizing that the constituent BLUE ROBOT may be modified as a whole by THE. The parser looks for "higher" structural relationships that combine the simple binary relationships found at the "lowest" level. Thus, the form class sequence DET ADJ N is parsed from the bottom up, from form classes to abstract rules.

One bottom-up system, designed by Colby, Parkison, and Faught (1974), uses pattern matching devices to recognize "idiomatic" sequences of English lexeme strings. Like the ELIZA system (Weizenbaum, 1966), it assumes that a limited corpus of such patterns can accommodate a reasonable subset of English. The pattern-matching process permits a semantic mapping of the string from syntactic patterns to the conceptual representation itself. This represents a bottom-up parse in which the mapping moves directly from the surface string to the semantic properties of that string. This sort of system works well in limited semantic environments (witness the success of ELIZA); however, in more complex environments it may become computationally intractable. A vast collection of patterns would be required.

Another bottom-up system based on more traditional lines has also been developed. Von Glasersfeld and Pisani (1970) describe their system as a multistore parser. It is based on the correlational grammar described in von Glasersfeld (1969). This is a grammar that correlates morpheme strings with their semantic interpretations. The grammar has some three hundred "correlators" to do this task. A correlator is the specification of some relation between two morphemes that may be syntactic or, on a more abstract level, semantic. Thus the syntactic relations between determiners and nouns are specified by these two correlator types (from Palme, 1971):

1. DETNOUN::= DET NOUN
2. DETNOUN::= DET ADJNOUN

The first indicates the correlation of a determiner to a single noun; the second to the adjective-noun relation. In the example given above, correlator (1) specifies that for example, THE may enter DETNOUN relations that link determiners only to nouns. Correlator (2) specifies that THE may also enter DETNOUN relations that link determiners to the ADJNOUN relation. Note that all correlator rules are considered to be strictly ordered (e.g., a determiner must appear to the left of its noun).

During a parse the system selects the first word of the string, finds its form class or set of alternative classes, stores them and their potential relations to other correlators in the system, and goes to the second word. The same operation is performed on each subsequent word in the string. Each of the pairwise relations between the correlators derived from the words is then tested to see if it will join to form higher constituents. For example, the DETNOUN and ADJNOUN correlators may unite in the PHRASE correlator. By pursuing this line of attack and preserving all the parse information for easy recovery (the multistore aspect of the system), a structural analysis of the string will eventually emerge. The relative inefficiency of this operation is minimized by storing all the necessary information in easily recoverable tabular form in memory.

The most prominent criticism of such bottom-up approaches is that they are quite inefficient (see Anderson and Bower, 1973). This is a popular and, under certain conditions, a powerful argument against this sort of approach. Certainly, a large number of erroneous relations may be produced in the initial stages of the parse that do not appear in the final, correct, structural analysis. Even in our simple example above, the erroneous relation THE BLUE was initially produced before the correct structural relations were obtained. However, this evaluation of efficiency ignores the possibility that, in the long run, such relations may be quite useful. They may contribute to the flexibility of the parsing process. Siklossy, Rich, and Marinov (1973), in their study of breadth-first search processes in theorem-proving machines, have shown that if the space of such relations is well constrained, the performance of such devices can exceed those of other systems. Allowing the broad examination of many relationships early in the proof process increases the likelihood of obtaining unique and interesting solutions.

The issue of flexibility versus brittleness is at the heart of the problem of parser design. It rests on the question of the programmer's expectations regarding the system: To what degree will the program be expected to operate in unusual grammatical environments? Typically brittle ATN parsers can be quite efficient given restricted grammatical environments. But an interest in the simulation of human parsing capabilities requires that the demands lie heavily toward flexibility. A brittle system is not desirable. As Winograd (1974) has pointed out, if we expect a parsing or understanding system eventually to mimic human performance, it will have to be capable of parsing or under-standing strings like BANG CRASH HOSPITAL. These "asyntactic" expressions defy analysis in most parsing systems.

As a case in point, we might examine what an ATN system would do with such expressions. Characteristically, the brittleness of such systems would cause them to reject these strings out of hand as not possible (Kaplan, 1973). After all, where is the verb phrase in the expression BOY ROBOT HOME? This vio-lates the typical order of NP V NP expected by the simple network above. If the criterion for a successful parse were relaxed a bit and this string parsed solely as a noun phrase in the ATN, we could get an interpretation of the string as two adjectives, BOY ROBOT, modifying a noun, HOME. But then the interpretation BOY (verbs) ROBOT HOME would be missing, as well as numerous others. An ATN would have to be equipped with special heuristics to handle these strings.

An improvement might allow variables to be inserted in the string whenever a transition could not be made. Then the parser could use these variables to complete the parse in hypothetical ways. Thus it is possible that BOY $\underline{x}$ ROBOT HOME could eventually be one guess of the parser. But on what basis would the program make such a guess? If no proper parse exists at a given transition, then all possible parses for the words up to that transition must have been tested. Further, if a variable was to be then inserted, its form class would have to be guessed before the rest of the string could be processed. Presumably this would be done on the basis of previously occurring words in the string. The parser would be required to guess the missing form class and continue parsing in the hopes that the inserted variable's form class would itself not lead to another im-possible parse.

ATN parsers have problems in situations like these. Perhaps, as has been suggested by Farbens (1975), a metaparser is required, a parser that could change its parsing procedures to fit different contexts. This would then require the parser to identify all contexts in which particular parsing procedures would be required. Before going this far we would hope some simpler solution might be available. Whatever that simpler solution might be, it is certain that for a system to handle asyntactic expressions, neosyntactisms, *and* grammatical strings, considerable flexibility will be required. In an attempt to get at the problem of flexibility, let us return to top-down parsers.

One of the most elegant top-down parsing systems in the literature is that of Harris (1972). His interest was really in adaptive problem solving, not in pars-ing per se. Nonetheless, his work on the parsing mechanism, and its adaptive properties, shows quite clearly the problems of top-down parsers. These prob-lems are essentially two: The first regards the overall efficiency of such systems. The second, and more important, regards the introduction of constraining in-formation in the parse.

As we have mentioned before, it has often been noted that bottom-up parsers are inefficient. However, top-down parsers are not necessarily any more ef-ficient. The problem of combinatorial mechanics in parsing does not disappear simply because a different parsing strategy is introduced. The initial impres-sion, that top-down parsers may converge more rapidly on the proper structural description of a sentence because each successive rule selection dramatically constrains the number of possible sentences that can be generated from that point, is not a priori true. For it is information in the surface string itself that must be used to select these rules.

The difference in efficiency between bottom-up and top-down parsers is a matter of how constraints are introduced to guide the parsing process. And in this matter, top-down parsers may turn out less efficient than other parsing techniques. Thus Harris (1972) introduces a heuristic device to his top-down parser called the *bandwidth heuristic search*. This is a tree-trimming heuristic in which the class of alternative parses is narrowed as each parse that leads to too many or too few terminal nodes is rejected. The parse must account for all and only the proper number of words in the string. As such, this heuristic serves to effectively limit the large number of surface descriptions available from the root of the parsing tree. However, no such heuristic is required in a bottom-up parser. Only rules directly relevant to the actual words of the string are ever considered in the analysis. For example, in strings that do not contain prepositions, the prepositional phrase rule is never considered as an alternate path for a correct parse.

The second problem of top-down parsers follows from the first: A grammatical rule that meets the requirements of the bandwidth heuristic must also be selected for its appropriateness to the form classes in the surface string. Specific information, present only in the surface structure of the string, must be used to constrain rule selection early in the parse. Harris's (1972) use of "semantic disambiguators" in his model depicts the problems encountered in introducing such constraints to a top-down parse.

Harris presents semantic disambiguators as rules for selecting only semantically appropriate parses. Each attempted parse of a string is first generated and then semantically selected. That is, the semantic components of the surface string are matched to those generated by the parse. If the match fails, another parse is generated and tested. This creates a unique back-up problem peculiar to such processors. Considerable time must be spent generating the field of parses from which the appropriate member must be selected. This problem is difficult to avoid. Even with a closed set of syntactic form classes, parses must be generated and the derived form classes of the terminal nodes compared to the actual form classes of morphemes in the string.

Some serious problems attend the construction of parsers that attempt to approximate human performance. ATN parsers are brittle and require extensive backtracking for difficult strings. They cannot easily handle asyntactic expressions, as strict conformance to the ordered transition network is required to obtain a successful parse. Top-down parsers, on the other hand, do not necessarily have this difficulty but have two other problems: First, they are not more efficient than any bottom-up process and they require extensive tree-trimming operations. Second, as exemplified by the introduction of semantic disambiguators in Harris's (1972) parser, structural analyses must be produced *before* being tested against the surface string.

It seems clear that another parsing mechanism must be considered, one that can parse well-formed strings and also give enough information about neosyn-tactisms and asyntactic expressions to suggest reasonable structural analyses. Further, it should be one that will maximally use the information in the surface string as the parse is constructed. Such information should guide parsing, not select parses. Finally, the parser should be able to serve both as an interpretive grammar and as a descriptive grammar. In other words, it should offer an interpretation of a string as well as evaluate and manipulate its structural properties. These requirements are demanding, but at least some of them can be met by a bottom-up parser based upon a syntax crystal grammar.

Bottom-up parsers and the syntax crystal grammar

SCRYP can best be defined as a multipass bottom-up parser. The syntactic structure of a sentence is revealed a layer at a time, pass by pass, from the lowest to the highest points in its constituent structure. Each pass of the parser represents an examination of the syntactic relations between morphemes in the string at one level of the analysis. Thus the parser begins by examining each pair of morphemes in the string and selecting only those rules of the grammar applicable to describing direct syntactic relations between them. This is the first pass of the parser. Subsequent passes examine the relations across these rules and describe more complex aspects of the syntactic structure of the string. The final pass of the parser occurs when a complete description of the syntactic structure of the string is developed. SCRYP has a number of similarities to the multistore parser of von Glasersfeld and Pisani (1970), and the reader is encouraged to examine their system. Here we will first introduce some of the advantages of bottom-up processing using the syntax crystal grammar.

There are three important features of the parser: First, because of the nature of the syntax crystal grammar, there are no pure metarules in the system, no rule serves merely to coordinate other rules. Second, the system is capable of best-guessing missing constituents in incomplete strings. It can supply partial structural descriptions for asyntactic and neosyntactic expressions. Third, a bottom-up parser using syntax crystal rules suggests that a complete structural analysis of a sentence may not be necessary for its comprehension. Each of these properties will be discussed before the system is described.

The flexibility of the hierarchical structures produced by a syntax crystal grammar is very important. Figure A.2 compares a syntax crystal grammar with a traditional phrase structure. The syntax crystal grammar presented is a simplified version of that described in Chapter 5. Here, independent constituents are underlined. One difference between the grammars is the variety of possible connections allowed by the syntax crystal rules. Thus rule (1′) indicates that the string may be rewritten as a noun and a verb, a noun and a verb phrase, a noun phrase and a verb, or a noun phrase and a verb phrase. In the bottom-up parse, each of these syntactic relations is available as descriptions of the relation between surface constituents.

In the first parsing stage for both grammars, the morphemes of the string are connected to their appropriate form classes. For simplicity, we assume through-

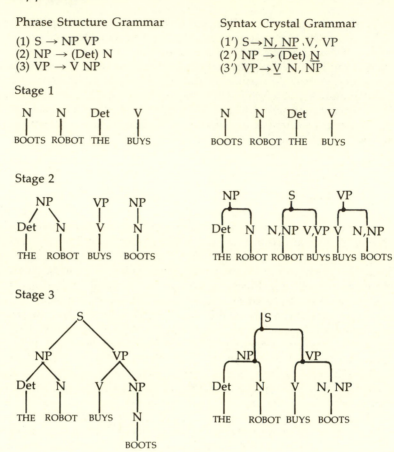

Figure A.2. Comparison of parses using phrase structure and syntax crystal grammars.

out this appendix that the form classes are correctly assigned in the first attempt. In practice this could fail to happen unless we consider that many parsing operations proceed in parallel. By the second stage, the differences between the two grammars can be observed. Stage 2 of the phrase structure parse provides a constituent structure relating the word pair THE ROBOT. The verb BUY is classified as a verb phrase and the noun BOOTS as a noun phrase. Stage 2 of the parse using syntax crystal rules, however, provides constituent structures for the word pairs THE ROBOT, ROBOT BUYS, and BUYS BOOTS. The redundant coding of syntax crystal connections allows each rule to connect constituent elements of the surface string.

One advantage of the syntax crystal description, then, derives from the fact that, typically, even the most abstract rules of the grammar, those most removed from the surface structure (e.g., rule 1' in Figure A.2), can directly connect to the simple constituents of the surface string (e.g., ROBOT BUYS). The comparable phrase structure rules (e.g., rule 1) may only provide descriptions of the relations between highly abstract sentence constituents (e.g., NP and VP). If bottom-up parsers search first for the simplest morpheme relations in a string and only then for higher constituent relations, this strict hierarchy of rules prevents simple relations such as ROBOT BUYS from appearing early in the parse. The flexible hierarchy of syntax crystal grammar promotes the discovery of such relations at an early point in the parse.

Like ATNs, bottom-up parsers have the advantage of being able to begin a parse before the entire string is received. Thus pieces of a parse may be assembled before the complete parse is obtained. As shown above, the syntax crystal grammar provides a convenient framework in which pieces of the constituent structure of a sentence may be derived. Unlike ATNs, however, bottom-up processors do not require contiguous links between successive pieces of all the input elements. If some relation fails to obtain between two morphemes, subsequent ones may still be processed.

Consider the neosyntactism DISASTERED BY A GOOF-OFF. ATN parsers would have a difficult time establishing a transition from the noun DISASTER to the verb ending -ED. In most grammars such a transition would simply not exist. In order for the ATN to continue parsing the string, an alternate route must be taken. Thus the parser must skip to the next constituent of the string, -ED, and continue the parse, attempting to derive the proper structural analysis of -ED BY A GOOF-OFF. As -ED is a constituent having no direct connection to the prepositional phrase BY A GOOF-OFF, the ATN parse will again fail. Skipping to the next constituent, a successful parse may be obtained for BY A GOOF-OFF. This would result in a structural analysis ignoring the existence of DISASTER and -ED, clearly an undesirable outcome.

The bottom-up parse is a natural alternative to an ATN parse. The flexibility afforded by syntax crystal rules combines with the processes of a bottom-up parse to produce fairly successful descriptions of the constituent structures of neosyntactisms. Thus the neosyntactism would first be analyzed into its simplest elements. The rules relating to each morpheme in the string would be examined for relations among the elements of surface structure. Two such rules connect DISASTER as a noun to a verb, $S \rightarrow N(NP) \underline{V}(VP)$ and the -ED as a morpheme associated with the past tense of a verb, $V \rightarrow \underline{V} T_p$. In the example, no verb exists for either of these rules to connect to. However, the bottom-up parse allows these rules to be connected to the remaining constituent structure of the sentence without requiring the existence of the verb form. Thus the structural analyses in Figure A.3 may be formed and the neosyntactism may be analyzed as three subparses: DISASTER BY A GOOF-OFF, a complete subparse suggesting that -ED be deleted; ————-ED BY A GOOF-OFF, an incomplete parse suggesting that the morpheme preceding -ED is a verb; and DISASTER ———— BY A GOOF-OFF, an incomplete parse suggesting that some verb form is missing from the structure.

This, then, is the second feature of a bottom-up parser using syntax crystal

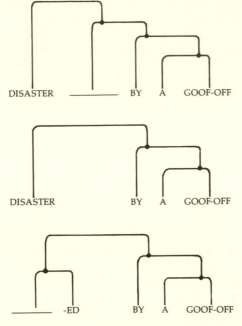

DISASTER ——————— BY   A   GOOF-OFF

DISASTER   BY   A   GOOF-OFF

——————— -ED   BY   A   GOOF-OFF

Figure A.3. Partial analyses of the neosyntactism DISASTERED BY A
GOOF-OFF.

grammar: Structural descriptions may be derived for neosyntactic expressions.
Successful parses include all surface elements in the string. Nodes that do not
connect directly to any surface constituent indicate the missing constituent's
proper location. In Figure A.3 the first parse has one terminal node of this type
pointing to the position in the string occupied by -ED. The third parse has a
single node indicating the position in the string occupied by DISASTER. These
parses suggest what types of constituents are missing from the string. They may
represent best guesses as to how the indicated elements are to be interpreted.
Given the human language user's reluctance to reject deviant strings as unacceptable (Gleitman and Gleitman, 1970), either of the parses could lead to an interpretable guess about the structure of the string. Thus the second subparse,
———————-ED BY A GOOF-OFF, suggests that DISASTER be interpreted as a verb form
(as the noun "trash" gives rise to the colloquial verb "trashed").
     Asyntactic expressions may be similarly analyzed. Take, for example, the
string given above, BOY ROBOT HOME. As we saw, an ATN parser could analyze
this adjective as an adjective-adjective-noun sequence. A bottom-up parser
would also arrive at this structural analysis. However, neither parser immediately produces a structural description suggesting the more likely *elliptical*
but asyntactic form, BOY ROBOT ——————— HOME. And, as suggested above, an ATN
parser would require some additional measures to determine where and what

the missing constituent of the string could be. A simple addition to the bottom-up parser will give this structural interpretation. Successive parsings of the string would be produced until the number of terminal nodes equaled the number of surface constituents of the string plus one. This extra terminal node, not connected to an element of the surface structure, would suggest what constituent is missing from the surface string.

This brings us to the third observation about a bottom-up parser using syntax crystal grammar: The notion of what it means to parse a sentence may be reconceptualized on the basis of such bottom-up processes. The question here is whether parsing need always go to completion in the analysis of sentence structure. The answer to this question bears upon the problem of structural complexity in sentence comprehension. This point is also related to the first observation regarding syntax crystal rules: Most rules can coordinate simple elements of the surface string. As pointed out above, in the execution of a parse these simple relations will be identified first, to be followed by the construction of more complex constituent structures. Thus, in Figure A.2, rule 1' will be examined early in the parse and found to directly relate the pair ROBOT BUYS in the string THE ROBOT BUYS BOOTS. Yet this rule will finally appear in the complete structural description of the string as the most abstract rule in the structure, relating the noun phrase THE ROBOT to the verb phrase BUYS BOOTS. This dual role of syntax crystal rules in sentence parsing has important implications for notions about sentence comprehension.

Consider the parse of the sentence, THE ROBOT BUYS BOOTS presented in Figure A.2. There we saw the noun-verb relation of ROBOT BUYS revealed in the earliest stages of the bottom-up parse using the syntax crystal grammar. This relation was obtained in the same stage as THE ROBOT and BUYS BOOTS. If comprehension of these relations is assumed to depend on their realization in the parse, each of them would appear equally available upon a reading of the string. That is, if a subject were presented with the string THE ROBOT BUYS BOOTS, verification of the relations THE ROBOT, ROBOT BUYS, and BUYS BOOTS would require an equal amount of processing. Verification of the more complex relations THE ROBOT BUYS and ROBOT BUYS BOOTS would require more processing because of the extra stage of parsing required to evaluate their structural descriptions in the string. Other things being equal, the amount of processing required to verify some particular syntactic relation, for example, ROBOT BUYS, will depend on which stage it appears during the bottom-up parse.

Verification of these same relations would be predictably different if a phrase structure grammar were assumed to underlie the parsing process. Again referring to Figure A.2, verification of the relation ROBOT BUYS would take longer than verification of THE ROBOT. This increase in processing is caused by the absence of any direct connections between the surface constituents in the phrase structure rules. Verification of the relation ROBOT BUYS would have to await stage 3 of the parse using the phrase structure grammar.

In terms of a bottom-up parser using a syntax crystal grammar, the comprehension of constituent relations in a string may thus be reconceptualized. The simple relations of surface constituents in the string became available first. Further analysis of the constituent structure depends upon the requirements of the listener. Thus, if the listener's concern is simply with "who buys?" an analysis of the simple relation ROBOT BUYS should be sufficient. However, if the listener's concern is with whether it is a particular ROBOT who BUYS BOOTS, then a complete structural analysis of THE ROBOT BUYS BOOTS may be required. Abstract relations among groups of surface constituents are examined only when necessary. The effects of structural complexity depend upon the depth of analysis required of each sentence, as in a verification task. If listeners do not need complete structural information about a sentence they will not go to the effort to obtain it. If the simple relations of surface string elements are sufficient for understanding a sentence in a particular context, deeper structural complexity will not affect the comprehension process. The parse may proceed only as far as the first elementary relations of morphemes in the surface string. Thus a complete analysis of THE ROBOT BUYS BOOTS is only necessary to verify that, indeed, THE ROBOT does BUY BOOTS, rather than A ROBOT BUYS BOOTS or THE ROBOT BUYS SNEAKERS.

In sum, these three points comprise the primary advantages of a bottom-up parser using a syntax crystal grammar:

1. As most rules can serve to relate surface elements in a string, the parser will supply these simple, immediately specifiable relations at the beginning of any parse.
2. In the context of a bottom-up procedure, this means that flexible descriptions may be afforded for the interpretation of asyntactic and neo-syntactic expressions. Simple, local-rule relations suggest these interpretations.
3. Finally, the mechanics of the bottom-up process suggest that the comprehension of a sentence may not necessarily entail a complete structural description. Partial processing of simple, local rule information may be sufficient for many language understanding situations.

Description of the syntax crystal parser

In what follows, a general outline of the form and operation of the syntax crystal parser will be presented. Emphasis will be placed upon an understanding of the general operations of the program rather than particulars of the program implementation. The program is a compiler, not an interpreter. It accepts the rules of the grammar as input, uses them in processing given strings, and outputs the results of the analyses. This particular structure is amenable to a simple description of the operations of the parser. The program was written in SPITBOL, a fast version of SNOBOL 4.

There are four types of data accepted as input by the program: (1) rules that specify the form classes of morphemes in the grammar, (2) structure rules that specify the relations between these rules and other structure rules of the grammar, (3) the strings to be parsed, and (4) control options for adjusting various parsing parameters.

Syntax crystal modules in Chapter 5

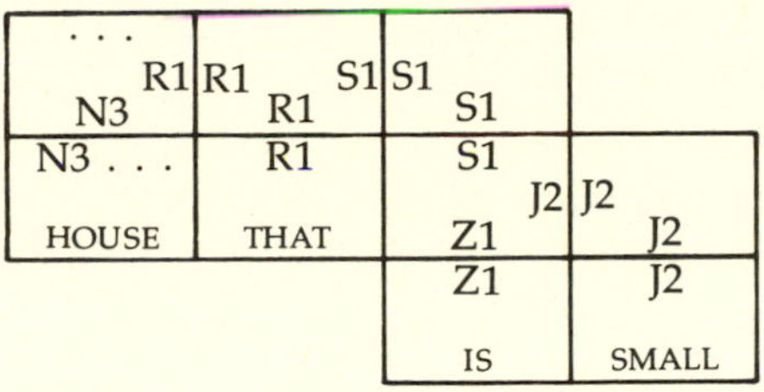

```
· · ·
      R1|R1    S1|S1
  N3      R1        S1
  N3 . . .    R1       S1
                          J2|J2
  HOUSE    THAT    Z1          J2
                          Z1        J2
                          IS     SMALL
```

N3 \ R1
R1 / R1 \ S1
S1 / S1
N3 → HOUSE
R1 → THAT
S1 → Z1\ J2
J2 /J2
Z1 → IS (BE)
J2 → SMALL

SCRYP modules

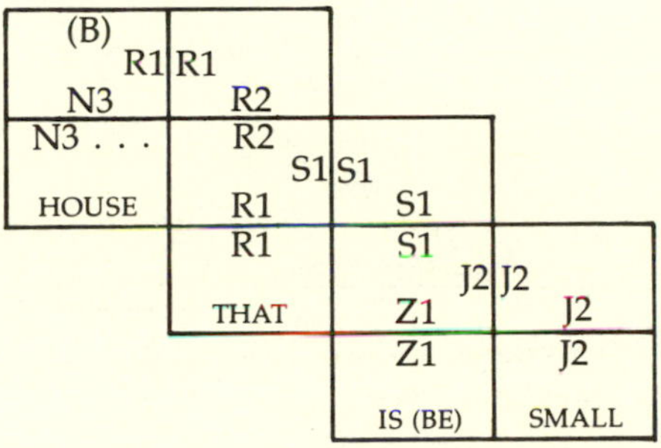

```
  (B)
      R1|R1
  N3      R2
  N3 . . .    R2
                 S1|S1
  HOUSE    R1        S1
              R1        S1
                          J2|J2
          THAT    Z1          J2
                          Z1        J2
                          IS (BE)  SMALL
```

(B) > N3 R2/C1 (top two
N3 > HOUSE   modules)
R2 > R1 S1/C2 (two
R1 > THAT   modules)
S1 > Z1 J2/C3
Z1 > IS (BE)
J2 > SMALL

Figure A.4. Comparison of rule structures in SCRYP and those in Chapter 5.

A simplified version of the syntax crystal rules of Chapter 5 was used in this implementation. Figure A.4 presents a comparison of rule forms between SCRYP and those presented in this book. The morpheme rules do not differ. However, there are two major differences between the structure rules used here and those used elsewhere in this text. The first is the use of a general connection code C to indicate dependencies in the rule structure. Thus, in the structure rule N > D∕C + N1, D∕C indicates that D (a code leading to the application of the rule D > THE) is dependent on N in the structure. In order to maintain a homogenous rule form throughout the parser, every rule must have a module top code. In other words, no rule of the form {R1∕R1\S1} may occur. This rule must be written as two rules: {B} > N R1∕C and R1 > R1 S1∕C. The advantages of this requirement will be explained below. The partial equivalence between rewrite rules and syntax crystal modules was discussed in Chapter 5.

Strings to be parsed by the system are expressed as a sequence of morphemes separated by blanks. Grammatical morphemes, that is, those with little semantic content, are indicated parenthetically, for example THE ROBOT WAS MO-VE(ING) THE PLANT. Control options will be specified as the program is explained further.

The bottom-up parser first defines a search space of possible relations among

The Grammar

The Lexicon

Vd > Va, W2   Vb, W1 /C
Vc > Va, W1 /C   Vb, W2
Vb > W1   W2 /C
Va > W1 /C   W2

W1 > M1
W2 > M2

Depth 1 Relations

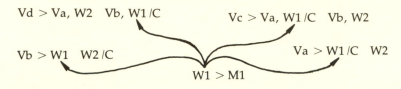

Vd > Va, W2   Vb, W1 /C

Vc > Va, W1 /C   Vb, W2

Vb > W1   W2 /C

Va > W1 /C   W2

W1 > M1

Depth 2 Relations

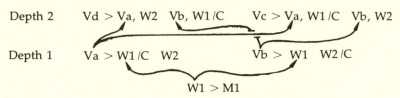

Depth 2   Vd > Va, W2 Vb, W1 /C   Vc > Va, W1 /C   Vb, W2

Depth 1   Va > W1 /C   W2   Vb > W1   W2 /C

W1 > M1

Figure A.5. Grammar, lexicon, and parses for two-morpheme language.

morphemes, using the rules of the grammar, then, trims this space heuristically to some manageable form (see Siklossy, Rich, and Marinov, 1973, for an excellent example of this approach in a theorem-proving machine). Consider, as a limiting case, a two-morpheme lexicon. The first problem is that of listing all the relations possible between these morphemes on the basis of the rules of the grammar. Figure A.5 presents the simple grammar of this example for parsing sentences containing two morphemes, (M1) and (M2). To begin with, the lexical rules for morphemes, W1>M1 and W2>M2, may link directly to each other through the connecting rules V_a, V_b, V_c, and V_d. These are depth 1 relations, that is, direct links between morpheme rules involving only a single structure rule (the simple relations discussed above). Figure A.5 presents the depth 1 relations available in the morpheme M1. Depth 2 relations are those in which links between morpheme rules involve two structure rules. In Figure A.5 morpheme rule W1>M1 connects to structure rule V_a>W1 W2/C (at depth 1), which in turn connects to rule V_d>(V_a, W2) (V_b, W1)/C (at depth 2). Depth 2 rules are obtained by searching the grammar for that set of rules which connect depth 1 rules directly. The grammar of the language may continue to be examined in this manner to any desired depth as long as rules remain available to link other rules together.

The result of applying this procedure to all morphemes in the lexicon is an extensive map of all possible relations between morphemes using all the structure rules for all specified depths. With even the simplest of recursive grammars this space is potentially infinite. As Siklossy, Rich, and Marinov (1973) point out, if no heuristics existed for constraining such a search space, it would be fruitless to search it for any specific relation. Fortunately, several heuristics are available.

The reader should by this time have some idea of what is meant by depth in the multipass parser. The term depth is used to indicate (a) the depth of the final structural analysis of a string, equal to the deepest constituent depth of the parse (see Figure A.6[a]), and (b) the depth of a particular rule with respect to a particular constituent in the surface string. At the top of Figure A.6(a), the depth of the whole structure is 4. The depth of rule 2 with respect to the constituent THE is 1; rule 2 is obtained in the first stage of search from THE. The depth of rule 2 with respect to constituent ROBOT is 2; rule 2 is obtained in the second search stage from ROBOT. The first definition above concerns the outcome of the parse, the depth that will have to be searched to successfully complete the parse. The second definition concerns the order of examination of relations for the parse, the stages of the parse discussed earlier.

Before a parse is attempted, two heuristics are immediately relevant. The first, and most obvious, is based on the observation that only the morphemes of the input string need to be considered in the parse. This limits the relations to be considered to those connecting the particular words used in the string. The second constraint on the search space is a consequence of insisting that every structure rule of the grammar be a well-formed formula of the type a>b d/C. Connections between rules of this sort specify a binary tree with the following properties: First, the number of rules required for a parse and the maximum depth possible in the description of an n word string is:

$$\text{DMAX} = n - 1$$

The top portion of Figure A.6(a) shows a crystal where the actual depth equals the maximum depth. Only in cases where right *or* left branching is used exclusively can this occur. Second, the minimum depth for an adequate parse of an n word string must be given by:

$$\text{DMIN} = \text{INT}(\log_2(n - 1) + 1)$$

where $\text{INT}(n)$ is a function specifying the integer value of n. If a parser does not examine relations to the DMIN depth, a complete description can never be obtained. The bottom portion of figure A.6(a) shows a crystal where the actual structural depth is equal to DMIN. Note, however, that the same number of rules is used in both structures in the figure.

The DMAX constraint in depth of processing is really quite weak. While it does define the upper limit of parsing depth, it does not indicate the probable parsing depth of a string. Any structure reaching a depth of $n - 1$ is unlikely, as it requires the use of *only* right- or left-branching structures. Normally, strings will more closely approximate the DMIN value for a limit on depth of processing. Thus, for a 40-word sentence, a depth of only 6 is likely, although a poten-

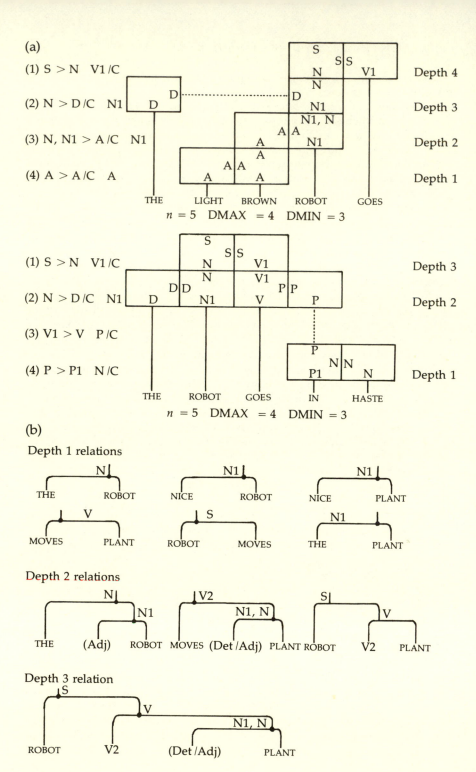

(a)

(1) S > N   V1 /C

(2) N > D /C   N1

(3) N, N1 > A /C   N1

(4) A > A /C   A

THE   LIGHT   BROWN   ROBOT   GOES

Depth 4

Depth 3

Depth 2

Depth 1

$n = 5$ DMAX $= 4$ DMIN $= 3$

(1) S > N   V1 /C

(2) N > D /C   N1

(3) V1 > V   P /C

(4) P > P1   N /C

THE   ROBOT   GOES   IN   HASTE

Depth 3

Depth 2

Depth 1

$n = 5$ DMAX $= 4$ DMIN $= 3$

(b)

Depth 1 relations

N
THE   ROBOT

N1
NICE   ROBOT

N1
NICE   PLANT

V
MOVES   PLANT

S
ROBOT   MOVES

N1
THE   PLANT

Depth 2 relations

N
N1
THE   (Adj)   ROBOT

V2
N1, N
MOVES (Det /Adj) PLANT

S
V
ROBOT   V2   PLANT

Depth 3 relation

S
V
N1, N
ROBOT   V2   (Det /Adj)   PLANT

tial depth of 39 is possible given the value of DMAX. For the purposes of the simulation, an arbitrary search depth limit of MAXD = 5 was used to constrain the search space.

Remaining heuristics controlling the search process are contained in the parsing procedures themselves and concern the elimination of unsuccessful relations, that is, those structure rules that do not lead to relations useful in the parse. There is nothing unique in these heuristics; in fact they are implicit or explicit in most, if not all, implementations of parsing grammars. We spell them out here to clarify the types of further constraints a parser of this sort has available.

The parse begins by examining all the depth 1 relations. From each of the words in the string, the search space is scanned for relations satisfying the properties of depth 1 rules. In the example, THE NICE ROBOT MOVES THE PLANT, THE and ROBOT are connected by a rule of the form $N > D / C$ N1 (its structural description). Examination of the relations takes place in left-to-right order through the morphemes of the string. Thus the first morpheme's relations to subsequent morphemes are evaluated, then the second's relation to subsequent ones evaluated, the third's, and so on. Each pass of the parser constitutes a scan of the relations in this order, finishing with the relations between the last and next-to-last morphemes in the string.

Rules must obey the following constraints to be accepted as appropriate connections between morphemes:

1. The two connected morphemes must maintain rule parity. Referring to our example, this means ROBOT, N1, must connect to one side of the rule (left or right) and THE, D, must connect to the other side.
2. The rule may or may not be ordered, according to a control option of the program. If ordered, THE, D, must occur to the left of ROBOT, N1, in the input string for the rule to be accepted. Rule order and surface structure order must concur.

These two constraints operate as active controls over rules admitted to the parse itself. Thus many rules in the search space may not be admitted to the parse space, leaving only that class of rules directly applicable to parsing the input string that also pass these heuristic tests.

The second pass of the parser examines depth 2 relations in the search space. As described above, these are relations in which a single rule intervenes between the connecting rule and the morpheme in the surface string. The rules connecting words at this depth are tested by the given heuristics and, if accepted, also admitted to the parse space. This procedure continues until all such connections are exhausted to the level specified by DMAX or MAXD. Figure A.6(b) contains a sampling of depth 1, 2, and 3 relations derived on successive passes of the parser for the string THE NICE ROBOT MOVES THE PLANT. For convenience, the nodes of the orreries are labeled in this figure.

The construction of the parse constitutes the organizing of relations in the

Figure A.6. (a) Examples of depth computation in SCRYP. (b) Depth relations between pairs of morphemes.

parse space. In Figure A.6(b) the depth 1 relation of THE ROBOT is described by the rule N > Det/ C N1 as well as the depth 2 relation of THE and ROBOT. Rule N > Det/ C N1 connects to rule N1 > Adj/ C N1, which in turn connects to ROBOT. Only one depth 3 relation is present, relating ROBOT to PLANT. As each of these relations is generated and passes the heuristic tests, it enters the parse space. As it enters, it is compared to the other relations in the space. If a connection between these structures is found, the relations are combined to form a new structure, which is also tested for membership in the parse space. Thus the structure describing the string ROBOT MOVES PLANT may be formed by combining the depth 1 relation of MOVES PLANT with the depth 2 relation of ROBOT and PLANT. As these new structures are generated they become members of the parse space itself. (This process is analogous to that of Siklossy, Rich, and Marinov, 1973, where proven theorems become part of the search space of the theorem-proving machine.)

At this point, an application of the positional priority heuristic comes into play (see Chapter 5). For, although some of these structures will pass the parity and local order tests, they may still violate order properties of the surface string. Consider the simple string SHINED THE ROBOT. Here the verb-noun relation SHINED ROBOT (as in I SHINED ROBOT) and the determiner-noun relation THE ROBOT will be produced. In addition, the adjective-noun relation SHINED ROBOT (as in A SHINED ROBOT) will be produced, as there are no a priori reasons in the first pass to suspect that this is not one of the simple relations that will be present in the final structure. During the second pass of the parser, a depth 2 relation between THE and ROBOT will be produced that will allow the insertion of an adjective into the structure. This will result in the string THE SHINED ROBOT, a string in which local order is preserved (THE ROBOT and SHINED ROBOT being the original relations) but which results in an incorrect description of the surface of the sentence (see Figure A.7). Obviously, some other constraint must be introduced to preserve word order. This may be accomplished by an application of the positional priority heuristic: As each relation is tested in the parse space, it must meet the criterion that all subordinate words of connected relations be properly ordered with respect to the superordinate word. Thus SHINED ROBOT, connected as a unit with THE, must reflect a surface structure in which SHINED as well as ROBOT is ordered to the right of THE.

By continuing to recombine relations in the parse space, eliminating those that fail the heuristic requirements, the parse of the entire structure will be realized. In general, such parses using SCRYP have been fairly readily obtained, at least before search goes beyond depth 3 relations. As pointed out before, a considerable number of surface constituents can be handled by relatively "shallow" structures. Further, in the recombination of such relations in the parse space, additional depth is obtained by linking depth 2 and 3 relations. This results in structures of considerable depth.

For our purposes here, two types of parse outcomes are of interest: adequate parses and complete parses. Adequate parses are those that evolve structures incorporating all the words of the surface structure. Complete parses are those that completely describe any set (or subset when so defined) of the input

Depth 1 relations

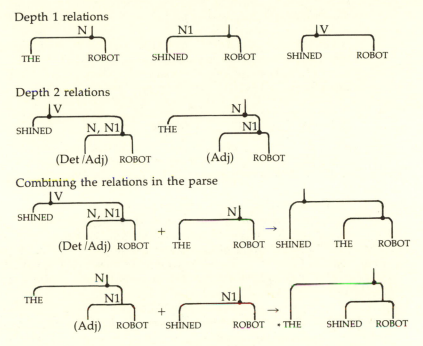

Figure A.7. Demonstration of the positional priority heuristic (★ indicates incorrect parse produced by two correct subparses).

string's constituents. They are complete in the sense that they only contain
structure rules that are completely used. The adequate *and* complete parse of a
surface string is its successful grammatical description: All the words of the surface string (adequacy) are incorporated in a complete structure (completeness).
Departures from the successful description can only be along these two dimensions. For example, in the neosyntactism discussed earlier, adequate but incomplete structures implicate missing form classes, for example, _____-ED BY
A GOOF-OFF.

The basic structure of the parser, then, is relatively straightforward:

1. Given an input sentence, form class rules, and structure rules, a search
   space is constructed consisting of the set of relations between morphemes potentially useful in the parse. The structure rules embody
   these relations. Initially, search through this space is constrained by an
   estimate of the depth to which the search need go (DMAX and DMIN)
   and the number of morphemes in the string.
2. The search itself proceeds from the bottom up, that is, from the morphemes to their connecting relations, the structure rules. Further, the
   search is performed in multiple left-to-right passes. As the relations

are selected, they are tested for parity and local order and, if passing, admitted to the parse space.

3. At this point, the relations are linked together to form larger structures, again with the parity and local order constraints. These structures are further subject to the positional priority constraint. By these procedures, a successful parse may be obtained.

SCRYP and the strategies of sentence processing

The success of SCRYP as a parser can best be measured by its ability to parse input strings. This is done in the following section. However, other measures of its success should also be considered. The system's modeling of human performance concerns us here.

Clark and Clark (1977) have presented a number of heuristics that appear to be used by language users in the process of understanding sentences. In particular, they present seven heuristics associated with syntactic aspects of the surface string (1977:57–72). Some of these heuristics are implicitly present in the current version of SCRYP and represent the joint operation of the bottom-up process and the local order and positional priority heuristics. We will briefly review them here.

The first "strategy," as Clark and Clark (1977) refer to these heuristics, is to use function words as signs of larger constituents. Hence, when THE, AN, TO, and so on, are found in a string they signal noun phrases, prepositional phrases, and other constituents. This heuristic was first proposed by Kimball (1973). In SCRYP, because most structure rules are coded for direct connection to morphemes, the presence of a function word immediately calls up those rules governing structures in which it characteristically occurs. Strategy 2, following from 1, suggests that once a function word is identified, content words appropriate to it may be expected. In SCRYP this means that once a grammatical morpheme, for example, THE, has occurred and its related constituent structures been identified, then other morphemes in the string may be examined in relation to these constituent structures. In any single pass of the parser this process takes place. Morphemes are selected and relations between them examined from left to right. Increased depths of the search involve larger and larger constituent structures. Strategy 3, similar to 2 involves the use of affixes (-ED, -ING, -NESS, and so forth) to signal form classes. Again, SCRYP can use the relations specified by syntax crystal structure rules to indicate the forms that must exist in the surface string when such affixes occur. (An example of this occurred in the parsing of DISASTERED BY A GOOF-OFF.) Strategy 4 involves the observation that certain verbs do not accept complementary clauses. For example, HIT requires a noun phrase as a complement, as in ROBOT HIT THE PLANT. On the other hand, BELIEVE accepts additional complements, allowing the sentence ROBOT BELIEVES THAT TODAY IS WEDNESDAY, as well as simple noun phrases, ROBOT BELIEVES THE RUMOR. Again, SCRYP allows this distinction to be made in parsing with such verb forms. Skipping over strategy 5, strategies 6 and 7 concern the signaling of clauses. Initial words of a clause identify the function the clause has in the sentence (the types of form classes to which it may be connected). For example, adverbial clauses are signaled by IF, BEFORE, SINCE, and BECAUSE when they are subordinate to the main clause.

These strategies are effectively implemented by SCRYP. Using morphemes that occur in the surface string, relations are suggested early (constituents identified) that may link larger units of the structure together (strategy 1). These relations further suggest the presence of other morphemes or structures that are likely to be found in the input string (strategy 2). Implicit in these strategies is the local order and positional priority heuristics, that is, that the morphemes indicating the presence of grammatical structures hold some easily specified orderly relation to these structures. Relative clauses, for instance, are usually preceded by relative pronouns. That is, relative pronouns appear to the left of other morphemes composing the relative clause. Merely knowing that a relative clause exists in a sentence is not as useful as knowing where in that sentence it is likely to be.

One strategy remains to be discussed, strategy 5. The basic notion behind strategy 5 is that the processing capacity of the system is limited. So a basic operating assumption should be to first try to attach each new element to the constituent that comes just before it in the string, thus associating the new element with a previously formed constituent structure instead of starting a new one. This would help explain the difficulties of understanding sentences of the type THE MAN THE ROBOT THE CAT BIT MET WAS NICE. Neither THE MAN, THE ROBOT, nor THE CAT are constituents that associate with preceding elements in the string. Here the basic assumption of strategy 5 fails, causing great difficulty in the parsing. Thus the import of strategy 5 arises from the fact that, while it is usually a useful strategy, it causes confusion in processing complex center- or left-embedded strings. Right-embedded strings fit the strategy well so they are very easy to process.

In SCRYP there are no local constraints on the connectedness of morphemes in the string as suggested by strategy 5. Thus no attempt is made to limit the relation of the current word to previous constituents in the string, or the last two words, or whatever. In fact, at the end of the first pass of the parser, all ordered relations available to the morphemes in the string have been produced. Consequently, there should be no difference on this basis between left-, center-, and right-embedded strings. However, on another, considerably more parsimonious basis the correct predictions can be made. The problem with left- and center-embedded structures is not that the processor gets locked into an erroneous parse but, rather, that too many relational possibilities are produced. Word-for-word, left- and center-embedded structures produce more potential connections, which the processor must operate upon, than right-embedded structures.

Compare THE MAN THE ROBOT THE CAT BIT MET WAS NICE with THE MAN WAS NICE WHO THE ROBOT MET WHICH THE CAT BIT. With the relative pronouns explicitly delineating the relative clauses, fewer relations need be considered. In the first, each of the mouns MAN, ROBOT, and CAT CAN BITE, MEET, or BE NICE (nine relations). In the second, only the CAT can BITE, the ROBOT can MEET or BITE, and the MAN can BE NICE, MEET, or BITE (six relations). Any time several potential subjects occur at the beginning of a string ahead of some verb or verbs, this confusion will result.

There does appear, then, to be an alternate explanation for the difficulty of processing left- and center-embedded structures. However, there remains some loss in elegance for SCRYP: In THE MAN WAS NICE WHO THE ROBOT MET WHICH THE CAT BIT, three erroneous subject-verb relations may still be produced. It should be obvious to the language user on pragmatic grounds that THE CAT BITES and not THE MAN BITES or THE ROBOT BITES is the most likely interpretation. And it is at this point that the design of the system is inadequate. In the process of developing the bottom-up parse of a sentence, many such erroneous relations are produced. As both Palme (1971) and Kaplan (1973) point out, this is the most crucial inefficiency of bottom-up parsers: The ratio of erroneous to proper relations immediately produced is quite large. This inefficiency might be remediable by employing additional heuristic strategies.

The strategies of Clark and Clark (1977) involve signaling the onset of noun phrases, relative clauses, and other constituents, but do not signal the *end* of these constituents. What is required is a set of rules that would help delineate the end of such constituents. Thus, in the example in the previous paragraph, each relative clause is opened by a relative pronoun and closed by a verb preceding another relative pronoun or a period. Perhaps a context-sensitive rule stating that the end of a relative clause occurs when a verb is followed by a relative pronoun would be adequate. Regardless of whether or not this is ultimately an adequate heuristic, it is sufficient to eliminate the erroneous alternative relations ROBOT BIT, MAN BIT, and MAN MET from the sentence above. Such demarcation of self-contained syntactic units would go a long way toward eliminating erroneous relations from the parse at an early stage.

Parsing with a syntax crystal grammar

The adequacy of a parsing system is best shown by examples. We have already presented a sample of SCRYP parses in the form of orreries derived from parser output, as illustrated in Figure A.7. However, these forms were not particularly demanding. SCRYP should also be capable of parsing more complex forms, such as structurally ambiguous sentences. One of these appears at the top of Figure A.8(a). As can be seen, the ambiguous relations among SERVED, YOUNG, and PLANTS are present in the simple relations of the parse. Two different subsets of these relations are incorporated in the two complete parses. At the bottom of the figure appears a disambiguated version of the sentence. Note that the same simple relations still exist early in the parse but result in only one complete parse, as other structural properties of the sentence eliminate the adjective-noun relation, YOUNG PLANTS. The determiner-noun relation, THE PLANTS, must be incorporated as a unit in the remaining structure. This is an excellent example of the signaling properties of determiners mentioned earlier as Clark and Clark's strategy 2. The order heuristics of SCRYP ensure this interpretation.

Other, more complex parsing problems may also be examined, for instance, sentences that create backtracking problems for ATN parsers. An example of this problem can be found by examining the difference in interpreting THE ROBOT SCRATCHES THE SOLENOID versus THE ROBOT SCRATCHES WERE MANY. In the first sentence, if SCRATCHES is first interpreted as a verb, the sentence is quickly parsed. But if the same assumption is made in parsing the second sentence, the interpretation of WERE fails (following the verb SCRATCHES, the ATN would expect a piece of some noun phrase). Since SCRATCHES must be interpreted as a noun and ROBOT as an adjective, the network is forced to backtrack to the initial word of the sentence, THE. In Figure A.8(b) appears the SCRYP analysis of these two sentences along with some partial parses. Obviously, no back-up problem occurs here, as the simple relations of the parse are available in the first pass. The only difference between the two parses is that the second sentence's noun phrase is deeper than the first and hence takes some additional time to be assembled.

The problems previously discussed have dealt with things parsers are typically expected to do within the bounds of grammatical form. However, such grammatical bounds may be too confining. A computer parser, like a human, should be able to at least partially process ill-formed strings. Above we discussed how the parser analyzes asyntactic and neosyntactic expressions. This serves as a partial demonstration that it is possible for the parser to make best guesses about the form classes of nonsense terms in a string.

Two criteria of a successful parse have been given: that the parse incorporate all the morphemes in the string and that the structural description be complete. In discussing asyntactic and neosyntactic expressions, the nearest approximations to a successful parse depended on best-guesses regarding missing or grammatically ill-formed elements in the strings. These approximations fail the adequacy and completeness criteria by either implying morphemes that are not present in the surface string or deleting improper forms from the parse. These are parallel to what humans do when confronted with ill-formed strings. Fillenbaum (1974) presented evidence that subjects confronted with uninterpretable sentences of this sort "normalize" their interpretation. That is, morphemes are ignored or interpolated in order to make some sense of the string.

Consider this paradigmatic nonsense sentence: ALL MIMSY WERE THE BOROGOVES. This string, along with one other, appears in Figure A.8(c). Again, we include a few partial parses. Note that, while neither is complete, each ambiguous nonsense term is incorporated. The first adequate structure for the upper sentence leaves two rules incomplete, indicating the places where the nonsense terms might connect to the remaining structure (denoted by dashed lines). Thus the rule connecting ALL to MIMSY is connected through another rule to WERE, giving it a reasonable place in the structure and serving as a place holder for the nonsense term. The partial parses indicate that this process occurs early in the parse. Examining the structure, MIMSY appears as a noun or adjective about which something is being stated in the predicate, and BOROGOVES subsequently becomes identified as a noun. Given this analysis and pragmatic information, the language user could make some rough guesses about what it means to be MIMSY and why that should or should not be said about BOROGOVES.

(a)

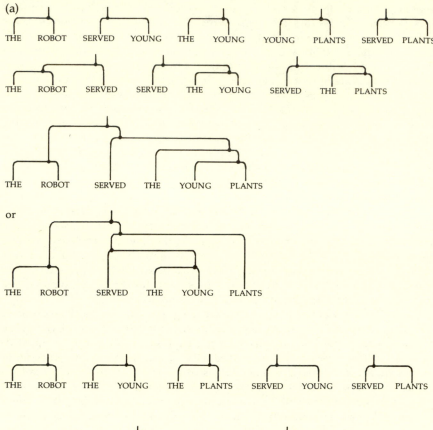

or

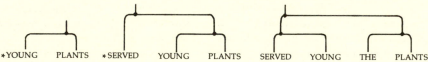

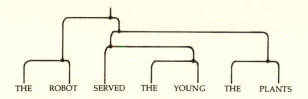

Figure A.8. (a) SCRYP parse of an ambiguous sentence, THE ROBOT SERVED THE YOUNG PLANTS, and an unambiguous version, THE ROBOT SERVED THE YOUNG THE PLANTS.

(b)

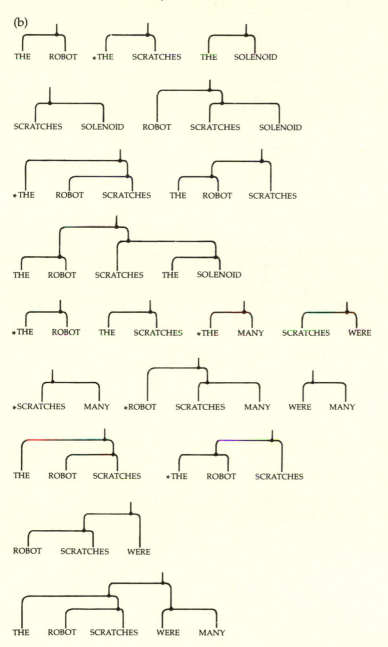

Figure A.8. (b) SCRYP analysis of THE ROBOT SCRATCHES THE SOLENOID and THE ROBOT SCRATCHES WERE MANY.

(c)

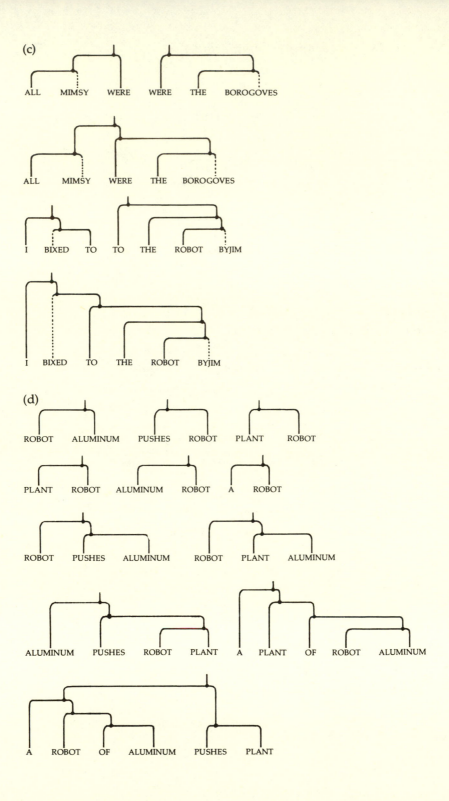

(d)

Consider now a more difficult problem, that of ungrammatical strings. Here the morphemes may not be nonsense, but their syntactic configuration is. The question now is whether the parser can handle syntactic nonsense as well. Here, the order heuristics of the parser come crucially to bear upon the problem.

In the analysis of neosyntactic expressions already presented, one variation of this problem was discussed. Given that the string is properly ordered, what is the best parse that can be made? As we saw, the parser can go so far as to indicate how words may be syntactically interpreted in the string in order to derive a proper structure. The ungrammaticality of the string is recognized before a possible parse is constructed, since the parse requires the recognition that at least one of the morphemes cannot fit any of the structurally required form classes. That is, it is impossible to interpret the morpheme in its position in the string and obtain a complete structural description. However, suppose the order requirement could be suspended. The morphemes might then be reordered into a structurally interpretable configuration.

Figure A.8(d) illustrates a special case of the problem of ungrammatical strings, sentence anagrams, where the morphemes are in a random sequence. Here the problem for the parser, as for any language user, is to find out what could be meant by an utterance such as ROBOT ALUMINUM A OF PUSHES PLANT. The morphemes of the string must be arranged to fit some interpretable structure. The figure presents some of the partial parses leading up to the complete parses available when the order heuristics of SCRYP are suspended. Thus one complete parse of ROBOT ALUMINUM A OF PUSHES PLANT is properly ordered as A ROBOT OF ALUMINUM PUSHES PLANT.

There are two effects of suspending the order heuristics: First, interpretations of incorrectly ordered strings can be made. Second, the efficiency of the parser drops greatly, since all possible unordered connections of morphemes must be considered. One possible way around this problem is to suspend order only with those particular rules that are most likely to yield the proper reordering. In ROBOT THE LIKES CATS, for example, since the determiner rule fails to find a proper noun phrase, its order constraint may be suspended to recover the relation THE ROBOT. It may well be that language users can selectively suspend order restrictions in order to interpret such strings. If an ordered interpretation fails, an unordered one is attempted. This somewhat artificial example can be supplemented by the observation that some standard grammatical forms have remarkable flexibility regarding the ordering of surface constituents. Thus LOBELIA CONSEQUENTLY WENT TO TOWN may be reordered as CONSEQUENTLY LOBELIA WENT TO TOWN, TO TOWN LOBELIA CONSEQUENTLY WENT, and so on, with only

Figure A.8. (c) SCRYP parses of two nonsense sentences: ALL MIMSY WERE THE BOROGOVES and I BIXED TO THE ROBOT BYJIM. (d) SCRYP parsing of the sentence anagram ROBOT ALUMINUM A OF PUSHES PLANT.

very subtle changes in meaning. Perhaps suppressing order restrictions on particular rules like that governing the adverbial may be advantageous. In the typically well-ordered environment of most parsers, in which strict order is usually required, a different order must be specified for each rule controlling these different forms. However, SCRYP can accomplish this by selectively suspending the order heuristic. This small change provides great economy in the structure. The selective suspension of the order constraint may also provide a more economical account of the abundance of alternative paraphrase forms in natural language. Instead of using a different transformation to derive each order, selective suspension on left-right order constraints in some rules could do the same thing much more simply. This remains to be explored.

Summary of SCRYP

The nature of the syntax crystal grammar enables the simple relations that occur in the first pass of the parser to specify the complete set of basic relations in the string. This eliminates most of the back-up problems found in other systems. Because these relations appear early and the parser proceeds from the bottom up in its analysis, a simple means of interpreting asyntactic and neosyntactic expressions is possible; complete and perfect information is not necessary for the specification of syntactic structure.

Parsing is like the problem of assembling a jigsaw puzzle (see Lindsey, 1971). Given the goal of assembling just the border of the puzzle, one must first specify the relevant class of pieces, evaluate their interrelationships, and assemble them under the control of some heuristic procedure. To parse a string, one must first specify the relevant class of structure rules, determine the types of relations they have to each other and the surface string, and assemble them, again, by some heuristic procedure. Important to the evaluation of the program as a simulation of human processes is the selection of appropriate heuristics. In our discussion of the Clark and Clark (1977) parsing strategies, we presented evidence that the operation of the left-to-right, bottom-up processes of SCRYP paralleled a variety of currently accepted heuristics in human language processing. Further, we found that a close examination of the order heuristics led to interesting suggestions regarding human performance in sentence anagram problems. This observation led to the suggestion that some heuristics could be selectively suspended in language-understanding situations.

This appendix assumes some specific goals for the construction of a parser beyond those normally expected of such mechanisms. This is because we want to develop a system that can imitate human performance. Besides this general criterion, there are several others:

1. Ultimately, a parser must be able to derive syntactic analyses for any and all grammatical strings of a language. This criterion for a parsing system is generally acknowledged.
2. The parser should eventually obtain all parses of an ambiguous sentence, find right-embedded sentences easier to process than left-embedded sentences, and so on.

3. Analyses of syntactically improper or incomplete strings should indicate what, if anything, is missing from the string, or what elliptical morphemes are required for interpretation of the string. One of the most challenging problems for any parser is how to deal with improper strings. Again, the processes for such interpretations should reflect those believed to be used by human language users.

4. Finally, the parser should be able to suspend normal parse processes when they do not lead to a proper structural solution. Thus, as we saw above, the selective suspension of the order heuristics could be quite valuable in correctly parsing grammatical distortions such as ROBOT ALUMINUM A OF PUSHES PLANT.

These desiderata for parser implementation all point to a single general requirement, flexibility. Any parser used as a simulation ideally should be capable of performing in as many language-understanding situations as a human. This requirement leads us to an additional criterion of adequacy: The parser must be able to account for language acquisition, which involves the application of incomplete grammars to the analysis of grammatically well-formed strings. Heuristics must be derived that can be used to generate a complete grammar from an incomplete one. A number of authors (Siklossy, 1971; Harris, 1972; Anderson, 1975; Reeker, 1976) have offered suggestions in this vein. While we cannot review them here, we can point out two aspects of SCRYP that may be of use in the design of a language acquisition system.

The first aspect is the importance of incomplete structural analyses to the development of grammatical rules. As we saw, guesses about the form classes of nonsense morphemes can be made on the basis of their relation to the known parts of a string's syntactic structure, the most complete and adequate parse available from the system. Thus, in ALL MIMSY WERE THE BOROGOVES, MIMSY could be classified as an adjective, since this permits a well-formed structure to be developed. By following the substitutivity and testing procedures described in Chapter 6, new rules of grammar may be developed.

SCRYP's use of partial processing to guide later stages also has advantages in accommodating alternative explanations of child language acquisition. The standard assumption (e.g., Reeker, 1976) is that there is a single primitive grammar which becomes elaborated into an adult grammar. However, it is possible that the child elaborates several independent partial grammars which are joined to form the adult grammar. The bottom-up processing of SCRYP makes this easier to do, since the surface structure initially determines which set of rules are called in for parsing.

In summary, SCRYP offers a number of contributions to understanding the parsing process: It is efficient as well as flexible because it uses bottom-up processing, which gives it immediate access to information in the entire surface string; it is promising as a simulation of human parsing performance, since it parallels many of the heuristics attributed to humans; finally, it deals with incomplete and ill-formed strings in a way that seems to parallel human performance.

Syntax crystal modules

This appendix is divided into two parts. First we provide a list of the modules given in Chapter 5 along with a description of the kinds of connections they can make and the grammatical constructions they allow. This list will be divided into four sections for heuristic purposes, and also to provide a method for testing the modules – the syntax crystal game. The second part describes additional grammatical constructions not mentioned in Chapter 5 but considered important for theories of grammar. We provide syntax crystal modules for these constructions and discuss how they can be handled.

It is important to point out that all the modules we describe are supposed to show only how the constructions *can* be handled by modules. We make no claim that grammatical constructions must be handled in exactly this manner. Our goal is only to show what the syntax crystal model can explain, how it can explain it, and occasionally, what it has difficulty explaining. We are saying: Given this sort of rule, with these sorts of properties, here are some of the constructions it can handle. We use English, as we have mentioned before, because it is a very complex and rich language. But we believe that the principles of the syntax crystal can be used to construct modules that will work for other languages.

The syntax crystal game

We are going to describe the modules of the syntax crystal grammar in four stages. To motivate the reader to get involved with the details of the rules, the modules are presented in the context of a simulation game as well as flow charts which may be used for reference. Unlike other forms of syntactic rules, the modules are very easy for a beginner to work with. In the game, the reader combines modules to produce crystals for English strings, thereby testing the power of the model and permitting the discovery of mistakes or inadequacies in the rules. For simplicity, the game allows strings to be generated by mechanically combining the modules without first determining underlying structure. The resulting crystals produce coherent structures that describe the scope and dependency relations of the concepts named by the lexemes in the string. The reader may also use the game to explore parsing and generating with the model.

The module rules are introduced in four stages of increasing complexity. Each stage constitutes a subgame. For the convenience of the player who generates strings randomly, we have provided four separate lexicons, one for each subgame, in order to allow the resulting strings to have some semantic coherence. Each subgame uses the structure and functor morpheme modules of the preceding subgames, adding additional modules to increase the complexity of the structures that can be assembled. The subgames, in increasing order of complexity, are labeled by the themes that characterize their lexicons: Delicatessen, Pornography, Politics, and Philosophy.

General instructions

The syntax crystal modules appear in Figure B.1. Photocopy them, making four or five copies. On your copies, lightly color the faces of the modules in each section with the color indicated. Use colored pencils, markers, or watercolor paints, anything as long as the markings on the modules are still legible. The colors are used to sort the modules into subgame groupings after they have been mixed up during play. Cement the pages of colored modules to light cardboard and cut them out along the lines provided.

As described in Chapter 5, one module can connect to another if it can be placed so that facing edges bear compatible codes and there are no intervening module(s). Compatible codes are matching pairs of letter-number combinations, or else identical letters with an overlapping range of numerals. For example, Z4 matches Z4, and J3 – 9 matches J5 – 11. A set of codes appearing in square brackets means that the choice of one of the codes in the brackets constrains the choice of codes from any other set of codes in brackets *on the same module*. The constraint requires that if the first code in brackets on one edge is chosen, the first code in brackets on the other edges must then be used, and similarly for the second, third, and so on. Blank edges may touch each other only as a consequence of other connections. A code in parentheses is optional; it may be treated either as a connection code or as a blank edge.

In more complex crystals, it is possible for modules to get in each other's way when they connect. As described in Chapter 5, there is a "positional priority" convention developed to handle this. Branches that grow from a column always have positional priority over branches that grow from higher up in that column. The higher branches must be detached and moved horizontally until they clear the growth from the lower branches. This detached connection is still a connection nonetheless – the separated codes that still face each other are considered to be matched and no other module may be attached between them. Beginning players may find it easier to keep track of these separated connections by bridging the gap with a row of blank rectangles. Again as described in Chapter 5, there are certain exceptions to the positional priority principle. Modules demanding this exception are marked with a downward arrow. The downward arrow means that the module to which it points has positional priority over any branch growing from the column lower down. Any branch that threatens to in-

"Delicatessen" structure modules (color these green)

A1 [B1, 2] / [B1, 2] / A1	B1 / N8 / B3	C1 C2 / C2	(J1) J1 / J1	N1	N2 –5, 7, 10 / J1, 4 / N2
N8 / N8	(C1) C1 / N12	N1, 7, 8 / C2 / N12	N1, 8 –12 / A1 / N4	N1, 4,7,8,12 / B1 / N7	

Morpheme modules (color these green)

A1	B3	B3	C2	J1	J1	J1
A(N)	WITH	ON	AND	HOT	DOUBLE	FRESH
N1 –12	N1 –12	N1 –12	N1 –12	N1 –12	N2	A1
MUSTARD	RYE	PASTRAMI	COFFEE	BLT	ORDER	SOME
N1 –12	N1 –12					
LOX	COLESLAW					

"Pornography" structure modules (color these pink)

G1 [↓] / G1	Z2 / J2, N8, Z2	J2 G2,B1, / J3 I1	[J4, 5] / [J4, 5]	A1 / O1 / N10	O1 / O1	P1 [↓] / P1
J4 / G1 / V0	J4 / P1 / V1 –3	[V4,9,10,8],V8 / N8 / [V1 –4]	V8 [B1, 2; / I1; / [V8 –10]^{T2}]	S1, 3 / V8	S1, 3 / G2, Z2 / Z1	S4 / Z2 / Z1
(T3) S1, 2 / N1	(X1) [S1, 2] / [S1, 2]	G2 G1 / S4, V8				

Morpheme modules (color these pink)

A1	A1	A1	A1, N8	B2	B2	B3
THE	A(N)	HIS	HER	HUNGRILY	BRUTALLY	INTO
C2	J1, 2	J1, 2	J1 –3	N2, 4	N2, 4	N1 –12
AND	HOT	MOIST	BUSY	NYMPH	INTRUDER	LIPS
O1	P1	V0, 4, 8	V0, 4, 8	V0, 4, 8	Z1	B3
'S	-EN, -ED	FONDLE(S)	DEVOUR(S)	NIBBLES	IS, ARE, BE	UNDER
B3	N4	G1				
WITH	HANDS	-ING				

"Politics" structure modules (color these purple)

	(X1)	Z2	N4	N1, 8, 12		P4	P4
I1 I2 I1	I2	J5 I3	R1, I1 N3	P4 N11		P4	P5
I1, N1, 8 I2 S1, V8	Z3 P1 S3, V8	I3 I2 V1 –4	[V17,16,15,ø], Z2 V13,P4 P1 [V1 –4]	(V13,P4) [B1,2; I1;T2; [V13,15,17] N8]	S1 Z3 Z3		S2 S1 Z4
P5 N8 R1 S1, 2 P6 R1		S2 S3 Z5				

Morpheme modules (color these purple)

A1	B2	B3, I2	B3, P6	C2	G1	J1, 2, 5
A(N)	QUIETLY	TO	BY	AND	-ING	EASY
J1 –3	N1 –12	N1-4,7,8,12	N1–4, 6–12	N1,3,4,6,8,12 V0–4,6	N1–4, 6–12	N1,3,4,6,8,12 V0, 4, 9
LIABLE	PEACE	HOSTILITIES	AGGRESSION	PROMISE	OPPOSITION	ATTEMPT
R1	Z1	Z3, V4, 6, 9	Z4	Z4	Z5	J1, 2, 5
WHO, WHICH	IS, ARE, BE	HAS, HAVE	MIGHT	COULD	DO(ES)	RISKY
J1, 2	O1	P1				
INTER-NATIONAL	'S	-EN, -ED				

"Philosophy" structure modules (color these gray)

J2 T3 J6	Q1 N1 ↓	N2 –7, 10 N5 N5 N5 N6	[S3; [E1 –3] I1; N8 G2]	[E4, 5] [I1, G2] P1	Q2 Q2
T2 (T1) T2, 3 (T1) T1 T1		(T3) S1, 2 T1 T2 T3	N1 –12 G1 V0	V8 [E1 –3] Z2 [V5 –7]	(V13,P4) [E4, 5] [V5, 7]
T2 I1 Q2	(X1) (Q2) Q1 S1, 2	X1 X1 X1 X2 ↓			

Morpheme modules (color these gray)

A1	B2	B3	B3	B3, I2	B3, P6	C2
ANY	NECESSARILY	BEFORE	BEYOND	TO	BY	AND
J1, 2, 5	J1, 2, 6	N1 –12	N1 –12	N1–4, 6–12	O1	P1
IMPOSSIBLE	CERTAIN	CERTAINTY	LOGIC	PRINCIPLES	'S	-EN, -ED
V0,2,4,6,10	V0, 4, 10	V0,1,3,4,6–8	X1	Z1	Z3, V4, 6, 9	Z4
KNOW	DEMONSTRATE	SHOW	NOT	IS, ARE, BE	HAS, HAVE	COULD
G1	J1, 2	Q2	R1, T1	Z5		
-ING	OPAQUE	HOW	THAT	DO(ES)		

Figure B.1. Syntax crystal modules.

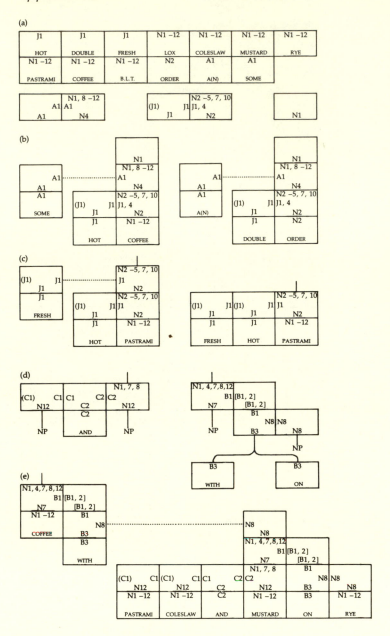

Figure B.2. (a) Deli vocabulary and some structure modules. (b) Some constructions with Deli modules. (c) Using some modules repeatedly. (d) Additional Deli modules. (e) A more complex crystal.

terfere with a module at the head of an arrow must detach and move horizontally to permit the arrowed connection positional priority.

The game may be played quite informally with one or more players attaching modules as their fancy suggests. More formal games are easily developed. One version we have enjoyed playing in groups is the syntactic analog of dominoes; each player selects a pile of modules at random and tries to attach them to the structure so as to use up as many as possible before the string is complete. Other variants offer prizes for the most interesting strings or the longest strings.

As mentioned above, the game may be used to exhibit the parsing and generating capabilities of the model as well as random generation. To parse, one first sets out the morpheme modules that make up the string so it reads in the ordinary fashion from left to right. Then the object is to add structure modules so that all the morphemes are combined into a single structure and there are no unmatched connection codes remaining. Syntactically ambiguous strings will of course have alternative structures. The scope and dependency relations underlying the string are then determined by tracing an orrery through the centers of the modules as described in Chapter 5. To generate a meaningful string, one starts with an orrery connecting the concepts to be expressed. The concepts may be in any order. Now, connect lexical morpheme modules together according to the connections of the orrery using any structure modules that will join them together. The structure modules will force the lexical morphemes into the correct left-to-right order and insert grammatical morphemes and functors where necessary. For more detail on the parsing and generating procedures, the reader should refer back to Chapter 5.

Playing the four subgames

The first subgame is played using only the green modules, which include the lexicon of a delicatessen. In a busy deli, language is mainly used for one purpose – to name something to eat. Verb phrases are not used because the people in a deli are too busy ordering or making sandwiches to tell stories about who did what to whom. Just say what you want. The first stage consists of simple noun phrases – nouns (which connect to modules whose bottom code contains an N), adjectives (connected to modules whose bottom code contains a J), articles or determiners (connected via a module coded A), prepositional phrases (the prepositions connect via a B code), and conjunctions (C codes) (see Figure B.2[a]). With the morpheme modules and structure modules for determiners (A), adjectives (J), and nouns (N), we can construct some simple noun phrases as in (b), and by repeating some of the modules, we can build the crystals of (c). The N1 module merely allows noun phrases to be complete strings. In the next stage it will be replaced by a module that connects noun phrases to verb phrases. Note that we are making no distinction between A and SOME in the modules. There are grammatical differences (A BOOK, ★A BOOKS, SOME BOOKS, ★SOME BOOK) that must either be made by using different modules (including

Table B.1. *Explanation of codes in Deli language*

A1	Determiners (articles, possessive pronouns)
B1	To prepositional phrase
B3	To preposition
C2	Conjunction
J1	Adjective modifying noun
N1	Connects to main noun of the phrase
N2	Noun that is modified by adjective
N4	Noun that is modified by determiner
N7	Noun that is modified by prepositional phrase
N8	Noun that is an object
N12	Noun that is part of a conjunction

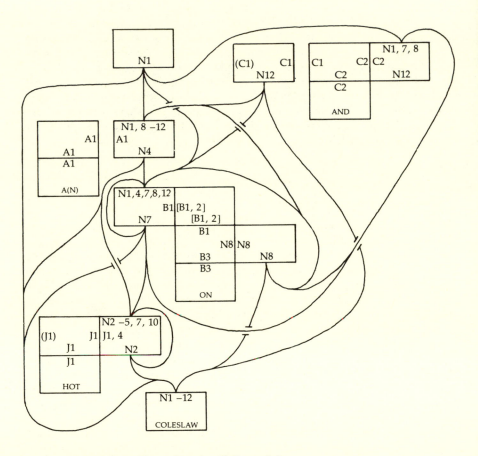

Figure B.3. Flow chart for Deli modules.

Table B.2. *Explanation of codes added for Porno language*

B2	Connects to adverbs
G1	Connects to suffix, -ING
J2	Connects to predicate adjectives
J3	Connects to predicate adjectives plus further modifiers
J4	Connects to participial adjectives
N1	Connects main NP to verb phrase
N10	Connects to possessive noun phrase
O1	Connects to possessive suffix, 's
P1	Connects to verb suffix, -EN or -ED
S1	Connects to copula, IS, BE, ARE
S4	Connects to copula in progressive tense, IS BEING
V0	Connects a verb to -ING suffix to form adjective
V1	Connections to verbs that take indirect objects either as main verb or as adjective with -EN or -ED suffix
V2	Connections to verbs that take direct objects plus infinitives (I1 connections), or as adjective with -EN or -ED suffix
V3	Connections to verbs that take direct objects plus propositional clauses (THAT clauses), or as adjective with -EN or -ED suffix
V4	Connections to verbs that take direct objects, but only adverbial modifiers in addition
V8	Connects main verb phrase to main noun phrase or to progressive tense
V9	Connects verb to infinitive phrases
V10	Connects verb to THAT clauses
Z1	Connects to copula

the intervening modules for adjectives and other noun modifiers) or by some system that goes outside the module connections. For simplicity we make no distinction here.

Now to complete the Deli stage we add prepositions and conjunctions (which were not given in Chapter 5 but are easy enough to show) shown in Figure B.2(d). Again, by repeating modules more complex structures can be built, as shown in (e). Other grammatical strings in a deli may include:

HOT COFFEE AND A BLT WITH COLESLAW ON RYE
A DOUBLE ORDER ON RYE AND COLESLAW

Figure B.3 gives a flow chart for the structure modules given so far, with some sample Deli morphemes for illustration. The bottom codes on the modules can be roughly identified by the kind of syntactic connections they allow. Table B.1 explains the grammatical role of each connection code.

The next stage adds simple verb phrases to the noun phrases. We also add the copula IS, the progressive tense, participial adjectives, and possessive construction. By retaining the previous structure modules, adding codes to the N1 module, and additional structure modules, a more complex grammar results. The

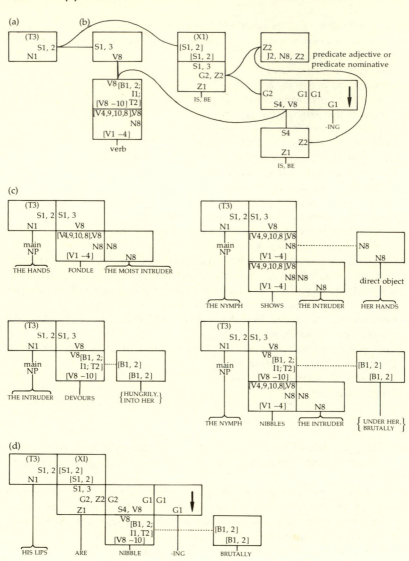

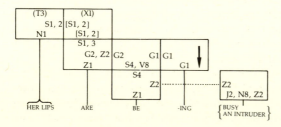

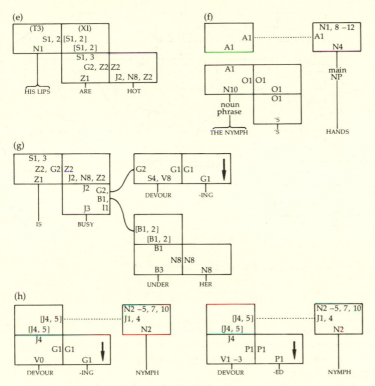

Figure B.4. Modules added to Deli language to get Porno language. (a) Add (T3) and S1, 2 codes to N1 module. (b) Additional structure modules for verb phrases. (c) Examples of simple verb phrases using new modules. The T3, I1, and T2 codes will be connected to modules at later stages. (d) Examples of progressive tense forms. (e) Example of simple copula. (f) Example of possessive NP. (g) Additional copula forms. (h) Examples of participial adjectives.

Deli vocabulary is replaced by a Porno vocabulary. There are no clauses, subjunctives, or anything to slow down the heart rate. Just simple direct action sentences: Subject noun does something to object noun.

To begin (1) replace the green Deli morpheme modules with the pink Porno morphemes, retaining the green structure modules. Table B.2 explains the syntactic function of the codes. (2) Add the codes to the N1 module as shown in Figure B.4(a). (3) Add the pink structure modules for verb phrases as in (b). We can now get simple-verb phrases such as those in (c) and progressive tense forms such as those in (d). We can use some of the above modules for a simple copula as shown in (e). The possessive form connects to the determiner (A1) module as in (f). Additional copula modifiers are illustrated in (g). Participial

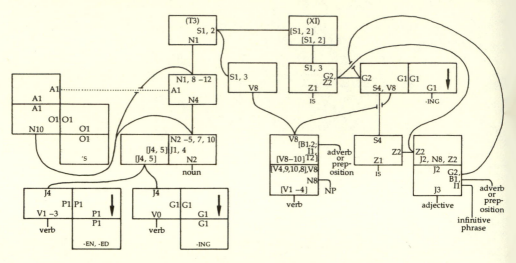

Figure B.5. Flow chart for Porno modules.

Table B.3. *Syntactic function of codes in Politics language*

I1	Connects verb phrase or infinitive to main verb phrase
I2	Connects to infinitive TO
I3	Connects infinitive phrase to predicate adjective as in EASY TO ATTEMPT
J5	Connects predicate adjective to infinitive phrase
N3	Connects main noun phrase to relative clause
N11	Connects noun phrase to BY prepositional phrase of passive, as in THE ATTEMPT BY THE OPPOSITION
P4	Connects passive verb phrase to BY prepositional phrase that corresponds to the subject of the active form
P5	Connects BY prepositional phrase of the passive to the verb phrase
P6	Connects preposition BY to the BY prepositional phrase of the passive
R1	Connects to relative pronoun
S1	Connects to perfect, progressive tenses, and the copula
S2	Connects to modal and DO auxiliaries
S3	Connects to the copula, forming the perfect tense
V13	Connects verbs in the passive to adverbs and prepositional phrases
V15	Connects passive verbs to infinitive phrases
V16	Connects passive verbs to THAT clauses
Z2	Connects to predicate adjective plus infinitive
Z3	Connects to HAS, HAVE of the perfect tense
Z4	Connects to modal auxiliaries
Z5	Connects to DO auxiliary

adjectives are illustrated in (h). (The T3, I1, and T2 codes will be connected to modules in later stages.)

A flow chart for these modules is given in Figure B.5.

For a more interesting syntax, proceed to the next stage. Here we use modal auxiliaries, relative clauses (of a simple sort), infinitives, indirect objects, and the passive construction. The vocabulary for this syntax is that of politics, a language full of qualifications, hesitations, and sidesteppings. Replace the pink morpheme modules with the purple Politics morphemes. Add the purple structure modules as well. Table B.3 explains the syntactic function of the codes. Addition of the purple modules will allow the past perfect (Figure B.6[b]) and the passive constructions (Figure B.6[a]). Infinitives are constructed via the mod-

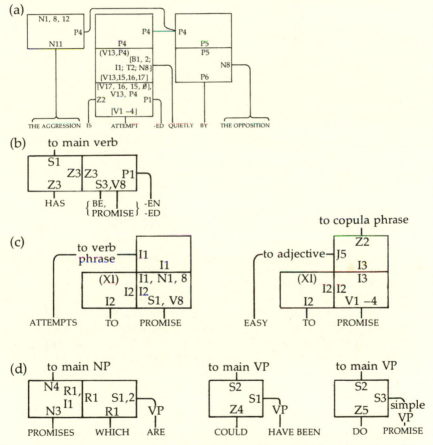

Figure B.6. (a) Example of modules used in passive construction. (b) Modules for past perfect. (c) Examples of infinitive constructions. (d) Modules for simple relative clauses, modal auxiliaries, and DO auxiliary.

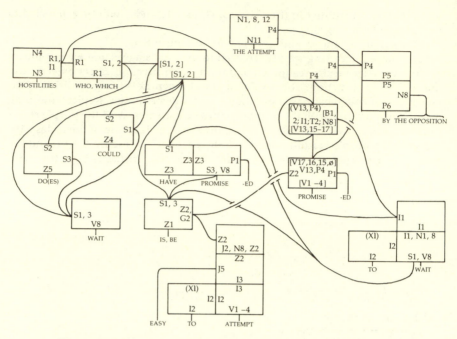

Figure B.7. A flow chart for the Politics language modules.

ules in (c), and simple relative clauses, and modal and DO auxiliaries use the modules illustrated in (d). A flow chart for these modules is given in Figure B.7.

To introduce even greater syntactic complexity, discard the purple Politics morpheme modules and add all the gray modules to the other structure modules. These represent Philosophy jargon. In addition to the structures allowed in the delicatessen, the soft porn literature, and the campaign rally, Philosophy has propositional verbs, questions, and negation. Table B.4 explains the syntactic function of the codes used for these modules. The structure modules for verbs that can be modified by propositions or proposition-like phrases are illustrated in Figure B.8(a). Modules for questions and negation are illustrated in (b), and modules for noun modifiers and gerunds are shown in (c). A flow chart for the Philosophy modules is given in Figure B.9.

Other syntax crystal modules

In this section we discuss constructions that were not covered in Chapter 5. In particular, we discuss differences in the structure of complements to the verbs EXPECT and PERSUADE, differences in the structures of EASY TO PLEASE and EAGER TO PLEASE, and present a partial analysis of how to handle different sentence forms such as:

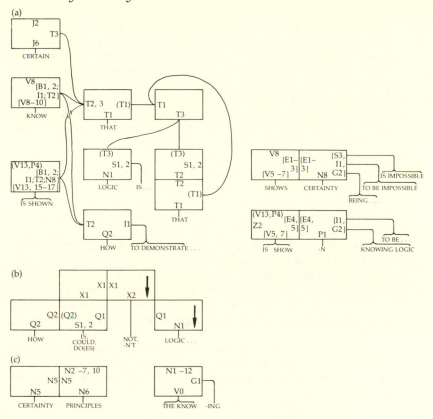

Figure B.8. (a) Modules for propositional verbs. (b) Modules for questions and negation. (c) Noun modifiers and gerunds.

WHAT THE DOG DID WAS EAT THE HAT

WHAT THE DOG ATE WAS THE HAT

IT WAS THE DOG THAT ATE THE HAT

IT WAS THE HAT THAT THE DOG ATE

WAS WHAT THE DOG ATE THE HAT?

WHAT DID THE DOG EAT?

We shall also supply modules for making participial adjectives, gerunds, and embedded clauses and discuss how to make some distinctions that other theories consider important.

Expect–persuade

First let us consider a pair of strings whose different structures can be represented by modules that have been described earlier. The following pair has

Table B.4. *Syntactic function of codes used in Philosophy language*

J6	Connects predicate adjective to proposition: HAPPY THAT IT IS SO
N1	Connects main noun phrase to declarative or interrogative form
N5	Connects modifier noun to main NP
N6	Connects main NP to modifier noun
N8	Connects NP to preposition as object, to verb as direct object, indirect object or object-of-verb/subject-of-phrase as in SEE HER SEWING THE DRESS, SEE HER SEW THE DRESS, I WANT HER TO LEARN
Q2	Connects to question adverb
S1, 2	Connects to verb auxiliary in declarative or interrogative form
T1	Connects to THAT which precedes or stands for embedded sentences, as in I KNOW THAT, I KNOW THAT THE PRINCIPLES ARE CERTAIN, or THAT THE PRINCIPLES ARE CERTAIN IS NOT KNOWN, THAT IS NOT KNOWN
T2	Connects to THAT clause which is subject of sentence
T3	Connects to main NP of embedded sentence, including to THAT clauses which function as main noun phrases
V0	Connects verb form to -ING and noun phrase modifiers to make gerunds
V5	Connects to verb which takes object plus simple verb phrase as modifier, as in I SAW (HER SEW THE DRESS), in the active form, and object-plus-infinitive phrase in the passive, as in SHE WAS SEEN TO EAT BY ME
V6	Connects to verb which takes object-plus-infinitive-phrase modifier in the active form, as in I WANT HER TO LEARN (no corresponding passive)
V7	Connects to verb which takes object plus participial phrase modifier in active and passive, as in I SAW HER SEWING THE DRESS and SHE WAS SEEN SEWING THE DRESS BY ME
X1	Connects auxiliary of verb to NOT
X2	Connects NOT to auxiliary of verb

been of interest to transformational grammarians because, although superficially similar, considerations of their paraphrases indicate that they have different structures. (Note, it is not merely that they *have* different paraphrases, for some strings with different paraphrases will be given similar deep structures by transformational grammars, but that the kinds of paraphrases they have indicate a difference in structure.)

> I EXPECTED THE DOCTOR TO EXAMINE JOHN
>
> I PERSUADED THE DOCTOR TO EXAMINE JOHN

Although the first implies: I EXPECTED JOHN TO BE EXAMINED BY THE DOCTOR, the second does not imply: I PERSUADED JOHN TO BE EXAMINED BY THE DOCTOR. These differences are explained in transformational theory in terms of subject-object relations, and different transformation rules are proposed to generate

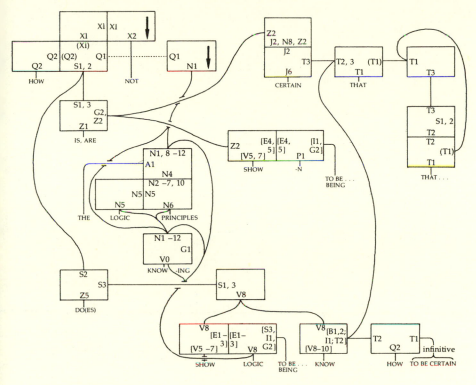

Figure B.9. Flow chart for Philosophy language modules.

them. The difference is that the phrase THE DOCTOR TO EXAMINE JOHN is not connected to the different verbs in the same way. What I *expected* was an event, described by THE DOCTOR TO EXAMINE JOHN. This event is related to the event described by JOHN TO BE EXAMINED BY THE DOCTOR. In contrast, what I *persuaded* was not an event but a person, the doctor. By mechanically transforming this string, the first noun phrase becomes attached to the verb so that the object of my persuasion is changed. In the orreries for the two strings, THE DOCTOR TO EXAMINE JOHN should connect as a whole to EXPECTED, while THE DOCTOR should connect to PERSUADED separately from TO EXAMINE JOHN (see Figure B.10[a]). When complementing EXPECTED, TO EXAMINE JOHN is connected directly to THE DOCTOR. When complementing PERSUADED, TO EXAMINE JOHN is connected to the unit PERSUADED THE DOCTOR. The modules for these constructions were given in Chapter 5 and are illustrated in Figure B.10(b).

A paraphrase of the first sentence should also connect THE DOCTOR and EXAMINE together directly, connecting them as a unit to EXPECTED. This is what

(a)

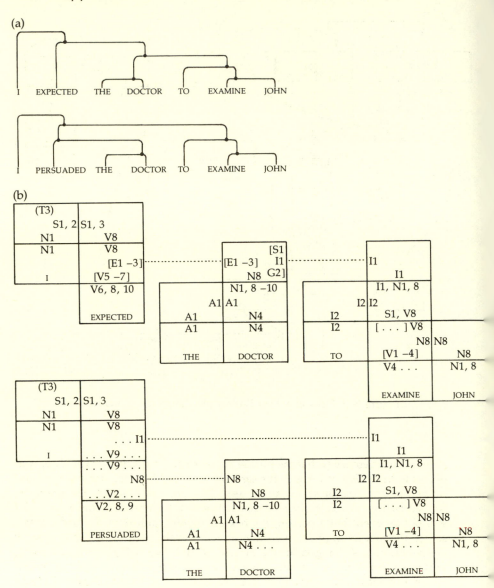

(b)

Figure B.10. (a) Different orrery connections to EXPECT and PERSUADE.
(b) Different crystals for connections to EXPECT and PERSUADE.

happens in THE DOCTOR'S EXAMINING OF JOHN WAS EXPECTED BY ME and in FOR THE DOCTOR TO EXAMINE JOHN WAS EXPECTED BY ME. However, a sentence whose underlying structure connected THE DOCTOR and EXAMINE together directly and then connected them as a unit to PERSUADED would *not* be a paraphrase of I PERSUADED THE DOCTOR TO EXAMINE JOHN.

Because the EXPECTED and PERSUADED modules have different codes, we could not attach EXPECTED to the structure now connected to PERSUADED, nor vice versa. However, it could be argued that these differences should not be attributed to a difference in the grammatical categories of the two verbs, but to the differences in their meanings. One can *persuade* only sentient beings (and objects in an extended sense), but one can (and usually does) *expect* events, states, activities. Therefore, it is natural to attach a description of an event, THE DOCTOR TO EXAMINE JOHN, directly to verbs like EXPECTED and to attach a description of a sentient being, THE DOCTOR, directly to verbs like PERSUADED. The two different structural descriptions of the different crystals would still characterize two sentences, but since the correct structure could be selected on semantic grounds, the individual verbs needs not be distinguished syntactically.

Easy to please–eager to please

A structural distinction can also be made in the way infinitive phrases connect to predicate adjectives (and predicate nominatives). There are differences in meaning among similar sentences that can be ascribed to differences in the way the infinitive phrase connects to a predicate adjective. The differences in meaning are indicated by differences in appropriate paraphrase. For example, consider the possible paraphrase of the superficially similar strings, JOAN IS EASY TO PLEASE and JOAN IS EAGER TO PLEASE, given in Table B.5. Transformationalists explain this difference by saying that in JOAN IS EASY TO PLEASE, JOAN is the object of PLEASE and in JOAN IS EAGER TO PLEASE, JOAN is the subject of PLEASE; that is, the first sentence says that others find it easy to please Joan, and the second says that Joan is eager to please others.[1]

If we construct orreries for the main terms in the paraphrases JOAN PLEASE, and EASY or EAGER, we get a systematic difference in the scope and dependency

Table B.5. *Paraphrases of* EASY TO PLEASE *and* EAGER TO PLEASE

JOAN IS EASY TO PLEASE	JOAN IS EAGER TO PLEASE
Joan pleases easily	?Joan pleases eagerly
It is easy to please Joan	*It is eager to please Joan
Pleasing Joan is easy	*Pleasing Joan is eager
*Joan's easiness to please	Joan's eagerness to please
*Joan is easy that she please others	Joan is eager that she please others

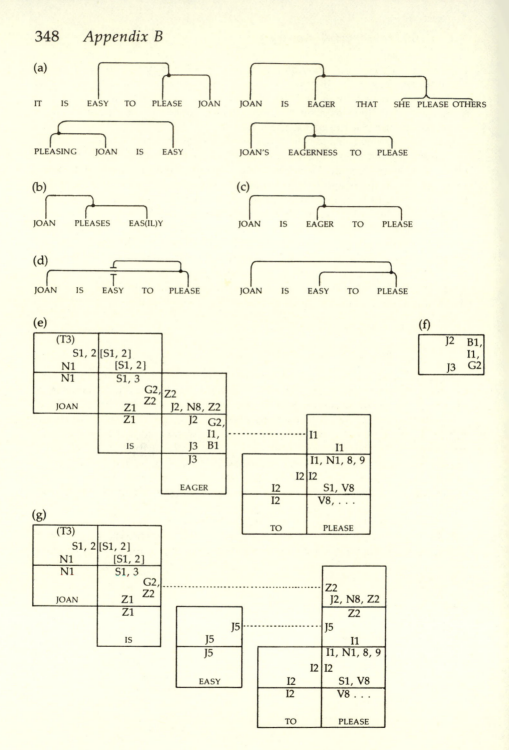

(a)

IT   IS   EASY   TO   PLEASE   JOAN   JOAN   IS   EAGER   THAT   SHE   PLEASE   OTHERS

PLEASING   JOAN   IS   EASY   JOAN'S   EAGERNESS   TO   PLEASE

(b)

JOAN   PLEASES   EAS(IL)Y

(c)

JOAN   IS   EAGER   TO   PLEASE

(d)

JOAN   IS   EASY   TO   PLEASE   JOAN   IS   EASY   TO   PLEASE

(e)

(T3)						
S1, 2	[S1, 2]					
N1	[S1, 2]					
N1	S1, 3					
		G2, Z2	Z2			
JOAN	Z1		J2, N8, Z2			
	Z1		J2	G2, I1,		I1
	IS		J3	B1		I1
			J3			I1, N1, 8, 9
					I2	I2
			EAGER		I2	S1, V8
					I2	V8, . . .
					TO	PLEASE

(f)

J2	B1, I1,
J3	G2

(g)

(T3)						
S1, 2	[S1, 2]					
N1	[S1, 2]					
N1	S1, 3					
		G2, Z2				Z2
JOAN	Z1					J2, N8, Z2
	Z1					Z2
			J5			J5
	IS		J5			I1
			J5			I1, N1, 8, 9
					I2	I2
			EASY		I2	S1, V8
					I2	V8 . . .
					TO	PLEASE

relations (see Figure B.11[a]). The lexemes PLEASE and JOAN connect as a unit to EASY, where PLEASE is the main term. In contrast PLEASE and EAGER connect to JOAN as a unit, with EAGER the main term. Now consider the orrery for JOAN PLEASES EASILY in (b). In this CASE EASILY connects to PLEASE, and JOAN connects to PLEASE, but the scope relations are different. In order for EASILY to modify the unit JOAN PLEASES, it would have to have the same orrery as for SURPRISINGLY, JOAN PLEASES, or POSSIBLY, JOAN PLEASES. In the case of JOAN PLEASES EAGERLY there is a difference in meaning from the original JOAN IS EAGER TO PLEASE. Being eager to please does not imply pleasing eagerly. One may be eager to please but not want to have to work at it, therefore the actual pleasing might be done in a begrudging, reluctant way. The differences in the two strings can be expressed by saying that JOAN IS EAGER TO PLEASE is about Joan's eagerness, her eagerness to please, while JOAN PLEASES EAGERLY is about Joan's pleasing, her pleasing eagerly. If this is correct, the scope and dependency relations should be different.

These considerations suggest that while the orrery for JOAN IS EAGER TO PLEASE should be the one in Figure B.11(c), the orrery for JOAN IS EASY TO PLEASE should be different, either of two illustrated in Figure B.11(d). The decision that with respect to JOAN, EAGER is the independent constituent while EASY is not, is strengthened by noticing that JOAN IS EAGER but not JOAN IS EASY seems to capture part of the main idea of their respective strings. So the constituent relations are different for the two strings. Syntax crystal modules for JOAN IS EAGER TO PLEASE are shown in Figure B.11(e).

The module shown in Figure B.11(f) allows a variety of modifiers to come after the predicate adjective, such as in IS HAPPY READING DICKENS, as well as IS EAGER TO PLEASE.

Modules for JOAN IS EASY TO PLEASE would be those in Figure B.11(g). These modules can be be rearranged to produce the orrery of JOAN PLEASES EASILY as in (b) but not the orrery of PLEASING JOAN IS EASY as in (a). We shall tentatively adopt these modules instead of introducing another arrowed module, unless we find further evidence that it is the scope rather than the dependency relations that distinguish these EASY/EAGER examples.

Other sentence forms

I EAT FRUIT   WHAT I DO IS EAT FRUIT
              WHAT I EAT IS FRUIT
              IT IS FRUIT THAT I EAT

Figure B.11. Comparison of EASY TO PLEASE and EAGER TO PLEASE. (a) Systematic differences in scope relations between EASY and EAGER connections. (b) Difference in scope from EASY orreries in (a). (c) Orrery for JOAN IS EAGER TO PLEASE. (d) Orreries for JOAN IS EASY TO PLEASE. (e) Crystal for JOAN IS EAGER TO PLEASE. (f) Module for modifiers following predicate adjective. (g) Crystal for JOAN IS EASY TO PLEASE.

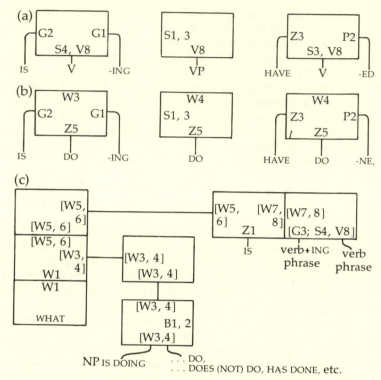

Figure B.12. WHAT-forms. (a) Modules for declarative sentences NP VP. (b) Modules for WHAT NP DO IS VP forms, replacing those in (a). (c) Other structure modules for this form.

We want structure modules for these forms that use as many of the modules for other constructions as possible, that represent the correct scope and dependency relations, that do not allow any ungrammatical constructions and do allow all the varieties of these forms.

For the first form, WHAT *noun phrase* DO (*adverb*) IS *verb phrase*, we need modules for DO that can be used in place of modules for other verb forms. In addition we need to make sure that the progressive form of DO is matched by an -ING suffix on the verb at the end. (WHAT I AM DOING IS EATING FRUIT.) To get this form, we can replace the modules for regular declarative sentences shown in Figure B.12(a) with the modules shown in (b).[2] The verb supplanted by DO need not be the main verb of the sentence: WHAT (I SAW IRA DO) IS EAT FRUIT or WHAT (I WANTED TO DO) WAS EAT FRUIT. The other structure modules for these connections are shown in (c).

In order to match the progressive DO with the -ING suffix on the verb, ordered multiple codes need to be carried through the structure. When there are a number of such codes needed, it becomes tempting to try to coordinate the disparate parts with global rules, for efficiency. The point of presenting modules is to show what can be done with local rules and to minimize the use of global processing in the model, not to deny that there are any global rules or strategies used in language processing.

Now let us consider the form for WHAT I ATE WAS THE FRUIT. In this form a complement to a verb, or part of one, that can answer the question WHAT? appears as a predicate nominative at the end of the sentence, with certain restrictions. We want to be able to construct the corresponding sentences:

> I EAT FRUIT WITH A KNIFE
>> (WHAT I EAT WITH A KNIFE) (IS)(FRUIT)
>> (WHAT I EAT FRUIT WITH) (IS)(A KNIFE)

> JOYCE HAS BEEN A PITCHER FOR TWENTY YEARS
>> (WHAT JOYCE HAS BEEN FOR TWENTY YEARS) (IS) (A PITCHER)
>> ? (WHAT JOYCE HAS BEEN A PITCHER FOR) (IS) (TWENTY YEARS)

> I TOLD HIM {THE STORY, THAT IT RAINED, TO EAT CABBAGE}
>> (WHAT I TOLD HIM) (WAS) {THE STORY, THAT IT RAINED, TO EAT CABBAGE}
>> (WHAT I TOLD HIM TO EAT) (WAS) (CABBAGE)

> I AM HAPPY
>> (WHAT I AM) (IS) (HAPPY)

> I WANTED HER TO SING
>> (WHAT I WANTED) (WAS) (HER TO SING)

An orrery for these WHAT forms is shown in Figure B.13(a). Modules to make these connections must match the correct kind of complement to the verb (or preposition) in the embedded sentence. The modules on the left of Figure B.13(b) have to be replaced by the modules on the right. The modules on the right of (b) along with the modules (c) can be used to join to other modules to produce the WHAT form. The module with the T3 code prevents a WHAT form from being generated from a question (∗ WHAT DID THE DOG EAT WAS THE HAT?) Additional restrictions are needed to rule out the possibility of operating on noun phrases that are within noun phrases: ∗ WHAT (THE DOG WITH) WAS THE HAT . . .

Questions that correspond to some of the WHAT forms are well-formed: IS WHAT YOU EAT WITH A KNIFE FRUIT? But other such questions seem less acceptable:

> WHAT I SAW WAS THE DOG RUNNING
> ?WAS WHAT I SAW THE DOG RUNNING?
> WHAT I DID WAS EAT THE FRUIT:
> ?WAS WHAT I DID EAT THE FRUIT?

(a)

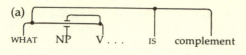

WHAT   NP   V . . .   IS   complement

(b)

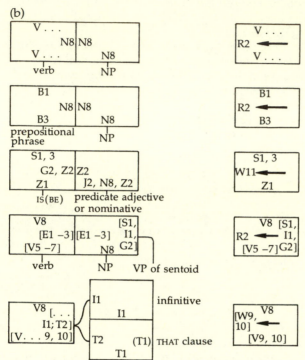

(c)

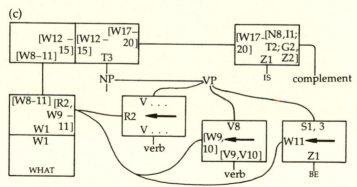

WHAT (NP   V) IS (V-complement)

WHAT THE DOG ATE WAS THE HAT
WHAT THE DOG WANTED WAS TO EAT
WHAT THE DOG IS IS MISCHIEVOUS
WHAT THE DOG KNEW WAS THAT THE HAT WAS THERE

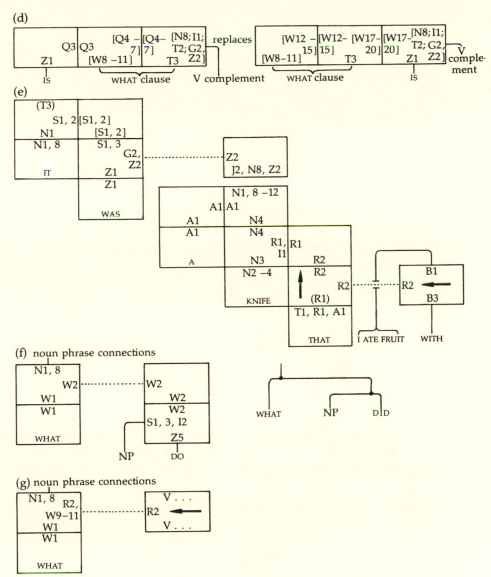

Figure B.13. WHAT NP V . . . IS V *complement* form. (a) Orrery for WHAT forms. (b) Modules for regular declarative sentences and corresponding modules for the WHAT form. (c) Additional modules for this WHAT form. (d) Modules for WHAT-form questions and corresponding modules for regular questions. (e) Using WHAT-form modules for IT WAS A NP THAT. . . form. (f) Modules for using WHAT NP DID as a noun phrase. (g) Modules for using WHAT NP VP as a noun phrase.

We will not make these distinctions but present modules for questions of all forms in Figure B.13(d).

Now let us consider yet another sentence form. Corresponding to I ATE THE FRUIT WITH A KNIFE and the other forms, WHAT I ATE THE FRUIT WITH WAS A KNIFE, WHAT I DID WAS EAT THE FRUIT WITH A KNIFE, is a sentence of the form IT WAS A KNIFE THAT I ATE THE FRUIT WITH. The modules from Chapter 5 will produce this structure along with arrowed modules introduced for the WHAT forms as shown in Figure B.13(e).

In addition, the WHAT forms are similar to ordinary relative clauses and noun phrases:

$$\text{WHAT IRA DID} \quad \begin{cases} \text{IS CRIMINAL,} \\ \text{HURT HIS CONSCIENCE} \end{cases}$$

$$\text{WHAT IRA ATE} \quad \begin{cases} \text{IS CRIMINAL,} \\ \text{HURT HIS LIVER} \end{cases}$$

Modules for treating WHAT IRA DID forms as simple noun phrases are shown in (f) and for treating WHAT IRA ATE forms as simple noun phrases in (g). The N1 top code connects the structures as subjects, and N8 as objects, to the rest of a crystal to form a sentence.

Discontinuous constituents

Almost any syntactic theory can correctly portray scope relations when the terms to be connected together (as constituents) are next to each other in the string. However, many phrase structure theories cannot connect two terms to form a constituent when there is an intervening term that does not belong to that constituent. Transformational grammars handle discontinuous constituents by first generating the parts of a constituent together and then moving them apart for the string.[3] We would like to show that the syntax crystal can also handle discontinuous constituents without the need to build one structure and then rearrange it to achieve sentence order.

An example of a discontinuous constituent is the relation of the two parts of the verb PUT and DOWN in PUT THE BOOK DOWN. The parts PUT and DOWN seem to connect together and form a constituent that connects as a unit to THE BOOK. This sort of discontinuous constituent has other special properties. We can say: PUT DOWN THE BOOK and PUT THE BOOK DOWN; PUT DOWN FIDO and PUT FIDO DOWN; PUT IT DOWN but not *PUT DOWN IT.

The syntax crystal modules for verb plus particle, such as LOOK AT and RUN AFTER, which allow a modifying noun phrase to follow, are shown in Figure B.14(a) These could be used for V + Particle + NP strings, but they do not prevent V + Particle + Pronoun. Modules that would allow only the correct structures are shown in (b). Now we must add a V12 code to other modules for other structures such as the passive, relative clauses, and WHAT forms (see [c]).

(a)

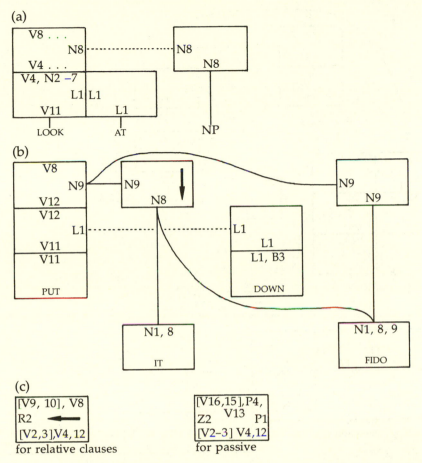

(b)

(c)

for relative clauses   for passive

Figure B.14. (a) Modules for verb plus particle. (b) Modules for discontinuous constituents: verb, object NP, and particle. (c) Addition of V12 code to other modules to take particles.

Embedding sentences

We have mentioned in several places how THAT clauses can be connected to a structure, but we have not yet shown in detail how this is done. A sentence can be embedded in another sentence through the T3 code on top of its noun phrase column. Modules for such connections are shown in Figure B.15(a). Sentences of the forms I KNOW THAT, I KNOW HOW, I KNOW THAT SNOW IS WHITE, I KNOW HOW TO SPELL, THAT SNOW IS WHITE SURPRISES RABBITS, THAT SURPRISES RABBITS, I KNOW THAT SNOW IS WHITE SURPRISES RABBITS, I KNOW THAT I KNOW THAT SNOW IS WHITE can be constructed with these modules. Any other sentence using

(a)

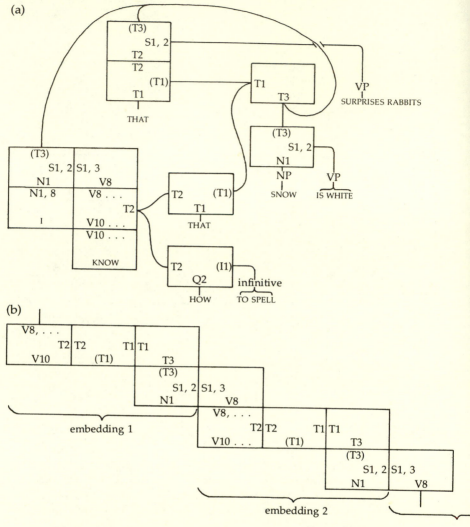

Figure B.15. Embedding sentences. (a) Modules that allow embedded
sentences. (b) Repeated modules allow multiple embeddings.

these modules could also be embedded. Multiple embedding would occur if the
modules were repeated as in (b).

Gerunds and participial adjectives

Verbs and verb phrases can appear in other roles in sentences, as adjectives or
nouns, for example: SWIMMING, MENDING. Participial adjective forms, such as

(a)

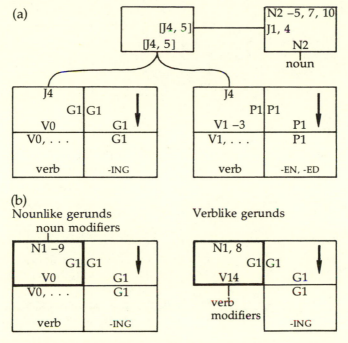

(b)

Nounlike gerunds   Verblike gerunds

Figure B.16. (a) Modules for verb forms that appear as adjectives. (b) Modules for verb forms that appear as nouns.

THE HEATED ARGUMENT, THE THINKING COMPUTER, are given in Figure B.16(a). Gerunds (verbs that act like nouns) can take noun modifiers or verb modifiers, but not both. For example, MENDING DRESSES CAREFULLY, or THE CAREFUL MENDING OF DRESSES can both be noun phrases, but not ⋆ THE MENDING DRESSES CAREFULLY. The article THE is a noun modifier, so MENDING cannot connect to DRESSES as if DRESSES were a direct object if it also connects to THE. We need modules for nounlike and verblike gerunds as shown in Figure B.16(b). The new V0 and V14 codes will be entered on the top of the relevant morpheme and structure modules.

Conjunctions

A conjunction may connect two or more words. In the Deli language given earlier in this appendix, the modules for an AND connection to noun phrases are shown in Figure B.17(a). All the noun phrases in the conjunction have the same scope, but the last noun, by having the top codes for connections to other modules, is the main term. There are probably good reasons for making some other term such as the conjunction itself the main term. Then the top codes that connect to other modules would appear on the C1╱C2╲C2 module top. For con-

(a)

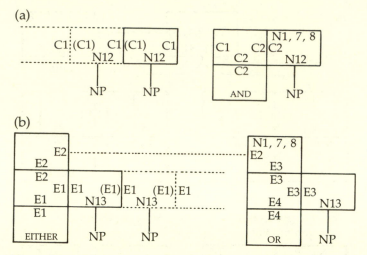

(b)

Figure B.17. (a) Modules for AND connections of noun phrases. (b) Modules for EITHER . . . OR connection of noun phrases.

junctions of other parts of speech – verbs (STOP, LOOK, AND LISTEN) and prepositional phrases (BY THE PEOPLE AND FOR THE PEOPLE) – we would need new modules.

Modules for connecting two or more noun phrases with EITHER . . . OR are given below. As with AND, other modules are needed for other parts of speech. All the noun phrases will have the same scope, and the optional E1 code allows an unlimited number of noun phrases to be connected. But this time the main term is the conjunction. We have made it the OR, but it could have been the EITHER (see Figure B.17[b]).

There are many other grammatical forms in English and grammatical forms in other languages that could have been included as illustrations of the syntax crystal. Constructing appropriate modules for some forms will be straightforward. In other cases one has to be careful to find modules that do not allow other ungrammatical forms. And for some regularities in language a different sort of rule may give a better account of what seemed at first to be merely a structural regularity. In still other cases, what at first seemed to be a regularity governed by an automatically applied rule may be best accounted for by a strategy or heuristic. More investigation is needed to see how the syntax crystal model can handle other regularities of language and to discover other sorts of rules or ways of accounting for the regularities that exist in language.

The language acquisition game

Here we describe a simulation in the form of a game of how a child learns to use language as it learns about its world. The central idea is that language is acquired in the context of nonlinguistic information, that pragmatic, lexical, and syntactic information processing work together. Playing the game takes only about an hour or less. In our experience, we have found that it is a very good way to convey a sense of the problems and strategies involved in language learning and teaching. Necessarily, an hour's experience cannot capture every aspect of a process that takes years to complete. There are shortcomings of the simulation, for example, that adults already know that linguistic signals are meaningful whereas a baby must discover this fact. Nevertheless, we highly recommend that readers experience the game. A simplified version is presented here. Modifications are easy to add for research or entertainment purposes.

The game is played by one or more teams of two players each. Competition requires at least two teams but the game may be played by a single pair. Each team represents a family, a baby player and a parent player. Initially the parent player is informed as to the lexicon and syntax of a simple artificial language while the baby player remains naive. The object of the game is to have the baby player learn the language and achieve competence sooner than the babies of other families.

The game is played on a table top with material convenient at hand. Since we often use the game in a classroom, we found that a supply of white and yellow paper is very convenient. Each team manufactures its materials by rolling and folding the paper. Here is a list of the materials needed for each team: large cone (either color), small cone (either color), large yellow tube, small white tube, small white ball, large white ball, small yellow ball, large yellow ball.

The large cone is the token representing the parent player. The small cone represents the baby player. Once the game has begun, players may touch only their respective tokens, since these represent their corporeal manifestations in the world of the game. Using their token they may manipulate the other game materials as long as their hands touch nothing but their own token. The balls and tubes are passive pieces; they don't move on their own but may be manipulated by the cones.

359

When the game has begun, either or both players may perform actions in the world. They also may transmit messages to each other. A message consists of a string of words, each represented by a capital letter, written on a piece of paper and handed to the other player. The words stand for concepts that are relevant to the world of the playing surface. The baby player must discover what each of the letters stands for. Since baby players are not provided with a list of concepts, they must discover *what* concepts the language encodes as well as which letter represents each concept. This simulates an important aspect of language acquisition: Language helps a child to learn about the conceptual distinctions made by its culture.

The artificial language, as well as having its lexemes represented by arbitrary capital letters, has a syntax that the baby player must learn. Often the ability to understand the strings depends upon knowledge of the syntax. Since it would be cheating for parent players to use English syntax to arrange the strings of symbols, this is not allowed. Although parent players will communicate in well-formed strings most of the time, there may be an advantage in simplifying the syntax in the beginning of the game, reducing it to a kind of "baby talk" in order for the naive baby player to more easily understand.

Since either or both players may transmit a message while one or both are moving, the type of message may vary considerably. The baby may move and the parent transmit a description of the move. The parent may move and provide a description of what it is doing. The parent may command the baby to perform some kind of activity and wait to see how well the message was understood. The baby may describe its own move and await a confirming or correcting message. No spoken or written English may be used during the game. Smiles of approval and frowns of disapproval are the only communication permitted outside of the artificial language. So that the game doesn't prove to be a test of memory, baby players may keep a notebook. However, parent players are not permitted to see it, since this would be the equivalent of looking inside a child's head to see what information was missing.

Here are the materials necessary to play the game. Table C.1 contains a sample lexicon. It can easily be expanded or changed. Table C.2 contains the syntax for a sequence encoding language; call it Conelish. Table C.3 contains the syntax for an inflected language; call it Cone-latin. Parent players, but not baby players, are provided with a copy of the lexicon and a copy of one of the syntaxes. Table C.4 contains part of a condensed protocol based on our experience with the game.

When a parent player believes the baby player is competent in the language, the baby player submits to an examination conducted by competing parents. This can either be a series of commands for the baby to act out or the request that the baby describe the actions of the examiners. The first team to have its baby player pass the examination is the winner.

People interested in language acquisition will find that the game is a useful way to explore the problems of language training strategies in miniature. The researcher must carefully consider the disanalogies involved in using adults to simulate children. We have used the game to explore (1) the value of simplify-

Table C.1. *Lexicon: Concepts and their English names*

F = parent	E = pushes
H = baby	L = goes, moves
B = tube	J = slowly
D = ball	R = N = fast (note synonym)
K = thing or person	V = near, up to
P = yellow	W = big
M = you (addressee)	
T = white	

Table C.2. *Syntax for Conelish*

All strings must have their symbols in the following order from left to right:

Verb	adverb	preposition	Noun obj of prep	Adj mod obj of prep	Noun direct obj	Adj mod direct obj	Noun subject	Adj mod subject

Example: To express PARENT PUSHES YELLOW TUBE, write EBPF
Note that not every part of speech must be used in each string.

Table C.3. *Syntax for Cone-latin*

Rule 1: All strings must have symbols in alphabetical order
Rule 2: Indicate grammatical role in string by using the following numerical superscripts:

1 Verb
2 Direct object of verb
3 Subject (also any noun presented alone)
4 Adjective modifying subject
5 Adjective modifying direct object
6 Object of preposition
7 Adjective modifying object of preposition
8 Preposition
9 Negative (place on last symbol in string)

Example: To express PARENT PUSHES YELLOW TUBE, write $B^2E^1F^3P^5$

ing the syntax into a "baby talk" as opposed to exposing the baby to full, well-formed sentences from the beginning; (2) the role of expansion, elaboration, and correction of the child's utterances; (3) receptive versus productive versus combined modes of language learning; (4) the advantages of having more than one parent and teaching styles simultaneously and more than one child; (5) experienced versus first parents; (6) training and learning strategy differences between inflected and sequence encoding languages.

Table C.4. *Part of a condensed protocol for language acquisition game using Conelish*

Move no.	Move description	Message transmitted	By whom	Parent's feedback	Baby's notes	Comments
1	Parent wiggles in place	F	Parent		F = Parent	Alternative hypotheses are "wiggles," "you"
2	Baby wiggles in place	H	Parent		H = Baby	Alternatively, "me"
3	Parent moves across table	LF	Parent		L = Goes?	Possibly "moves," "walks"
4	Baby moves across table	LH	Parent		L = Goes!	
5	Parent goes up to small white ball	LVDF	Parent		VD = small white ball?	
6	Parent goes up to large white ball	LVDF	Parent		VD = white ball?	
7	Parent goes up to small yellow ball	LVDF	Parent		VD = up to ball?	
8	Parent goes up to large yellow tube	LVBF	Parent		V = up to! D = ball! B = tube!	
9	Baby goes up to small white ball	LVDH	Baby	Smiles	Confirmation	

Notes

Chapter 1. Introductory perspectives

1 The simple metaphysics we use here for explanation is not crucial to our account.

2 Some readers may prefer to consider the meaning of a lexeme to be that part of a concept shared by other language users, or all instantiations of a concept only part of which may correspond to the concepts of individual language users (cf. Putnam, 1975). The meaning of a lexeme then may be something more or something less than the corresponding concept of a language user.

3 It might be argued that frequent experience with the same relation of concepts leads to the formation of the complex idea as a single concept.

4 In an exegesis sympathetic to Skinner, Segal (1977) does an excellent job of reconciling the operant view of language and the arguments for underlying structure.

5 We use the term *recursive* as the linguist (e.g., Lyons, 1968) uses it and not the mathematician, who would prefer *iterative*. In linguistics, *iterative* is a technical term reserved for aspect.

6 In recent years there has been a movement toward a simpler and leaner transformational grammar, allowing lexical and pragmatic information to do the jobs once thought to be the domain of transformation rules. For arguments on this trend within the transformational grammar tradition, see Jackendoff (1972); Chomsky (1972, 1975); and Bresnan (1978). We welcome this trend and hope it continues to move in a direction compatible with our model.

7 Hierarchical organization is not unique to language. The recursive procedure for constructing hierarchical connections presented in this book could easily be adapted to explain the acquisition of other cognitive and motor skills considered to be hierarchically organized (Lashley, 1951; Miller, Galanter, and Pribram, 1960).

Chapter 2. Underlying conceptual structure

1 Even this statement would be disputed by those who would equate thought with language. We are not going to argue about what counts as thinking, ex-

363

cept to claim that some cognitive operations must precede language for it to be learnable. And this would be so even if much of the ability to learn language were innate.

2 Alternatively, we could suppose that their positions represent their relative proximities in "semantic space" as assessed by multidimensional scaling techniques. Thus GIRL is closer to BOY than to other concepts.

3 This arrangement of scope and dependency is not the only one possible for this particular relation of concepts. However, it is the one that fits the intuitions of linguists and of subjects in psycholinguistic experiments (e.g., Levelt, 1970). Later, we will provide an argument for why it is the preferred arrangement. However, alternative arrangements could be substituted without lessening the plausibility of the model we are presenting. In fact, there may well be different arrangements for different people. This problem is discussed more fully later in the chapter.

4 The introduction of the dependency feature in the scope hierarchy permits this variety of structures. If N = number of concepts connected by the structure, then the number of structures possible with dependency as well as scope is 2^{N-2} times the number of different structures possible with scope alone. Later we will describe how other theories increase the resolving power of their conceptual structures by introducing semantic features.

5 However, Gleitman and Gleitman (1970) found that people with enough determination and imagination can find an interpretation for almost any relation of concepts no matter how bizarre.

6 To make them easy to read, this orrery and the ones that follow have the concept names in the order they would be expressed in a language string.

7 In English, questions can be expressed by uttering the affirmative sentence form with a rising intonation contour. In this case the orrery mode governs the intonation instead of the appearance of the morpheme DO.

8 This could be true just because the underlying representation for syntactic encoding is not the only aspect that contributes to meaning – our first point. But we are making a stronger claim here.

9 In this case, though, because of the similarity of lexemes, there is a systematic relation between passive and active forms: Both express a two- or three-place ordered relation, the same relation except with the order reversed.

10 However, partial correspondences would not be surprising (cf. McNeill, 1975).

11 The only other place this information could come from is the concepts themselves. But since a given set of concepts can typically be combined into more than one orrery structure, each of which would be expressed by a different sequence of lexemes, it cannot always be the set of concepts by themselves that yields the sequence information.

12 Chomsky now (1975, for example) advocates a theory in which transformation rules play a very minor role in interpreting conceptual relations. He now believes that lexical information and the "surface" hierarchical structure is almost all that is needed for interpretation of a string. Since this is moving closer to our theory, we are pleased with the change in his thinking.

However, many linguists do not agree with Chomsky's present position and still hold theories quite close to Chomsky's 1965 version of transformational grammar. See, for example, Akmajian, Demers, and Harnish (1979), a new text in linguistics from MIT Press; and Katz (1977).

13 In Chapter 6 we will discuss how syntactic information, such as the grammatical category of a word, might be used to supplement scope and dependency to make finer distinctions among relations of concepts.

14 There have been proposals to suspend the order in the underlying structure of transformational theory. However, these are rejected by Chomsky (1965, p. 221) because they were not accompanied by substantive plans for how to go between the unordered structure and the ordered string.

15 A theory that treats one- or two-word strings as ellipses of full sentences renders itself incapable of explaining how the syntactic structures of full sentences could be acquired by learning to combine smaller phrases. Such a theory is congenial with a theory that would attribute much of syntax to innate structure. In contrast, we do not suppose that the relations of SAD sentences are necessarily basic syntactic relations. Other, simpler, more general relations may be able to do the same job.

16 Lakoff and Ross (1967:2), in an informal paper that began generative semantics, argued that several of the properties of syntactic deep structure were actually semantic. But unlike our claim, they said that "subject of" and "object of" were irrelevant for semantic interpretations. "All that is necessary is that subject and object be kept distinct."

17 The LNR model and several others use a linear (rather than hierarchic) syntactic mechanism known as an *augmented transition network* (Woods, 1970). This will be discussed in Appendix A.

18 Sometimes the transformational model is considered lean compared with case theory because the latter has a structure filled with explicitly semantic information. However, because the syntactic information contained in the nodes and features of the transformational model is needed by the projection rules to develop the idea expressed by the string, it is appropriate to call it a rich model. Other, more recent versions of transformational theory are leaner than the standard version.

19 See, for example, Matthews (1968) and Stockwell, Schachter, and Partee (1969:947 ff.).

Chapter 3. Experimental evaluation of models underlying conceptual structure

1 Of course, there is some linear association working also. Thus a serial position effect could explain the data for this particular sentence. However, Johnson eliminated this alternative explanation by using another set of seven-word sentences where the major constituent break came later in the string. The TEP curve was shifted accordingly.

2 Weisberg (personal communication) pointed out that some of the associations did show asymmetry. Since lexical information is being processed as

well as syntactic, these may be attributed to asymmetries of word association. It is still possible that there are asymmetries of word association that are just balancing out the syntactic asymmetries to account for the data supporting our claim. However, it is unlikely that word associations would develop opposite to the normal syntactic order.

3 The experiment reported in this section was done in collaboration with John Gregory. It was both fortunate and frustrating that Gregory at the time was an advocate of case theory. We acknowledge his collaboration with gratitude.

4 Thank you, Harold Schiffman, for psychometric advice.

5 This pilot study was done in collaboration with M. A. Wheeler.

Chapter 4. Syntax: background and current theories

1 We are not arguing that redundancy per se means that a criterion does not exist.

2 In the following discussion both parentheses and brackets are used alternately to make it easier to see what goes with what.

3 However, McCawley (1968) has pointed out that linguistic gender may be determined by the whole phrase, not just one morpheme alone. For example, THE PATIENT TAKING ORAL CONTRACEPTIVES, THAT PREGNANT SHOPKEEPER, and until recently, RHODES SCHOLARS. Thus a feature might have to be assigned to units larger than morphemes.

4 Chomsky (1965) divided features into "strict subcategorization rules" and "selectional restrictions" but later said this distinction was not necessary. Some features are redundant. For example [−animate] implies [−human], so if [−animate] is listed, [−human] does not have to be. In order to avoid redundancy, Chomsky listed only positively marked subcategorization rules and negatively marked selectional restrictions. Stockwell, Schachter, and Partee (1969) give redundancy rules for features and list positively and negatively marked nonredundant ones.

5 To allow WE WENT UP THE MOUNTAIN IN THE MORNING and exclude WE WENT IN THE MORNING UP THE MOUNTAIN, time and place adverbials (which include prepositional phrases that connect to verbs) must be distinguished for order. And if one wants to rule out ⋆PSYCHOLOGY LEARNED FRENCH, ⋆THE PHONE DIRECTORY HAS A HEADACHE, and ⋆THE CARS WHO FRIGHTENED THE DOG . . . then the classification of nouns into [±human], [±animate], and other categories is necessary.

6 Using surface structure to supplement semantic interpretation reduces the complexity of the syntactic rules (see Jackendoff, 1972).

7 Some linguists do not treat COULD as the past of CAN, preferring instead to treat it as a distinct modal. In these treatments, the rules are slightly different, but the general principles are the same.

8 Not all transformation rules need to be ordered, and of those that must be, it is not always clear exactly where they must go, except that they must come before some rules and/or after others.

9 Recall the explanation of local and global in Chapter 1.

Chapter 5. The syntax crystal model

1 This distinction could be controversial in the case where an occurrence of a lexical morpheme could be explained by pragmatic information while the occurrence of a grammatical morpheme with no conceptual content would have to be accounted for by syntax (e.g., prepositions).

2 Since the arrows may point in any direction, a more general formulation of the positional priority exception is: The module to which the arrow points moves in the direction of the arrow until the modules connected to it are not interfered with by any modules connected in the structure. Other parts of the structure that interfere must move out of the way in directions perpendicular to the arrow. By allowing the syntax crystal more than two dimensions, this global operation would be much simplified. Since it would be difficult to draw the diagrams, we elected not to do this.

3 Note that the syntactic roles of the morphemes are not distinguished at this stage. This is illustrated, for example, by the HOUSE module having five different connection code alternatives.

4 We could incorporate context sensitivity in the syntax crystal and thus provide a precise description of the operations required. This is how it would work: Let each module be extended upward from the plane so that it is three dimensional. The third dimension is divided into discrete levels like the stories of a rectangular building. Structure modules carry the same information on every one of their levels. Morpheme modules that require coordination carry different information on each level. Each level corresponds to one of the morpheme modules in Figure 5.4(a). The levels are arranged so that coordinated forms are on the same levels. A crystal is constructed by matching codes as usual, except that construction is performed by operating at only one level. This ensures that, for example, once a singular subject form is chosen on semantic grounds, the coordinated verb form from the same level will be selected.

5 Models like the syntax crystal that map hierarchical organization into abstract regions of other psychological spaces may be applied to any cognitive skill that requires complex processing of input or output. Just as inflections are detectable features distributed over the parts of a sentence, so are other types of features distributed over perceptual fields and complex behaviors. To the extent that extracting and combining general properties of the configuration of features is relevant in explaining pattern learning and motor performance, this method of analysis may be useful.

6 Stockwell, Schachter, and Partee (1969) consider some relativizations of this sort grammatical, such as: THE PRIZE WHICH THE WINNER OF WAS A NAVAHO and use case categories to distinguish acceptable from unacceptable forms, both in subject and object position. However, cases do not distinguish satisfactorily the differences between:

THE GARDENIA I SAW THE DOG WITH
★ THE GARDEN I SAW THE HOUSE WITH

THE SKETCH I SAW THE ARTIST WITH
★ THE SKETCH I KNEW THE ARTIST WITH

7 In transformational grammar these similarities are claimed to be the result of similarities in the rules of an ordered base structure. In the syntax crystal the similarities are attributed to similarities in the scope and dependency relations exhibited by the rules, but not necessarily to similarities in the rules themselves.

8 But unlike transformational grammar, the syntax crystal does not contain rules that convert one form to another, either directly or through a base structure.

9 Chomsky (1968) defends the standard version of transformational grammar against case theory with this argument in slightly different words.

10 This criticism might arise more often in linguistics than in other fields because Chomsky (1957, 1965) did much to define the domain of syntax at the same time he proposed a theory to explain it. Thus people suppose that any theory that explains what transformational grammar does must be a transformational grammar. But this presupposes that transformational theory is the *only* way to account for the phenomena Chomsky claimed were important. We acknowledge the importance of the phenomena but present an alternative solution.

Chapter 6. Syntax acquisition

1 Fodor could not dismiss these counterexamples of learning-without-hypothesis-testing on the grounds that they are mechanical examples of learning since he himself cites artificial intelligence research to support his claim.

2 For this to be strictly true, the physicist would add some qualifications. Nevertheless, the analogy is heuristically (and historically) valid.

3 In Chapter 1 we argued that natural languages must have *some* system of syntactic categories in order to be learned. Without them the information to be processed becomes impossibly large. Badlish was an example.

4 Some of these lexemes may be composed of more than one word in adult language, such as GIMME, or GO-BYE, or even longer phrases, but they are treated as a single unit by the child.

5 Of course, this account is enormously oversimplified. Children apparently recognize relations of concepts well before they combine lexemes (Moskowitz, 1978).

6 Brown (personal communication) has recently become disenchanted with case theory.

7 For simplicity, we assume that early in language acquisition, the child does not confront the rarer uses of DOG and CHAIR as verbs.

8 It is not clear that the scope of the plural is appropriately above the connection to the verb, but at any rate, it includes the whole noun phrase, so the connection belongs high up on the noun column.

9 Perhaps no morpheme is identical to any other in its distribution privileges when all contexts are considered. To allow the reuse of structure modules, i.e., to permit them generality, substitution tests must be limited to some

reasonable number of trials. The number of tests may facilitate or hinder the learner's syntactic development just as any generalization may be too broad or too narrow. And there is the burden of performing the tests. Some heuristic shortcuts are probably used: for example, varying the number of substitution tests inversely as the number of corrections required increases or using semantic similarity to locate appropriate test contexts. Such procedures will produce a unique set of syntactic subclassifications for each learner, but there will be considerable overlap to the extent that each learner is exposed to competent language users who themselves share syntactic rules. But this is as it should be. The range of acceptability varies considerably with different dialects and even idiolects (Lyons, 1968:152). Although the algorithm performs tests of syntactic acceptability one at a time, real language learners probably do much parallel processing.

10 These conditions take the place of the conditionals of steps 5–7.

Appendix B. Syntax crystal modules

1 The explanation in terms of subject and object does not quite characterize the relations of JOAN to PLEASE because the relation between the verb PLEASE and a single noun phrase connected to it is ambiguous. The sentence JOAN PLEASES EASILY may mean that she is easily pleased and therefore be a paraphrase of JOAN IS EASY TO PLEASE. Or JOAN PLEASES EASILY may mean that JOAN is a winning sort of person and pleases others easily. In either case JOAN is the subject of PLEASE. The ambiguity can be disambiguated syntactically only by relating PLEASE to another noun phrase and seeing whether it has larger or smaller scope than JOAN.

2 It is in principle possible for modules to be created that can be then connected to another structure so that there is no way to figure out how they should be arranged. This can happen when WHAT-form modules are combined with relative clause modules. There is no rule to decide which of the modules should move aside (see Figure N.1[a]). A similar problem can arise if more than one relative pronoun were to be related to a single relative clause. The existing modules allow such a structure to be begun, but there is no procedure for deciding which of the arrowed modules moves to make room for the other (see Figure N.1[b]). It would be possible to add a global rule to say how to arrange such conflicts, but without one, such structures cannot be completed, and strings that give rise to such structures cannot be parsed. This may be a sufficient explanation for why such structures do not exist. We do not have to posit additional restrictions on the modules to prevent such structures, rather the modules themselves produce unstable structures corresponding to THE COAT THAT TORE WAS MINE, such as ★WHAT THE COAT THAT DID WAS TEAR WAS MINE or ★WHAT THE COAT THAT DID WAS MINE WAS TEAR, preventing such strings from being parsed.

3 Bresnan (1978) treats some verb-particle relations (RELY ON, ARRIVE AT [A CONCLUSION]) as being connected in a lexical rule that makes the verb transitive, rather than as structural units.

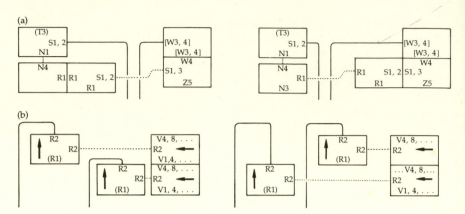

Figure N.1. Problems with some connections of modules. (a) Indeterminacy in the structure of WHAT form and relative clause modules. (b) Indeterminacy in the structure of relative clause modules.

References

Adjukiewicz, K. (1935). Die syntaktische Konnexität. *Studia Philosophica* 1:1–28.

Akmajian, A., Demers, R., and Harnish, R. (1979). *Linguistics*. Cambridge, Mass.: MIT Press.

Anderson, J., and Bower, G. H. (1973). *Human Associative Memory*. Washington, D.C.: Winston.

Anderson, J. R. (1975). Computer simulation of a language acquisition system: A first report. In R. L. Solso (ed.). *Information Processing and Cognition*. Hillsdale, N.J.: Erlbaum.

Arbib, M. (1972). *The Metaphorical Brain*. New York: Wiley.

Bach, E. (1974). *Syntactic Theory*. New York: Holt, Rinehart and Winston.

Barlow, H., and Pettigrew, J. (1971). Lack of specificity of neurons in the visual cortex of young kittens. *Journal of Physiology* 218:98P–99P.

Bellugi, U. (1967). The acquisition of negation. Ph.D. dissertation, Harvard University.

Blakemore, C., and Cooper, G. (1970). Development of the brain depends on the visual environment. *Nature* 228:477–478.

Blakemore, C., and Mitchell, D. (1973). Environmental modification of the visual cortex and the neural basis of learning and memory. *Nature* 241:467–468.

Block, H. (1965). Learning in some simple nonbiological systems. *American Scientist* 53:59–79.

Block, H., Moulton, J., and Robinson, G. (1975). A robot to use natural language. *International Journal of Man-Machine Studies* 7:571–608.

Bloom, L. (1971). Why not pivot grammar? *Journal of Speech and Hearing Disorders* 36:40–50.

(1973). *One Word at a Time: The Use of Single-Word Utterances before Syntax*. The Hague: Mouton.

Bloom, L., and Lahey, M. (1978). *Language Development and Language Disorders*. New York: Wiley.

Bobrow, D. (1970). Memory for words in sentences. *Journal of Verbal Learning and Verbal Behavior* 9:363–372.

Bolinger, D. (1965). The atomization of meaning. *Language* 41 (4):555–573.

(1975). *Aspects of Language*, ed. 2. New York: Harcourt Brace Jovanovich.

371

Braine, M. (1963). The ontogeny of English phrase structure: the first phase. *Language 39:*1–14.

Braine, M., and Wells, R. (1978). Case-like categories in children: the actor and some related categories. *Cognitive Psychology 10:*100–122.

Brame, M. (1976). *Conjectures and Refutations in Syntax and Semantics.* New York: North Holland.

Bransford, J. D., and Franks, J. J. (1971). The abstraction of linguistic ideas. *Cognitive Psychology 2:*331–350.

Bresnan, J. (1978). A realistic transformational grammar. In M. Halle, J. Bresnan, and G. Miller (eds.). *Linguistic Theory and Psychological Reality,* pp. 1–59. Cambridge, Mass.: MIT Press.

Brown, R. (1973). *A First Language.* Cambridge, Mass.: Harvard University Press.

Brown, R., and Fraser, C. (1963). The acquisition of syntax. In C. Cofer and B. Musgrave (eds.). *Verbal Behavior and Learning: Problems and Processes,* pp. 158–201. New York: McGraw-Hill.

Caroll, J. B. (1971). Pp. 140–150 in D. L. Horton and J. J. Jenkins (eds.). *The Perception of Language.* Columbus, Ohio: Charles E. Merrill.

Carroll, L. (1872). *Through the Looking Glass.* Baltimore: Penguin (1946 reprint).

Chomsky, N. (1957). *Syntactic Structures.* The Hague: Mouton.

(1959). Review of Skinner's *Verbal Behavior. Language 35:*26–58.

(1964). "Degrees of grammaticalness." In J. Fodor and J. Katz (eds.). *The Structure of Language,* pp. 384–389. Englewood Cliffs, N.J.: Prentice-Hall.

(1965). *Aspects of a Theory of Syntax.* Cambridge, Mass.: MIT Press.

(1968). Deep structure, surface structure and semantic interpretation. In pamphlet, Indiana University Linguistics Club, Bloomington. Reprinted in D. Steinberg and L. Jacobovitz (eds.). *Semantics: An Interdisciplinary Reader in Philosophy, Linguistics and Psychology,* Cambridge: Cambridge University Press, 1971.

(1970). Remarks on nominalization. In pamphlet, Indiana University Linguistics Club, Bloomington. Reprinted in R. Jacobs and P. S. Rosenbaum (eds.). *Readings in English Transformational Grammar,* pp. 184–221. Waltham, Mass.: Ginn.

(1972). *Language and Mind.* New York: Harcourt Brace Jovanovich.

(1973). Conditions on transformations. In S. R. Anderson and P. Kiparsky (eds.). *A Festschrift for Morris Halle.* New York: Holt, Rinehart and Winston.

(1975). *Reflections on Language.* New York: Pantheon.

Clark, H., and Clark, E. (1977). *Psychology and Language: An Introduction to Psycholinguistics.* New York: Harcourt Brace Jovanovich.

Cofer, C., and Bruce, D. (1965). Form-class as the basis for clustering in the recall of nonassociated words. *Journal of Verbal Learning and Verbal Behavior 4:*386–389.

Colby, K. M., Parkison, R. C., and Faught, B. (1974). Pattern matching rules for the recognition of natural language dialogue expressions. *American Journal of Computational Linguistics,* microfiche no. 5.

Davidson, D. (1967). Truth and meaning. *Synthese 17*:304–323.

(1975). Thought and talk. In S. Guttenplan (ed.). *Mind and Language,* pp. 7–24. Oxford: Clarendon.

Descartes, R. (1641). *Meditations on First Philosophy.* Reprinted in E. Anscombe and P. Geach (eds.). *Descartes.* London: Nelson (1954).

Emonds, J. (1976). *A Transformational Approach to English Syntax.* New York: Academic Press.

Farbens, W. (1975). PEDAGLOT and understanding natural language processing. *Proceedings of the 13th Annual Meeting of the Association for Computational Linguistics.*

Feldman, C., and Rodgon, M. (1970). The effects of various types of adult responses in the syntactic acquisition of two to three year olds. Unpublished paper. Department of Psychology, University of Chicago.

Fillenbaum, S. (1974). Pragmatic normalization: further results for some conjunctive and disjunctive sentences. *Journal of Experimental Psychology 102*:574–578.

Fillmore, C. (1968). The case for case. In E. Bach and R. Harms (eds.). *Universals in Linguistic Theory.* New York: Holt, Rinehart and Winston.

(1969). Toward a modern theory of case. In D. Reibel and S. Schane. *Modern Studies in English.* Englewood Cliffs, N.J.: Prentice-Hall.

Fodor, J. (1971). Recognition of syntactic structures. In D. L. Horton and J. J. Jenkins (eds.). *The Perception of Language,* pp. 120–139. Columbus, Ohio: Merrill.

(1975). *The Language of Thought.* New York: Crowell.

Fodor, J., Bever, T., and Garrett, M. (1974). *The Psychology of Language.* New York: McGraw-Hill.

von Frisch, K. (1967). *The Dance Language and Orientation of Bees.* Cambridge, Mass.: Harvard University Press.

Gardner, R. A., and Gardner, B. (1969). Teaching sign language to a chimpanzee. *Science 165*:664–672.

von Glasersfeld, E. (1969). Semantics and the syntactic classification of words. International Conference on Computational Linguistics, Sanga-Säby, Sweden, September 1–4.

(1975). The yerkish language for non-human primates. *American Journal of Computational Linguistics,* microfiche no. 12.

von Glasersfeld, E., and Pisani, P. (1970). The multistore parser for heirarchical syntactic structures. *Communications of the ACM 13*:74–82.

Gleitman, L., and Gleitman, H. (1970). *Phrase and Paraphrase: Some Innovative Uses of Language.* New York: Norton.

Goodman, N. (1955). *Fact, Fiction and Forecast.* Indianapolis, Ind.: Bobbs Merrill.

Greene, J. (1972). *Psycholinguistics: Chomsky and Psychology.* London: Penguin.

Grice, H. P. (1975). Logic and conversation. In P. Cole and J. L. Morgan (eds.). *Syntax and Semantics,* vol. 3, *Speech Acts,* pp. 41–58. New York: Seminar Press.

Gullikson, H. (1950). *Theory of Mental Tests.* New York: Wiley.

Harris, L. R. (1972). A model for adaptive problems solving applied to natural language acquisition. Ph.D. dissertation, Cornell University.

Hayes, K., and Hayes, C. (1952). Imitation in a home-raised chimpanzee. *Journal of Comparative and Physiological Psychology 45:450–459.*

Hebb, D. O. (1949). *The Organization of Behavior.* New York: Wiley.

(1972). *Textbook of Psychology.* Philadelphia: Saunders.

Hinde, R. (1972). *Non-verbal Communication.* Cambridge: Cambridge University Press.

Hirsh, H., and Spinelli, D. (1970). Visual experience modifies distribution of horizontally and vertically oriented receptive fields in cats. *Science 168:869–871.*

Hubel, D., and Wiesel, T. (1962). Receptive fields and functional architecture in the cat's visual cortex. *Journal of Physiology 160:106–154.*

Hume, D. (1739). *A Treatise of Human Nature.* Oxford: Oxford University Press (1888 reprint).

Hutchinson, J. W., and Lockhead, G. (1977). Similarity as distance: a structural principle for semantic memory. *Journal of Experimental Psychology: Human Learning and Memory 3:660–678.*

Jackendoff, R. (1972). *Semantic Interpretation in Generative Grammar.* Cambridge, Mass.: MIT Press.

Johnson, M. (1967). Syntactic position and rated meaning. *Journal of Verbal Learning and Verbal Behavior 6:240–246.*

Johnson, N. F. (1965). The psychological reality of phrase structure rules. *Journal of Verbal Learning and Verbal Behavior 4:469–475.*

Kaplan, R. M. (1973). A general syntactic processor. In R. Rustin (ed.). *Natural Language Processing.* New York: Algorithmics Press.

Katz, J. (1964). Semi-sentences. In J. Fodor and J. Katz (eds.). *The Structure of Language.* Englewood Cliffs, N.J.: Prentice-Hall.

(1966). *The Philosophy of Language.* New York: Harper & Row.

(1977). *Propositional Structure and Illocutionary Force: A Study of the Contribution of Sentence Meaning to Speech Acts.* New York: Crowell.

Katz, J., and Fodor, J. (1963). The structure of a semantic theory. *Language 39:170–210.*

Katz, J., and Postal, P. M. (1964). *An Integrated Theory of Linguistic Descriptions.* Cambridge, Mass.: MIT Press.

Kimball, J. (1973). Seven principles of a surface structure parsing in natural language. *Cognition 2: 15–47.*

Kintsch, W. (1972). Notes on the structure of semantic memory. In E. Tulving and W. Donaldson (eds.). *Organization of Memory.* New York: Academic Press.

Labov, W. (1973). The boundaries of words and their meanings. In C.-J. N. Bailey and R. W. Shuy (eds.). *New Ways of Analyzing Variation in English,* pp. 340–373. Washington, D.C.: Georgetown University Press.

de Laguna, G. (1927). *Speech: Its Function and Development.* New Haven, Conn.: Yale University Press.

Lakoff, G. (1968). Instrumental adverbs and the concept of deep structure. *Foundations of Language 4:4–29.*

(1970). Global rules. *Language 46:* 627–639.

(1973). Deep language: a letter to the editors. *New York Review of Books 20:* (1):34.

Lakoff, G., and Ross, J. (1967). Is deep structure necessary? Indiana University Linguistics Club. Reprinted in J. McCawley (ed.). *Syntax and Semantics: Notes from the Linguistic Underground 7:*159–164. New York: Academic Press, 1976.

Lashley, K. (1951). The problem of serial order in behavior. In L. Jeffress (ed.). *Cerebral Mechanisms in Behavior: The Hixon Symposium.* New York: Wiley.

Leibniz, G. W. (1704). *New Essays Concerning Human Understanding.* Trans. A. G. Langley. Chicago: University of Chicago Press (1916).

Lenneberg, Eric (1964). The capacity for language acquisition. In J. Fodor and J. Katz (eds.). *The Structure of Language,* pp. 579–603. Englewood Cliffs, N.J.: Prentice-Hall.

— (1967). *Biological Foundations of Language.* New York: Wiley.

Leonard, L. (1976). *Meaning in Child Language: Issues in the Study of Early Semantic Development.* New York: Grune and Stratton.

Levelt, W. (1970). A scaling approach to the study of syntactic relations. In G. B. Flores d'Arcais and W. J. M. Levelt (eds). *Advances in Psycholinguistics.* New York: American Elsevier.

(1974). *Formal Grammars in Linguistics and Psycholinguistics,* vol. 3, *Psycholinguistic Applications.* The Hague: Mouton.

Lindsay, P., and Norman, D. (1972). *Human Information Processing.* New York: Academic Press.

(1977). *Human Information Processing: An Introduction to Psychology.* New York: Academic Press.

Lindsey, R. (1971). Jigsaw heuristics and a language learning model. In N. V. Findler and B. Meltzer (eds.). *Artificial Intelligence and Heuristic Programming.* New York: American Elsevier.

Linn, W., and Reitman, W. (1975). AUTONOTE: Network mediated natural language communication in a personal information retrieval system. *American Journal of Computational Linguistics,* microfiche no. 23.

Lord, C. (1974). Variations in the pattern of acquisition of negation. *Papers and Reports on Child Language Development* (Stanford University) *8:*78–86.

Lorenz, K. (1957). Der Kumpan in der Umwelt des Vogels. *Journal of Ornithology 83:*137–213, 239–413. Trans. and reprinted in C. Schiller, *Instinctive Behavior.* New York: International Universities Press.

Lyons, J. (1968). *Theoretical Linguistics.* Cambridge: Cambridge University Press.

Lyons, J. (ed.) (1971). *New Horizons in Linguistics.* Middlesex, England: Penguin.

McCawley, J. (1968). Concerning the base component of a transformational grammar. *Foundations of Language 4:*243–269.

MacKay, D. M. (1972). The structure of words and syllables: evidence from errors in speech. *Cognitive Psychology 3:*210–227.

McNeill, D. (1966). Developmental psycholinguistics. In F. Smith and G. A. Miller (eds.). *The Genesis of Language: a Psycholinguistic Approach,* pp. 15–84. Cambridge, Mass.: MIT Press.

(1970). *The Acquisition of Language*. New York: Harper & Row.

(1975). Semiotic extension. In R. Solso (ed.). *Loyola Symposium on Cognition*. Hillsdale, N.J.: Erlbaum.

Marchand, H. (1966). *The Categories and Types of Present-Day English Word-Formation*. University: University of Alabama Press.

Matthews, G. H. (1968). Le Cas échéant, parts 1 and 2. Unpublished paper.

Miller, G. (1962). Some psychological studies of grammar. *American Journal of Psychology 17*:748–762.

(1967). *The Psychology of Communication*. Baltimore: Penguin.

Miller, G., Galanter, E., and Pribram, K. (1960). *Plans and the Structure of Behavior*. New York: Holt, Rinehart and Winston.

Miller, G., and Johnson-Laird, P. (1976). *Language and Perception*. Cambridge, Mass.: Belknap Press.

Miller, G., and Stein, M. (1963). Grammarama, I. Preliminary studies and analysis of protocols. *Science Report CS-2*. Center for Cognitive Studies, Harvard University.

Moeser, S., and Bregman, A. (1972). The role of reference in the acquisition of a miniature artificial language. *Journal of Verbal Learning and Verbal Behavior 11*:759–769.

Moskowitz, B. A. (1978). The acquisition of language. *Scientific American 239*:92–108.

Neisser, U. (1967). *Cognitive Psychology*. New York: Appleton-Century-Crofts.

von Neumann, J. (1966). *The Theory of Self-Reproducing Automata*. Ed. and completed by A. W. Burks. Urbana: University of Illinois Press.

Norman, D., Rumelhart, D., and the LNR Research Group (1975). *Explorations in Cognition*. San Francisco: Freeman.

Osgood, C. (1963). On understanding and creating sentences. *American Psychologist 18*:735–751.

Osherson, D. N., and Wasow, T. (1976). Task-specificity and species-specificity in the study of language: a methodological note. *Cognition 4*:203–214.

Palme, J. (1971). Making computers understand natural language. In N. V. Findler and B. Meltzer (eds.). *Artificial Intelligence and Heuristic Programming*. New York: American Elsevier.

Partee, B. (1978). Semantics – mathematics or psychology? Address given at Chapel Hill Colloquium. To appear in *Semantics from a Different Point of View*. Berlin: Springer-Verlag.

Premack, D. (1971). Language in chimpanzee? *Science 172*:808–822.

Putnam, H. (1975). The meaning of "meaning." *Mind, Language and Reality*. Philosophical Papers, *2*:215–271. Cambridge: Cambridge University Press.

Reeker, L. H. (1976). *The computational study of language acquisition*, vol. 15, *Advances in Computers*. New York: Academic Press.

Robinson, G. (1977). Procedures for the acquisition of syntax. In V. Honig and J. Staddon (eds.). *The Handbook of Operant Behavior*, pp. 619–627. Englewood Cliffs, N.J.: Prentice-Hall.

(1979). Syntactic prostheses and the underlying structure of language. Paper presented to the Psychonomic Society, Phoenix, Ariz.

Rosenblatt, F. (1962). *Principles of Neurodynamics.* Washington, D.C.: Spartan Books.

Ross, J. (1967). Constraints on Variables in Syntax. Ph.D. dissertation, MIT.

Rumelhart, D., Lindsay, P., and Norman, D. (1972). A process model for long-term memory. In E. Tulving and W. Donaldson (eds.). *Organization of Memory,* pp. 197–246. New York: Academic Press.

Schank, R. (1973). Identifications of conceptualizations underlying natural language. In R. Schank and K. Colby. *Computer Models of Thought and Language.* San Francisco: Freeman.

Schank, R. (ed.) (1975). *Conceptual Information Processing.* Amsterdam: North-Holland.

Scollon, R. (1974). One child's language from one to two: the origins of construction. Ph.D. thesis, University of Hawaii.

Segal, E. (1977). Toward a coherent psychology of language. In W. K. Honig and J. E. R. Staddon. *Handbook of Operant Behavior,* pp. 628–653. Englewood Cliffs, N.J.: Prentice-Hall.

Shafto, M. (1973). The space for case. *Journal of Verbal Learning and Verbal Behavior* 12:551–562.

Siklossy, L. (1971). A language-learning heuristic program. *Cognitive Psychology* 2:479–495.

Siklossy, L., Rich, A., and Marinov, V. (1973). Breadth-first search: some surprising results. *Artificial Intelligence* 4:1–27.

Skinner, B. F. (1957). *Verbal Behavior.* New York: Appleton-Century-Crofts.

Slobin, D. (1971). *Psycholinguistics.* Glenview, Ill.: Scott, Foresman.

Stockwell, R., Schachter, P., and Partee, B. (1969). *Integration of Transformational Theories on English Syntax.* Department of Linguistics, University of California, Los Angeles. Reprinted as *Major Syntactic Structures of English.* New York: Holt, Rinehart and Winston, 1973.

Taylor, I. (1976). *Introduction to Psycholinguistics.* New York: Holt, Rinehart and Winston.

Tinbergen, N. (1951). *The Study of Instinct.* Oxford: Oxford University Press.

Tolman, E. (1948). Cognitive maps in rats and men. *Psychological Review* 55:189–208.

Walter, W. cited by H. D. Block (personal communication).

Weisberg, R. (1969). Sentence processing through intrasentence word association. *Journal of Experimental Psychology* 82:332–338.

Weizenbaum, J. ELIZA – a computer program for the study of natural language communications between man and machine. *Communications of the Association for Computing Machinery,* January 1966, pp. 36–45.

Whorf, B. (1956). *Language, Thought and Reality.* Cambridge, Mass.: MIT Press.

Winograd, T. (1972). *Understanding Natural Language.* New York: Academic Press.

(1974). Five lectures on artificial intelligence. *Computer Science Department Report,* STAN CS 74–759. Stanford University, September.

Winokur, S. (1976). *A Primer of Verbal Behavior: An Operant View.* Englewood Cliffs, N.J.: Prentice-Hall.

Woods, W. A. (1970). Transition network grammars for natural language analysis. *Communications of the ACM 13.*

Wundt, W. (1901). *Sprachgeschichte und Sprachpsychologie,* Leipzig: W. Engelmann.

Ziff, P. (1964). On understanding "Understanding Utterances." In J. A. Fodor and J. Katz (eds.). *The Structure of Language,* pp. 390–400. Englewood Cliffs, N.J.: Prentice-Hall.

Name Index

Subject Index

acceptability of language strings, 124–31, 285

  feedback about, 263–7

accidents and substance of language, 250–1

acquisition of language, 1, 3, 6, 17, 19, 29–30, 34, 36, 38, 111–12, 123, 168, 180, 187, 229, 329, 358, 359–62, 363, 364, 365, 368–9

  see also child language acquisition; primate language acquisition; syntax crystals, in language acquisition

  experimental evidence on, 91, 108–13, 234–99

active sentence mode, *see* passive sentence mode, paraphrase similarity

adequacy, 71, 102, 118–19, 123, 130, 138, 167, 183, 260

  of language data in learning, 241–5

  levels of, 119, 248

  of linear associations, 239, 261

  see also criteria

agent-action-object relations, 3, 42, 77–9

  experimental studies of, 106–13

  innate claims for, 252

  see also case grammar

agreement between modules in syntax crystal, 197–202

algorithm, 21, 36

  for coding syntax crystal modules, 295–9, 369

ambiguity, 6, 41, 49, 69–70, 71, 76–7, 83, 120, 122–3, 126–31, 164, 169

  problems for phrase structure grammars, 133

  representation by SCRYP, 322, 329

  representation by syntax crystal, 183–5, 335

  with same structure, 67, 155, 233

analysis-by-syntheses, 115

artificial miniature language

  for criticizing associationist principles, 175, 239–40

  for experiment, 112–13

  see also Badlish and Goodlish

associationist principles, *see* associative connections

associative connections, 175–7

  hierarchical, 176, 271–4, 299; in empiricism, 237

  word-word (linear), 176, 236–40, 243–5, 261, 365

asyntactic expressions, 305, 310–11, 323, 329

ATN, *see* augmented transition network

augmented transition network, 365

  parsers, 300–5

  top-down parsing, 300–3, 309

autoclitic frame, 17–18

automatic rules, 119, 120, 145, 196, 246, *see also* computer simulation

backtracking in computer parsing mechanisms, 300–1, 306, 328–9

Badlish artificial language, 14–15, 135, 368

bandwidth heuristic search in top-down parsers, 306

base structure, 150–5, 158, 161, 164, 204, 214, 216, 219, 231, 365, 368

  for paraphrases, 226

  universals in, 251, 254

  see also underlying structure(s), and phrase markers

behaviorism, 236, 238, 256

"bootstrap" problem in language acquisition, 245–8, 256

bottom-up parsing system, *see* parsers

bracketing

  to represent constituents, 132–5, 366

  to represent ordered connections, 188–9, 199